THE ESSENTIALS OF RESPIRATORY THERAPY

THE ESSENTIALS OF RESPIRATORY THERAPY

Robert M. Kacmarek, R.R.T.
Instructor, Department of Health Sciences and Arts,
Northwestern University Medical School
Program Director, Northwestern University Medical School,
Department of Anesthesia, Respiratory Therapy Programs
Program Director, Northwestern Memorial Hospital,
Respiratory Therapy Program

Steven Dimas, R.R.T.
Clinical Coordinator, Northwestern University Medical School,
Department of Anesthesia, Respiratory Therapy Programs
Instructor, Northwestern Memorial Hospital,
Respiratory Therapy Program

Craig W. Mack, R.R.T.
Instructor, Northwestern University Medical School,
Department of Anesthesia, Respiratory Therapy Programs
Instructor, Northwestern Memorial Hospital,
Respiratory Therapy Program

YEAR BOOK MEDICAL PUBLISHERS, INC.
CHICAGO • LONDON

Library of Congress Cataloging in Publication Data
Kacmarek, Robert M
The essentials of respiratory therapy.
Includes index.
1. Inhalation therapy. 2. Respiration. I. Dimas, Steven,
joint author. II. Mack, Craig W., joint author. III. Title.
[DNLM: 1. Respiratory therapy. WB342 K113e]
RC735.I5K32   615'.836   79-14683
ISBN 0-8151-4953-0

To Darla, Carol and Karen

Preface

Over the years the field of respiratory therapy has expanded significantly and become increasingly complex. Along with this maturing of the profession has come an increase in the level and diversity of knowledge required of the respiratory care practitioner. In order to keep abreast of the educational needs of the field, many texts have been developed by a myriad of authors, each highlighting various aspects of the field.

The purpose of this text, *The Essentials of Respiratory Therapy,* is to unite in a simple and logical presentation areas in which the respiratory care practitioner must develop expertise. In format the text is an extensive presentation of the essential aspects of respiratory therapy; the basic sciences, anatomy and physiology, and the therapeutic aspects of the field are organized in an easily followed outline. As this format indicates, the text is intended as a secondary rather than a primary text; that is, a certain level of overall understanding of respiratory therapy is assumed. The individual requiring in-depth, detailed discussion on a topic should refer to texts of a primary nature.

The text begins with a presentation of the chemistry and gas physics related to respiratory therapy, followed by an extensive, detailed outline of the anatomy and physiology of the respiratory, cardiovascular and nervous systems. Pharmacology, pulmonary functions, neonatal comparative anatomy and obstructive and restrictive pulmonary diseases are then presented. A description of specific therapeutic methods, ventilators, analyzers, microbiology and sterilization techniques completes the text.

At the end of each chapter, references are provided for those interested in pursuing the topic in greater detail.

The general organization of the text makes it an excellent tool for the individual preparing for the registry or certification examinations.

Acknowledgments

A very sincere and special thank you to those respected colleagues whose assistance, criticism and guidance over the years has made this text possible: Terry L. Alfredson, R.R.T., Judy Alman, R.R.T., R.P.T., M. Darnetta Baker, R.R.T., Michael F. Callahan, R.R.T., Pam Harman, R.P.T., Diane E. Leamy, R.R.T., James M. Ludwig, R.R.T., Patricia M. McMahon, R.R.T., Robert F. Molina, R.R.T., Dionne M. Rodi, R.R.T., Merl Wallace, R.R.T., John R. Walton, R.R.T. and Susie Wheeler, R.P.T.

Also, a special thank you to Barry A. Shapiro, M.D., Ronald A. Harrison, M.D., Roy D. Cane, M.D., Michael Steiner, R.R.T., Carole A. Trout, R.N., R.R.T., Kurt Stauff, R.R.T. and Camille Woodward, R.N., R.R.T. for their continued interest, support and guidance.

A special thank you to Albert Hara for his fine graphics.

We are sincerely indebted to Patti Hara for her perseverance, loyalty and tremendous patience in the preparation of this manuscript.

ROBERT M. KACMAREK
STEVEN DIMAS
CRAIG W. MACK

Contributing Authors

ALAN C. HALFEN, R.R.T.
Instructor, Northwestern University Medical School,
Department of Anesthesia, Respiratory Therapy Programs
Instructor, Northwestern Memorial Hospital,
Respiratory Therapy Program

DAVID J. HAUPTMAN, R.R.T.
Instructor, Northwestern University Medical School,
Department of Anesthesia, Respiratory Therapy Programs
Clinical Coordinator, Northwestern Memorial Hospital,
Respiratory Therapy Program

NORMAN P. PUCILO, R.R.T.
Instructor, Northwestern University Medical School,
Department of Anesthesia, Respiratory Therapy Programs
Instructor, Northwestern Memorial Hospital,
Respiratory Therapy Program

Contents

1 / Basic Chemistry

I. Atomic Structure
  A. Atom: The smallest subdivision of a substance that still maintains the properties of that substance. An atom is composed of the following:
    1. Nucleus: Central portion of an atom, which contains protons and neutrons.
      a. Proton: Positively charged particle with a mass of one atomic mass unit
      b. Neutron: Neutral particle with a mass of one atomic mass unit
    2. Electron: Negatively charged particle that revolves around the nucleus of the atom with a mass of about 1/1000 of an atomic mass unit.
    3. Normally, in its nonreactive state, an atom contains the same number of protons and electrons. The number of neutrons of the same substance may vary from one atom to another.
  B. Element: General term applied to each of the 106 different types of atoms.
  C. Isotope: Atom of a substance with the same number of protons but with a varying number of neutrons.

TABLE 1–1–ATOMIC WEIGHTS AND VALENCES
OF 13 COMMON ELEMENTS

ELEMENT	SYMBOL	ATOMIC NUMBER	ATOMIC WEIGHT	VALENCE
Calcium	Ca	20	40.08	+2
Carbon	C	6	12.0	±4
Chlorine	Cl	17	35.5	−1
Fluorine	F	9	18.99	−1
Hydrogen	H	1	1.00	+1
Iron	Fe	26	55.84	+1 or +2
Lithium	Li	3	6.94	+1
Magnesium	Mg	12	24.31	+2
Oxygen	O	8	15.99	−2
Phosphorus	P	15	30.97	−3
Potassium	K	19	39.09	+1
Sodium	Na	11	22.98	+1
Sulfur	S	16	32.06	−2

D. Atomic weight: Average weight of an atom of a particular substance based on atomic weight of the carbon 12 isotope. The atomic weight is about equal to the sum of the weights of protons and neutrons in the nucleus of an atom (Table 1-1).

E. Gram atomic weight: Mass in grams of an element equal to its atomic weight (see Table 1-1).

F. Atomic number: Number equal to the number of protons in the nucleus of an atom.

G. Ion: Charged species of an element resulting from a gain or loss of electrons in a particular atom.

II. Molecular Structure

A. Molecule: Particle that results from chemical combination of two or more atoms.

B. Compound: Molecule formed from two or more elements.

C. Molecular formula: Expression indicating types of atoms and their numbers in the molecule.

   Examples:

   C_6H_{12} = 6 carbon atoms and 12 hydrogen atoms contained in the molecule

   H_2SO_4 = 2 hydrogen atoms, 1 sulfur atom and 4 oxygen atoms contained in the molecule

D. Molecular weight: Sum total of all individual atomic weights of atoms that make up a molecule.

   Example (H_2SO_4):

Atom	No. of Atoms		Atomic Wt.	Total Contributing Wt.
H	2	×	1	2
S	1	×	32	32
O	4	×	16	64
			Molecular wt.	98

   Example (CO_2):

Atom	No. of Atoms		Atomic Wt.	Total Contributing Wt.
C	1	×	12	12
O	2	×	16	32
			Molecular wt.	44

E. Gram molecular weight: Mass in grams of a molecule equal to its molecular weight.

III. Valence

A. Valence: Number given to an atom that indicates its tendency to gain or lose electrons in a chemical reaction.

Example (see Table 1–1):

Na (sodium): Valence of $+1$ indicates that it will react so as to lose one electron.

Ca (calcium): Valence of $+2$ indicates that it will react so as to lose two electrons.

F (fluorine): Valence of -1 indicates that it will react so as to gain one electron.

B. Generally, valences of elements allow predictions of their reactivity with each other.

IV. Chemical Compounds

A. Ionic compound: Compound formed as a result of atoms in the compound gaining or losing electrons.

Examples:

$NaCl$: Na has valence of $+1$, and Cl has valence of -1.

CaF_2: Ca has valence of $+2$, and each F atom has a valence of -1.

1. Properties
   a. Ionic compounds have high boiling points.
   b. Ionic compounds have high melting points.
   c. Ionic compounds dissolve readily in polar solvents.
   d. Ionic compounds are strong electrolytes. They dissociate readily in polar solvents.

$$NaCl + H_2O \rightarrow Na^+ + Cl^- + H_2O$$
$$CaF_2 + H_2O \rightarrow Ca^{+2} + 2F^- + H_2O$$

B. Covalent compound: Compound formed by sharing electrons between the various atoms in the compound.

Examples:

$$O^{-2} + O^{-2} \rightarrow O_2$$
$$N^{-3} + N^{-3} \rightarrow N_2$$

1. Properties
   a. Pure covalent compounds exist only between atoms of the same element.
   b. Covalent compounds have low melting points.
   c. Covalent compounds have low boiling points.
   d. Covalent compounds dissolve poorly in polar solvents.

C. Polar covalent compound: Compound intermediate between a pure covalent compound and an ionic compound and characterized by incomplete sharing of electrons.

Examples:

$$H_2O \leftrightarrows H^+ + OH^-$$
$$H_2CO_3 \leftrightarrows H^+ + HCO_3^-$$

1. Properties
   a. Vary according to the particular compound.
   b. These compounds normally are weak electrolytes. Only a small percentage of ionization takes place when polar covalent compounds are added to a polar solution.

V. Volume Percent and Gram Percent
   A. Volume percent (vol%): Method of indicating the number of milliliters of a substance in 100 ml of solution
   B. Gram percent (gm%): Method of indicating the number of grams of a substance in 100 ml of solution

VI. Chemical Solutions
   A. Solution: Homogeneous mixture of two substances.
   B. Solute: Substance dissolved in a solution.
   C. Solvent: Substance that is the dissolving agent.
   D. Effects of a solute on physical characteristics of water
      1. Solutes cause an increase in boiling point of water at one atmosphere (atm) pressure.
      2. Solutes cause a decrease in freezing point of water at 1 atm pressure.
      3. Osmotic pressure of a solution containing a solute is lower than that of pure water.
   E. As the temperature of the solvent increases, the volume of solute that can be dissolved in the solvent also increases.
   F. Dilute solution: A small amount of solute dissolved in each unit of solvent at a particular temperature.
   G. Saturated solution: Maximum amount of solute dissolved in each unit of solvent at a particular temperature. In a saturated solution a precipitate is seen at the bottom of the solution.
   H. Supersaturated solution: A greater amount of solute than the solvent would normally hold, dissolved at a particular temperature.

VII. Solution Concentrations
   A. Ratio solution: Solution concentration represented in ratio form.
      Examples:
         2:500 reads 2 gm to 500 ml: 2 is equal to the number of

grams of solute and 500 equals the number of milliliters of solvent.

1:1000 reads 1 gm to 1000 ml: 1 is equal to the number of grams of solute and 1000 equals the number of milliliters of solvent.

1. Problems

    a. How many milligrams are there in 1 ml of a 1:200 solution?

$$1:200 \text{ means 1 gm to 200 ml}$$
$$1 \text{ gm equals 1000 mg, thus}$$
$$\frac{1000 \text{ mg}}{200 \text{ ml}} = \frac{x}{1 \text{ ml}}$$
$$x = 5 \text{ mg.}$$

    b. How many milligrams are there in 5 ml of a 1:500 solution?

$$1:500 \text{ means 1 gm to 500 ml}$$
$$1 \text{ gm equals 1000 mg, thus}$$
$$\frac{1000 \text{ mg}}{500 \text{ ml}} = \frac{x}{5 \text{ ml}}$$
$$x = 10 \text{ mg.}$$

B. Percent W/V: Solution concentration where the actual percentage indicates the number of grams of solute per 100 ml of solution.

Example:

1% W/V solution means 1 gm of solute contained in 100 ml of solution.

1. Problems

    a. How many milligrams are there in 10 ml of a 3% W/V solution?

$$3\% \text{ W/V means 3 gm per 100 ml}$$
$$1 \text{ gm equals 1000 mg, thus}$$
$$3 \text{ gm equals 3000 mg}$$
$$\frac{3000 \text{ mg}}{100 \text{ ml}} = \frac{x}{10 \text{ ml}}$$
$$x = 300 \text{ mg.}$$

    b. How many milligrams are there in 3 ml of a 0.5% W/V solution?

0.5% W/V means 0.5 gm per 100 ml
1 gm equals 1000 mg, thus
0.5 gm equals 500 mg

$$\frac{500 \text{ mg}}{100 \text{ ml}} = \frac{x}{3 \text{ ml}}$$

$$x = 15 \text{ mg.}$$

C. True percent solution: Solution concentration where *both* solute and solvent are expressed in either weight or volume. The solute is expressed as a true percentage of the solution. *Examples:*

10% solution with a total solution of 100 gm means 10 gm of solute and 90 gm of solvent.

3% solution with a total solution volume of 100 ml means 3 ml of solute and 97 ml of solvent.

1. Problems

    a. How many grams of solute are there in 250 gm of a 5% solution (5% indicates the percent by weight that the solute makes up of the total solution)?

$$(250)(0.05) = 12.5 \text{ gm}$$
$$\text{solution} \qquad \text{solute}$$

$$(250 - 12.5) = 237.5 \text{ gm}$$
$$\text{solvent}$$

    b. How many milliliters of solute are there in 500 ml of a 10% solution (10% indicates the percent by volume that the solute makes up of the total solution)?

$$(500)(0.10) = 50 \text{ ml}$$
$$\text{solution} \qquad \text{solute}$$

$$(500 - 50) = 450 \text{ ml}$$
$$\text{solvent}$$

VIII. Dilution Calculations

A. The following formula is used to determine the concentration that will result when a solution is diluted:

$$V_1 \times C_1 = V_2 \times C_2 \qquad\qquad (1)$$

where

V_1 is the volume before dilution
C_1 is the concentration before dilution

V_2 is the volume after dilution
C_2 is the concentration after dilution.

B. In order to use Eq. 1, three of the four variables must be known.
C. Problems
    1. What volume of water should be added to 50 ml of a 40% W/V solution of alcohol to dilute it to a 20% W/V solution?

$$V_1 \times C_1 = V_2 \times C_2$$
$$(50)(40) = (x)(20)$$
$$x = 100 \text{ ml}$$
$$100 \text{ ml} = V_2$$
$$V_2 - V_1 = \text{added volume}$$
$$100 \text{ ml} - 50 \text{ ml} = 50 \text{ ml of water to be added.}$$

    2. If 4 ml is added to 0.5 ml of a 15% W/V solution, what will be the solution's final concentration?

$$V_1 \times C_1 = V_2 \times C_2$$
$$(0.5)(15\%) = (4.5)(x)$$
$$x = 1.67\% \text{ W/V}$$

IX. Gram Equivalent Weights
  A. Gram equivalent weight: Amount of a substance that will react completely with a mole of H^+ or OH^-.
  B. Gram equivalent weight of an element: Its gram atomic weight divided by its valence. The valence charge is disregarded.
  C. Gram equivalent weight of an acid: Its gram molecular weight divided by the number of replaceable hydrogen ions.
  D. Gram equivalent weight of a base: Its gram molecular weight divided by the number of replaceable hydroxyl ions.
  E. Gram equivalent weight of a salt: Its gram molecular weight divided by the total valence of the positive ion or radical in the molecule.
  F. Gram equivalent weight of a free radical: Its gram molecular weight divided by its valence.
  G. Milliequivalent weight (numerically equal to gram equivalent weight): Weight of a substance that will react with one millimole (mM) of hydrogen or hydroxyl ions.

X. Temperature Scales
  A. Temperature scales (in degrees) in general use

      1. Fahrenheit (F)
      2. Celsius or Centigrade (C)
      3. Rankine (R)
      4. Kelvin (K)
  B. The Rankine and Kelvin scales are absolute zero scales, i.e., zero on their scales represents the point where all molecular activity stops.
  C. Conversion formulas for temperature scales
      1. $C = 5/9 \ (F - 32)$
      2. $F = (9/5 \ C) + 32$
      3. $K = C + 273$
      4. $R = F + 460$

XI. Osmosis
  A. Osmosis: Net movement of water caused by concentration difference of water.
  B. Osmosis usually is seen when two compartments of fluid are separated by a membrane that is selectively permeable.
  C. Osmosis will proceed in a system until the concentration of water in the involved compartments is equal.
  D. Osmotic pressure of a solution is the amount of pressure required to stop osmosis completely. It is the force "pulling" water into a solution with nondiffusible particles.
  E. Osmosis can be stopped by exerting a force equal to and opposite to the osmotic pressure.

XII. Hydrostatic Pressure
  A. This is the amount of force exerted by the weight of a column of water.

XIII. Expressions of H^+ Ion Concentration
  A. pH: Negative log of the H^+ concentration per liter (L) of solution
      1. $pH = -\log_{10} [H^+]$ or $\log_{10} \dfrac{1}{[H^+]}$
      2. pH of 7.0: Neutral
      3. pH greater than 7.0: Basic or alkalotic
      4. pH less than 7.0: Acidic or acidotic
      5. pH scale: 1 to 14, equivalent to an $[H^+]$ of 10^{-1} to 10^{-14} M/L
  B. Nanomoles per liter (nM/L): H^+ concentration in number of billionths of moles of H^+ per liter
      1. The $[H^+]$ is expressed as a number multiplied by 10^{-9}.
      2. A pH of $7.0 = 3.98 \times 10^{-8}$ M/L or 39.8×10^{-9} M/L or 39.8 nM/L.

3. Nanomole expressions normally are used for [H⁺] in normal physiologic range.
    a. pH of 6.90 = 126 nM/L
    b. pH of 7.70 = 20.1 nM/L

XIV. Acids and Bases
    A. Acid: A compound that donates H^+ ions when placed into solution
        1. The active compound responsible for the properties of acids is the hydronium ion (H_3O^+).
        2. In solution the liberated H^+ reacts with H_2O to form the H_3O^+ ion.

$$H^+ + H_2O \rightarrow H_3O^+$$

    B. Base: A compound that accepts H^+ ions when placed into solution
        1. The active compound responsible for the properties of bases is the OH^- (hydroxide) ion.
    C. Neutralization reaction: The reaction between an acid and a base, where the results are salt plus water.

$$NaOH + HCl \rightarrow NaCl + H_2O$$

XV. Oxidation and Reduction
    A. Oxidation: Process in a chemical reaction whereby a substance loses electrons.
    B. Reduction: Process in a chemical reaction whereby a substance gains electrons.

XVI. Metric System
    A. Length
        1. The basic unit of length is the meter (m). One meter is equal to 39.37 inches (in.).
        2. One meter is equal to all of the following, and they are thus equal to each other:
            a. 100 centimeters (10^2 cm)
            b. 1000 millimeters (10^3 mm)
            c. 1,000,000 microns ($10^6 \mu$)
            d. 10,000,000,000 angstroms (10^{10} Å)
        3. Basic factors used in converting from the metric to the British system or British to the metric system:
            a. 1 m = 39.37 in.
            b. 1 in. = 2.54 cm

B. Weight
   1. The basic unit of weight in the metric system is the kilo-
      gram (kg). One kilogram is equal to 2.2 pounds (lb).
   2. One kilogram is equal to all of the following, and they are
      thus equal to each other:
      a. 1000 grams (10^3 gm)
      b. 1,000,000 milligrams (10^6 mg)
   3. Basic factors used in converting from metric to British
      system or British to metric system:
      a. 1 kg = 2.2 lb
      b. 1 lb = 454 gm
C. Volume
   1. The basic unit of volume in the metric system is the liter
      (L), which is equal to 1.057 quarts (qt).
   2. One liter is equal to 1000 milliliters (10^3 ml) and also to
      1000 cubic centimeters (10^3 cc).
      a. The volume of 1 cc is 1 ml
      b. 1 ml of water weighs 1 gm
   3. One cubic meter contains 10^3 L.
   4. Basic factors used in converting from the metric to
      British system or British to metric system:
      a. 1 L = 1.057 qt
      b. 1 cu ft = 28.3 L

BIBLIOGRAPHY

Beckenback, E. F., Drooyar, I., and Wooton, W.: *College Algebra* (4th ed.;
   Belmont, Calif.: Wadsworth Publishing Co., Inc., 1966).
Brooks, S. M.: *Integrated Basic Sciences* (3d ed.; St. Louis: C. V. Mosby Co.,
   1970).
Egan, D. F.: *Fundamentals of Respiratory Therapy* (3d ed.; St. Louis: C. V.
   Mosby Co., 1977).
Johnson, R. H., and Grunwald, E.: *Atoms, Molecules, and Chemical Change*
   (2d ed.; Englewood Cliffs, N.J.: Prentice-Hall, Inc., 1965).
Masterton, W. L., and Slowinski, E.: *Chemical Principles* (4th ed.; Philadel-
   phia: W. B. Saunders Co., 1977).
Sackheim, G. I.: *Chemical Calculations, Series B* (8th ed.; Champaign, Ill.:
   Stipes Publishing Co., 1962).
Young, J. A., and Crocker, D.: *Principles and Practice of Respiratory Therapy*
   (2d ed.; Chicago: Year Book Medical Publishers, Inc., 1976).

2 / General Principles of Gas Physics

I. States of Matter
   A. All matter exists in one of three basic states:
      1. Solid
      2. Liquid
      3. Gas
   B. The state of a molecular substance is determined by the relationship of two forces.
      1. Kinetic energy of the molecules.
      2. Intermolecular attractive forces among the molecules.
   C. The kinetic energy of a substance is directly related to temperature.
      1. The greater the kinetic energy of a substance the greater its tendency to exist as a liquid or gas.
      2. All molecules of every substance are in constant motion as a result of kinetic energy.
      3. At absolute zero the kinetic activity of a substance is theoretically zero.
   D. Intermolecular attractive forces oppose the kinetic energy of molecules and tend to force them to exist in a solid or liquid state. Basically there are three types of intermolecular attractive forces: dipole, hydrogen bonding and dispersion.
      1. Dipole forces: Forces that exist between molecules that have electrostatic polarity; the negative aspect of one molecule is lined up and attracted to the positive aspect of another molecule, as seen with NaCl.
      2. Hydrogen bonding: A force that exists between molecules formed by hydrogen reacting with fluorine, oxygen or nitrogen.
         a. As a result of the electronegative difference between hydrogen and fluorine, oxygen or nitrogen, the hydrogen atom in the molecule appears as a pure proton.
         b. The hydrogen of one molecule is thus attracted to the negative aspect of another molecule of the substance.
         c. Hydrogen bonding occurs only with compounds of fluorine, oxygen and nitrogen because of their

11

(1) Strong electronegativity

(2) Small atomic diameter

3. Dispersion forces (London or van der Waals forces): Forces between molecules of relatively nonpolar substances.

     a. In nonpolar substances the electron cloud normally is distributed equally among all of the atoms in the molecule.

     b. However, at some point in time the electron cloud may be instantaneously concentrated at one end of the molecule. When this occurs, a polarity is set up on the molecule.

     c. This instantaneous polarity allows attraction between adjacent molecules.

E. Units of heat

1. Calorie: Unit of heat in metric system. Essentially it is the amount of heat necessary to cause a 1 degree Celsius increase in the temperature of 1 gm of water.

2. British thermal unit (BTU): Unit of heat in the British system. Essentially it is the amount of heat necessary to cause a 1 degree Fahrenheit increase in the temperature of 1 lb of water.

3. One BTU is equal to 252 calories of heat.

4. Heat capacity: Number of calories needed to raise the temperature of 1 gm of a substance 1 degree C.

5. Specific heat: Ratio of heat capacity of a substance compared to heat capacity of water.

F. Change of state

1. A specific amount of heat is needed to cause the molecules of a substance to change their state.

2. Latent heat of fusion is the amount of heat necessary to change 1 gm of a substance at its melting point from a solid to a liquid without causing a change in temperature.

     a. The melting point is the temperature (at 1 atm of pressure) at which a substance will change from a solid to a liquid.

     b. The total volume of a substance must change from a solid to a liquid before its temperature will change.

     c. Latent heats of fusion and melting points for various substances.

SUBSTANCE	HEAT OF FUSION (CALORIES/GM)	MELTING POINT (C)
Water	80	0
Hydrogen	13.8	−259.25
Carbon dioxide	43.2	−57.6
Nitrogen	6.15	−210
Oxygen	3.3	−218.8

3. The latent heat of vaporization is the amount of heat necessary to change 1 gm of a substance at its boiling point from a liquid to a gas without causing a change in temperature.
   a. Boiling point is the temperature at 1 atm pressure at which a substance will change from a liquid to a gas.
   b. The total volume of a substance must change from a liquid to a gas before its temperature will change.
      (1) In order for a substance to boil, its vapor pressure must equal the pressure of the atmosphere above it.
      (2) Evaporation is a surface phenomenon whereby individual molecules of a substance gain enough heat to change their state. Boiling, on the other hand, occurs throughout the entire volume of the substance.
   c. Latent heats of vaporization and boiling points for various substances

SUBSTANCE	HEAT OF VAPORIZATION (CALORIES/GM)	BOILING POINT (C)
Water	540	100
Hydrogen	40	−252.5
Carbon dioxide	83	−78.5
Nitrogen	−	−196
Oxygen	50	−183

G. Effects of pressure on melting and boiling points
   1. In general, the greater the pressure over a substance the higher the temperature necessary to cause the substance to change its state. Pressure has a greater effect on the boiling point of a substance than on its melting point.
   2. Critical temperature: The highest temperature at which a substance can exist as a liquid regardless of the amount of pressure applied to it (O_2 = −118.8 C).

       3. Critical pressure: The lowest pressure necessary at the critical temperature of a substance to maintain it in its liquid state ($O_2 = 49.7$ atm pressure).

       4. Critical point: Combination of critical temperature and critical pressure of a substance.

  H. Triple point: Specific combination of temperature and pressure in which a substance can exist in all three states of matter in equilibrium.

  I. Sublimation: Transition of a substance from a solid directly to a gas without existence in a liquid state. The heat of sublimation equals the heat of fusion plus the heat of vaporization.

II. Kinetic Theory of Gases

  A. The kinetic theory normally is applied to relatively dilute gas volumes.

  B. Principles of kinetic theory

       1. Gases are composed of molecules that are in rapid continuous random motion.

       2. The molecules undergo near collisions with each other and collide with the walls of their container.

       3. All molecular collisions are elastic, i.e., as long as the container is properly insulated, the temperature of the gas will remain constant.

       4. The kinetic energy of molecules of a gas is directly proportional to the absolute temperature.

         a. An increase in temperature will cause an increase in kinetic energy of the gas.

         b. The increased kinetic energy will cause an increase in the velocity of the gas molecules.

         c. The increased velocity will cause an increase in the frequency of collisions.

         d. The increased frequency of collisions will cause an increase in the pressure in the system.

         e. With an increase in temperature, the velocity of gas molecules is indirectly related to their molecular weight.

III. Avogadro's Law

  A. One gram molecular weight, 1 gm atomic weight, 1 gm ionic weight, etc., of a substance will contain 6.02×10^{23} particles of that substance.

  B. The above mass of any substance is referred to as a mole (M).

  C. One mole of a gas at 0 C and 760 mm Hg (standard temperature and pressure; STP) occupies a volume of about 22.4 L. There is a small percent variation in this number for individual gases.

D. An equal number of moles of gases at a specific temperature and pressure will occupy the same volume and contain the same number of particles.

IV. Density

A. Density is the mass of an object per unit volume and usually is expressed as grams per liter:

$$D = \frac{M}{V}. \qquad (1)$$

B. On the surface of the earth, mass in Eq 1 may be replaced by weight.

C. Calculation of densities of solids and liquids is straightforward since their volumes are relatively stable at various temperatures and pressures.

D. Gases, on the other hand, have volumes severely affected by temperature and pressure.

E. For this reason, the standard density of all gases is determined at STP conditions where the volume used is 22.4 L and the weight used is the gram molecular weight (GMW) of the particular gas:

$$\text{Density of gas} = \frac{\text{GMW}}{22.4 \text{ L}} = \times \text{ gm/L}$$

$$\text{Density of oxygen} = \frac{32 \text{ gm (GMW)}}{22.4 \text{ L}} = 1.43 \text{ gm/L}. \qquad (2)$$

F. Standard densities of various substances:
1. Oxygen: 1.43 gm/L
2. Nitrogen: 1.25 gm/L
3. Carbon dioxide: 1.965 gm/L

G. The density of a mixture of gases is determined by the following equation:

$$D = \frac{(\text{conc. A})(\text{GMW}_A) + (\text{conc. B})(\text{GMW}_B) + (\text{conc. C})(\text{GMW}_C)}{22.4 \text{ L}}. \qquad (3)$$

Example: Density of a gas containing 40% oxygen, 55% nitrogen and 5% carbon dioxide would be computed as follows:

$$D = \frac{(0.4)(32) + (0.55)(28) + (0.05)(44)\text{gm}}{22.4 \text{ L}}$$

$$D = \frac{(12.8) + (15.4) + (2.2)gm}{22.4 \text{ L}}$$

$$D = \frac{30.4 \text{ gm}}{22.4 \text{ L}}$$

$$D = 1.36 \text{ gm/L}.$$

H. Specific gravity: Comparison of the density of a substance with the density of a standard. The specific gravity of solids and liquids is determined using water as the standard; for gases, oxygen is used as the standard. Specific gravity is expressed purely as a ratio.

V. Gas Pressure

A. Pressure (P) in any sense is equal to force per unit area:

$$P = \frac{gm}{sq \text{ cm}}; \quad P = \frac{lb}{sq \text{ in.}} \tag{4}$$

B. The pressure of a gas is directly related to the kinetic energy of the gas (see Section II) and to the gravitational attraction of the earth.

C. With an increase in altitude, the gravitational attraction of the earth on molecules of gas in the atmosphere decreases.

1. This causes a decrease in density of the atmospheric gases.

2. Decreased density causes fewer molecular collisions.

3. Thus with increasing altitude there is basically a linear decrease in pressure of the total atmosphere and of individual gases.

4. Even though there is a steady decrease in pressure of the atmosphere with altitude, the concentration of gases in the atmosphere remains stable to an elevation of about 50 miles.

5. Concentration of atmospheric gases
   a. Oxygen: 20.95%
   b. Nitrogen: 78.08%
   c. Argon: 0.93%
   d. Carbon dioxide: 0.03%
   e. Trace elements: 0.01%

D. The barometric pressure (PB) of the atmosphere is equal to the height of a column of fluid times the fluid's density:

$$P_B = (\text{height of column of fluid})(\text{fluid's density}). \tag{5}$$

If the fluid used is mercury (psi = pounds per square inch):

$$14.7 \text{ psi} = (29.9 \text{ in. Hg})(0.491 \text{ lb/cu in.}).$$

E. Mercury's density in the metric system is 13.6 gm/cc; in the British system it is 0.491 lb/cu in.
F. Gas pressure is frequently expressed as the height of a substance, i.e., mm Hg, cm H_2O. These are not true pressure expressions but they may be easily converted to the proper pressure notation by use of Eq. 5 if necessary.
G. Atmospheric pressure normally is determined by a mercury or an aneroid barometer.
H. Equivalent expressions of normal atmospheric pressure:
   1. 14.7 psi
   2. 760 mm Hg
   3. 1034 gm/sq cm
   4. 33 ft of salt H_2O
   5. 33.9 ft of fresh H_2O
   6. 29.9 in. Hg
   7. 76 cm Hg
   8. 1034 cm H_2O
VI. Humidity
   A. Water vapor content of the air under atmospheric conditions is variable. Temperature is the factor that most significantly affects water vapor content levels in the atmosphere.
   B. At a particular temperature, there is a maximum amount of water that a gas can hold.
   C. Since the boiling point of water (100 C) is considerably higher than the normal temperature of the atmosphere, the maximum water vapor content of the atmosphere varies with temperature.
      1. As the temperature increases, the rate of evaporation of water accelerates and the capacity of the atmosphere to hold water increases.
      2. All other standard gases in the atmosphere have boiling points much lower than atmospheric temperature. This causes stability in their concentrations.
      3. Water is the only standard atmospheric gas that responds to temperature changes in this manner.
   D. Expressions of water vapor content
      1. Partial pressure of water vapor (P_{H_2O}), maximum P_{H_2O} at 37 C, is equal to 47 mm Hg.

2. Absolute humidity is defined as the actual weight of water vapor contained in a given volume of gas.
   a. Absolute humidity may be expressed as grams per cubic meter or milligrams per liter.
   b. The maximum absolute humidity at 37 C is 43.8 gm/cu m or 43.8 mg/L.
3. Relative humidity (RH) is defined as a relationship between the actual weight or pressure (content) of water in air at a specific temperature and the maximum weight or pressure (capacity) of water that air can hold at that specific temperature. Relative humidity is expressed as a percentage.
   a. Expressions of actual and maximum amounts of water
      (1) mm Hg
      (2) gm per cu m
      (3) mg per liter
   b. Formula for calculating relative humidity:

$$RH = \frac{content}{capacity} \times 100. \qquad (6)$$

   Example: At 37 C, if the actual water vapor pressure is 20 mm Hg, what is the relative humidity?

$$RH = \frac{20 \text{ mm Hg}}{47 \text{ mm Hg}} \times 100 = 43\%.$$

   c. If water content is kept constant and temperature is increased, relative humidity decreases because capacity of air for water increases. As temperature decreases, the opposite effect is seen.

VII. Dalton's Law of Partial Pressure
   A. Dalton's law states that the sum of the individual partial pressures of the gases in a mixture is equal to the total barometric pressure of the system.
   B. The partial pressure (P) of a gas is equal to the barometric pressure (PB) times the concentration of the gas in the mixture:

$$(P) = (PB)(conc.). \qquad (7)$$

   Example: If the PB is 760 mm Hg and the concentration of O_2 is 21%, what is the P_{O_2}?

$$P_{O_2} = (760)(0.21) = 159.6 \text{ mm Hg.}$$

C. The concentration of a gas is equal to the partial pressure of the gas divided by the barometric pressure:

$$\text{Conc.} = \frac{P}{P_B} \times 100. \tag{8}$$

Example: If the P_B is 750 mm Hg and the P_{O_2} is 200 mm Hg, what is the concentration of O_2?

$$O_2 \text{ conc.} = \frac{200 \text{ mm Hg}}{750 \text{ mm Hg}} \times 100 = 26.7\%.$$

VIII. Effect of Humidity on Dalton's Law
   A. Water vapor pressure does not follow Dalton's law because under normal atmospheric conditions P_{H_2O} is dependent primarily on temperature.
   B. When calculating the partial pressure of a gas where water vapor is present, the total barometric pressure of the system must be corrected before the partial pressure of any other gas can be calculated.
   C. Following is a modification of Dalton's law to account for the presence of water vapor:

$$(P) = (P_B - P_{H_2O})(\text{conc.}) \tag{9}$$

Example: If P_B is 770 mm Hg, P_{H_2O} is 30 mm Hg and concentration of O_2 is 50%, what is the P_{O_2}?

$$P_{O_2} = (770 \text{ mm Hg} - 30 \text{ mm Hg})(0.50)$$
$$P_{O_2} = 370 \text{ mm Hg.}$$

   D. When the temperature is 37 C with barometric pressure at 760 mm Hg, the gas saturated with water vapor and the oxygen concentration 21%, the P_{O_2} is 149.7 mm Hg:

$$P_{O_2} = (760 \text{ mm Hg} - 47 \text{ mm Hg})(0.21) = 149.7 \text{ mm Hg}$$

IX. Ideal Gas Laws
   A. The ideal gas laws apply to dilute gases at temperatures above the boiling point of the individual gases.
   B. The closer the temperature to the boiling point of a gas the greater the error involved in the calculations.
   C. The *Ideal gas law* demonstrates the interrelationships among volume, pressure, temperature and amount of gas.
      1. According to the Ideal gas law, multiplying the pressure of the system by the volume of the system and dividing this by the product of the temperature (absolute) and

amount of gas in any gas system, yields a result that is a constant. This is referred to as Boltzmann's constant and is a constant that can be applied to all gas systems.

2. The Ideal gas law is normally expressed as

$$R = \frac{PV}{nT}$$

or

$$PV = nRT \tag{10}$$

where P = pressure, V = volume and n = amount of gas (expressed normally as moles), R = Boltzmann's constant and T = temperature (expressed in degrees Kelvin).

3. Boltzmann's constant is equal to
   a. 82.1 ml−atm/mole−degree K when pressure is expressed in atmospheres and volume in milliliters
   b. 62.3 L−mm Hg/mole−degree K when pressure is expressed in atmospheres and volume in liters

D. *Boyle's law* states that pressure and volume of a gas system will vary inversely if the temperature and amount of gas in the system are constant.

1. Boyle's law mathematically is

$$PV = nRT \tag{11}$$

where nRT is equal to a constant, thus

$$PV = K. \tag{12}$$

2. In a system where temperature and amount of gas are constant, the original pressure and volume will equal the final pressure and volume:

$$P_1V_1 = P_2V_2. \tag{13}$$

E. *Charles' law* states that temperature and volume of a gas system will vary directly if the pressure and amount of gas in the system are constant.

1. Charles' law mathematically is

$$\frac{V}{T} = \frac{nR}{P} \tag{14}$$

where nR/P is equal to a constant, thus

$$\frac{V}{T} = K. \tag{15}$$

2. In a system where pressure and amount of gas are constant, the original temperature and volume will equal the final temperature and volume:

$$\frac{V_1}{T_1} = \frac{V_2}{T_2}. \tag{16}$$

F. *Gay-Lussac's law* states that pressure and temperature of a gas system will vary directly if volume and amount of gas in the system are constant.

1. Gay-Lussac's law mathematically is

$$\frac{P}{T} = \frac{nR}{V} \tag{17}$$

where $\frac{nR}{V}$ is equal to a constant, thus

$$\frac{P}{T} = K. \tag{18}$$

2. In a system where volume and amount of gas are constant, the original pressure and temperature will equal the final pressure and temperature:

$$\frac{P_1}{T_1} = \frac{P_2}{T_2}. \tag{19}$$

G. The *Combined gas law* states that pressure, temperature and volume of gas are specifically related if the amount of gas remains constant.

1. The Combined gas law mathematically is

$$\frac{PV}{T} = nR \tag{20}$$

where nR is equal to a constant, thus

$$\frac{PV}{T} = K. \tag{21}$$

2. In a system where the amount of gas in a system is constant, the original pressure, temperature and volume are equal to the final pressure, volume and temperature:

$$\frac{P_1 V_1}{T_1} = \frac{P_2 V_2}{T_2}. \tag{22}$$

H. All gas law calculations must use temperature on the Kelvin scale for accurate results.
I. Water vapor does not react as an ideal gas; therefore, in a system where water vapor is present, water vapor pressure must be subtracted from total pressure before calculations are made.
J. When precision is needed, the barometric pressure reading should be corrected for expansion of mercury as affected by temperature.

X. Diffusion
A. Diffusion is movement of gas from an area of high concentration of a gas to an area of low concentration.
B. As diffusion occurs, a gas will occupy the total container as if it were the only gas present, i.e., a gas in a container will distribute itself *with time* equally throughout the whole container.
C. The rate of diffusion of a gas through another gas is affected by the following factors:
 1. The concentration gradient, which is directly related to the rate of diffusion.
 2. The temperature, which is directly related to the rate of diffusion.
 3. The cross-sectional area available for diffusion, which is directly related to the rate of diffusion.
 4. The molecular weight, which is indirectly related to the rate of diffusion.
 5. The distance the gas has to diffuse, which is indirectly related to the rate of diffusion:

$$\text{Rate of diffusion of a gas through a gas} = \frac{(\text{press.})(\text{temp.})(\text{cross-sectional area})}{(\text{MW})(\text{distance})}. \quad (23)$$

D. *Henry's law* states that the amount of a gas that can dissolve in a liquid is directly related to partial pressure of the gas over the liquid and indirectly related to temperature of the system.
 1. Henry's law expresses the solubility coefficients of gases in liquids.
 2. Solubility coefficients of oxygen and carbon dioxide in plasma at 37 C:
  a. 0.023 ml of O_2/ml of blood/760 mm Hg P_{O_2}
  b. 0.510 ml of CO_2/ml of blood/760 mm Hg P_{CO_2}

E. *Graham's law* states that the rate of diffusion of a gas through a liquid is indirectly related to the square root of its gram molecular weight (GMW).

F. Combining Henry's and Graham's laws, the rates of diffusion of carbon dioxide to oxygen can be compared in a situation of equal pressure gradient, equal distance, cross-sectional area and temperature.

   1. The above factors being equal, the only factors affecting the comparison would be the GMW of the gases and their solubility coefficients.

   2. The comparison may be mathematically represented as follows:

   Rate of diffusion of
   $$\frac{CO_2}{O_2} = \frac{(\text{sol. coef. } CO_2)(\sqrt{\text{GMW } O_2})}{(\text{sol. coef. } O_2)(\sqrt{\text{GMW } CO_2})}$$
   $$= \frac{(0.510)(5.66)}{(0.023)(6.66)}$$
   $$\approx \frac{19}{1}. \tag{24}$$

   3. Thus under the above mentioned conditions, carbon dioxide would diffuse about 19 times faster than would oxygen.

   4. At the alveolar capillary membrane, pressure gradients for oxygen and carbon dioxide are not equal.

      a. Diffusion gradient for oxygen is 60 mm Hg.

      b. Diffusion gradient for carbon dioxide is 6 mm Hg.

      c. As a result of the above pressure gradients, oxygen actually diffuses slightly faster than does carbon dioxide across the alveolar capillary membrane.

      d. With any type of pulmonary disease, the diffusibility of oxygen is affected significantly sooner than that of carbon dioxide. Hypoxemia normally is the first blood gas abnormality associated with onset of pulmonary disease (see Chapter 6, Section VII).

XI. Ideal Alveolar Gas Equation

   A. In addition to the effects of P_{H_2O} on partial pressure of gases in the alveoli, the carbon dioxide diffusing from the bloodstream into the alveoli will further decrease alveolar P_{O_2}.

   B. Since carbon dioxide is leaving the bloodstream, a closed system, and entering the respiratory tract, an open system, there is an indirect relationship between the pressures of carbon dioxide and oxygen. Increases in PA_{CO_2} result in decreases in PA_{O_2}.

C. This indirect relationship basically involves only carbon dioxide and oxygen because they are the only metabolically active gases.

D. Dalton's law must be modified to account for incoming carbon dioxide when applied to alveolar gas. The ideal alveolar gas equation is:

$$PA_{O_2} = (PB - PH_2O)(FI_{O_2}) - PA_{CO_2} + \left[PA_{CO_2} \times FI_{O_2}\left(\frac{1-R}{R}\right) \right] \quad (25)$$

where R is the respiratory quotient.

E. A modification of the above equation may be used with reasonably accurate results:

$$PA_{O_2} = (PB - PH_2O)(FI_{O_2}) - \frac{PA_{CO_2}}{0.8}. \quad (26)$$

In both Eq. 25 and 26, PA_{CO_2} is always considered equal to Pa_{CO_2} because of the rapid equilibration of carbon dioxide.

XII. Compliance

A. Compliance: The ease with which a system may be distorted from its original shape.

B. Compliance is inversely related to elastance.

C. Elastance: The tendency of a distorted object to return to its original shape.

$$C = \frac{1}{E}. \quad (27)$$

1. As compliance increases, elastance decreases; as compliance decreases, elastance increases.

D. Compliance is normally a static measurement so as to eliminate the effects of nonelastic resistance.

E. Compliance is determined by comparing the change in volume in a system to the pressure necessary to maintain the volume change:

$$C = \frac{\Delta V}{\Delta P}. \quad (28)$$

F. In the respiratory system, there are basically three types of compliance.

  1. Pulmonary
  2. Thoracic
  3. Total
G. In the lung-thorax system, the tendency of the lung is to collapse to its resting position, whereas the tendency of the thorax is to expand to its resting position (Fig 2–1).

Fig 2–1. —C represents the equal and opposite effects of lung and thoracic compliances at functional residual capacity (FRC). The pleural surfaces of lung and thorax link the two structures. A depicts effects of removing the lung from the thorax. Lung collapse will occur. B depicts effects of opening the thoracic cage to atmospheric pressure. The thorax would expand to its *unopposed* resting state. (From Shapiro, B. A., Harrison, R. A., and Trout, C. A.: *Clinical Application of Respiratory Care* [Chicago: Year Book Medical Publishers, Inc., 1975]. Used by permission.)

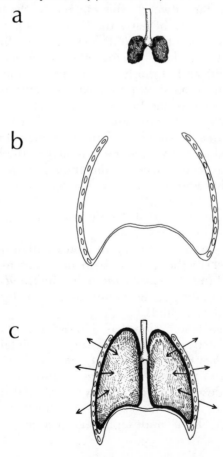

a

b

c

H. As a result of the elastic recoil of the lung and thorax (in opposite directions), a negative (subatmospheric) intrapleural and intrathoracic pressure is established.

I. The functional residual capacity (FRC) is that volume maintained in the lung at resting expiratory position as a result of the opposing effects of pulmonary and thoracic compliance.

J. Total compliance of the lung-thorax system is a result of the interaction of pulmonary and thoracic compliance.

K. Compliance is only linear at normal tidal exchange. As the lung volume exceeds or falls below tidal levels, the compliance decreases. Thus, the total compliance curve is significantly distorted as lung volume approaches residual volume (RV) or total lung capacity (TLC).

   1. When approaching TLC, the tendency of the lung to collapse far outweighs the tendency of the thorax to expand. This occurs because the thorax has moved closer to its resting point and exerts less force, tending to expand the lung. The lung, on the other hand, has been distorted significantly from its resting position and exerts a large force, opposing pulmonary expansion. At TLC, the tendency of the lung to collapse is so great that an individual cannot voluntarily inhale a larger volume.

   2. When approaching RV, the tendency of the thorax to expand far outweighs the tendency of the lung to collapse. This occurs because the lung is now near its resting point, whereas the thorax is significantly distorted from its resting point. At RV, the tendency of the thorax to expand is so great that the individual cannot voluntarily exhale a larger volume.

L. Total compliance is determined by dividing the tidal volume (VT) by the static pressure necessary to maintain the VT in the lung. *Pressure should be measured at the patient's mouth.* In the average young adult male, total compliance is equal to 0.1 L/cm H_2O.

M. Pulmonary compliance is determined by dividing the VT by the static pressure necessary to maintain the VT in the lung. *The pressure measured should reflect changes in intrapleural pressures.* A pressure reading taken at the level of the midesophagus is reflective of pleural pressure changes (the patient swallows a pressure transducer and its level is adjusted to a midesophageal position). In the average young adult male, pulmonary compliance is equal to 0.2 L/cm H_2O.

N. Thoracic compliance normally is a calculated value based on the following equation:

$$\frac{1}{C_{total}} = \frac{1}{C_{pulmonary}} + \frac{1}{C_{thoracic}}. \tag{29}$$

In the average young adult male, thoracic compliance is equal to 0.2 L/cm H_2O.

O. *Specific compliance* is a method of comparing the compliance of individuals of different sizes.
   1. The formula for its determination takes into consideration the patient's measured FRC.
   2. Specific compliance (Cs) is equal to pulmonary compliance divided by the patient's FRC and normally is equal to about 0.08 (dimensionless number):

$$Cs = \frac{pulmonary\ compliance}{FRC} \tag{30}$$

$$Cs = \frac{V/P}{vol} = 0.08.$$

P. Compliance determinations of ventilator patients
   1. Since compliance is a static measurement, an inspiratory hold must be incorporated into the system to allow a plateau effect to occur.
      a. Compliance determined by this method is referred to as *effective dynamic compliance* (CED):

$$CED = \frac{tidal\ volume}{plateau\ pressure}. \tag{31}$$

      b. This compliance measurement is not as accurate as a pure laboratory measurement, but it allows monitoring of compliance changes in ventilator patients.
   2. Compliance determined by using peak airway pressures is referred to as *dynamic compliance* (CD). Dynamic compliance is not reflective of pure elastic change because there is gas flow, and a higher pressure reading is noted owing to airway resistance:

$$CD = \frac{tidal\ volume}{peak\ pressure}. \tag{32}$$

XIII. Surface Tension
  A. Surface tension is a force that exists at the interface between a liquid and a gas or between two liquids.
  B. Surface tension is a result of like molecules being attracted to each other and thus moving away from the interface. This will cause the liquid to occupy the smallest volume possible.
  C. A specific force is necessary to cause a tear in the surface of the liquid because of the effects of surface tension.
  D. Surface tension is expressed in units of dynes per linear centimeter.
  E. Surface tension also is indirectly related to temperature.
  F. *LaPlace's law* allows calculation of the amount of pressure generated inside a system as a result of surface tension.
      1. The law states that the pressure (P) in dynes/sq cm as a result of surface tension (ST) in dynes/cm is equal to the surface tension of the liquid multiplied by one over the radii (r), in centimeters, of curvature:

$$P = ST\left(\frac{1}{r_1} + \frac{1}{r_2} + \frac{1}{r_3} + \ldots\right). \qquad (33)$$

      2. LaPlace's law as applied to a drop is

$$P = \frac{2\,ST}{r}. \qquad (34)$$

Here reference is made to a perfect sphere that has only two radii of curvature, one in the vertical plane and one in the horizontal plane.

      3. LaPlace's law as applied to a bubble is

$$P = \frac{4\,ST}{r}. \qquad (35)$$

There are two interfaces, one on the inside of the bubble and one on the outside; thus, there is a total of four radii. All are considered equal because the film of the bubble is only angstroms in diameter.

      4. LaPlace's law as applied to a blood vessel is

$$P = \frac{ST}{r}. \qquad (36)$$

When the radii of curvature in a blood vessel are viewed, the only radius that is used in the calculation is that of the vessel's width because the radius of length is so great. When the inverse of the radii of length is calculated, the number essentially goes to infinity and is meaningless in calculating the pressure as a result of surface tension.

5. It is important to remember that the pressure as a result of surface tension is indirectly related to the radius. *The smaller the sphere the greater the pressure as a result of surface tension.*

G. *Critical volume* is a volume below which the effects of surface tension are so great that the structure will collapse. Once the critical volume is reached, collapse is always eminent.

H. The surface tension of a fluid is reduced by chemicals referred to as surfactants. Surfactants are surface-active agents that interfere with the molecules of the fluid at the surface, causing a reduction in the force (ST) that draws the fluid centrally.

I. In the alveoli the relationship of surface tension of the fluid lining the alveoli to the surfactant produced by the Type II alveoli cells is extremely important.

1. The volume of surfactant produced by the respiratory tract is relatively constant. The effect the surfactant exerts is related to the surface area it covers.

2. At FRC there is a large amount of surfactant applied per unit area. This causes a significant reduction in pressure as a result of surface tension with the following results:

   a. Prevention of alveolar collapse on exhalation (preventing alveoli from reaching their critical volume).

   b. Reduction in pressure needed to overcome surface tension as inspiration begins.

3. At maximum inspiration a small volume of surfactant is applied per unit area, and the pressure as a result of surface tension tending to collapse the alveoli is great. This pressure assists in normal passive exhalation.

4. Pressure as a result of surface tension

   a. At maximal inspiration: About 40 dynes/sq cm

   b. At maximal exhalation: About 2–4 dynes/sq cm

XIV. Airway Resistance

A. Airway resistance is similar to the frictional forces that exist between solids. In other words, it manifests itself only under dynamic conditions.

  B. In order for gas movement to occur, there must be a pressure gradient. The magnitude of the pressure gradient is determined by the overall resistance of the system.

  C. Flow versus velocity

    1. Flow of gas normally is expressed in liters per minute or liters per second and is defined as the *volume* of a gas that passes a *single point* in a unit of time.

    2. Velocity of gas normally is expressed in centimeters per second and is the *speed* at which a volume of gas passes between *two points*.

  D. In general, resistance is defined as the force (pressure) necessary to maintain a specific flow in a particular system.

    1. In gas physics, airway resistance is equal to the change in pressure divided by flow:

$$R = \frac{\Delta P}{\dot{V}} \qquad (37)$$

where R = airway resistance, ΔP = change in pressure and $\dot{V}$ = flow.

    2. Airway resistance is a physical property of a system in which a particular gas is flowing.

    3. The change in pressure reflects the amount of pressure necessary to maintain a *specific flow* in the system.

    4. The resistance of a system is increased under the following situations:

      a. Decreased lumen of the system

      b. Directional changes in the system

      c. Branching of the system

  E. Types of flow

    1. *Laminar flow* is a smooth, even, nontumbling flow.

      a. A laminar flow system will proceed with a cone front. The molecules of gas in the center of the system will encounter the least frictional resistance and will move at a greater velocity than those at the sides of the system.

      b. In all laminar flow situations, the pressure necessary to overcome airway resistance is directly related to flow:

$$R = \frac{\Delta P}{\dot{V}}. \qquad (38)$$

2. *Turbulent flow* is a rough, tumbling, uneven flow pattern.
   a. A turbulent flow system will proceed with a blunt front. Due to a tumbling effect, all of the molecules in the system will encounter the walls of the vessel, the effects of resistance affecting them all.
   b. In a turbulent flow system, the pressure necessary to overcome airway resistance is directly related to the *square* of the flow:

$$R = \frac{P}{V^2}. \tag{39}$$

   c. *The pressure gradient necessary to maintain turbulent flow is much higher than that necessary to maintain laminar flow.*
3. *Tracheobronchial flow* is a combination of areas of laminar and turbulent flow. Tracheobronchial flow is believed to be the type of flow maintained throughout the respiratory system.

F. *Reynold's number*
   1. The Reynold's number (RN) is a dimensionless number that indicates whether flow through a system is laminar or turbulent.
   2. The Reynold's number is calculated as follows:

$$RN = \frac{(\text{diameter})(\text{velocity})(\text{density})}{(\text{viscosity})} \tag{40}$$

   where the diameter refers to the diameter of the system and velocity, density and viscosity refer to the gas that is flowing in the system.
   3. If the Reynold's number is 2000 or greater, the flow in the system will be turbulent. If it is less than 2000, the flow will be laminar.

G. *Bernoulli effect*
   1. Bernoulli effect: As a gas moves through a free-flowing system, transmural pressure is inversely related to velocity of the gas, i.e., as velocity of the gas increases, transmural pressure decreases.
   2. The above statement holds true because the total energy in a free-flowing system is equal at all points.
   3. In a gas flow system of limited size functioning essentially as a nongravity-dependent system, the total energy is

equal to the sum of the kinetic energy and the transmural pressure energy.

4. Transmural pressure energy is purely a measure of the force that gas flow exerts on the walls of the system.

5. Kinetic energy in this sense is equal to 0.5 times the gas density times the gas velocity squared:

$$\text{Kinetic energy} = 0.5\,(D)(\text{vel.}^2). \tag{41}$$

6. Thus, in a free-flowing system

$$\text{Total energy} = 0.5\,(D)\,(\text{vel.}^2) + P_{\text{transmural}}. \tag{42}$$

This illustrates the fact that velocity and transmural pressure are inversely related.

7. As the radius of the system decreases and velocity of the gas moving through the system increases, transmural pressure will decrease, per Eq. 41.

8. The lower the density of a gas the smaller the decrease in transmural pressure as the gas moves through a stenosis. This relationship demonstrates the effect of density on maintaining a more laminar flow.

9. *Venturi principle*
   a. The Venturi principle is an elaboration of the Bernoulli effect.
   b. It states that distal to a stenosis in a free-flowing system, prestenotic pressure can be restored if the angle of divergence of the system from the midline does not exceed 15 degrees.
   c. Also, if the stenosis in the system is small enough, subatmospheric transmural pressure can be developed and used to entrain a second gas or liquid.
   d. Venturi systems can be designed to deliver specific oxygen concentrations.
   e. All venturi systems designed to deliver a specific oxygen concentration will have the same entrainment ratio.
   f. The concentration of oxygen delivered by a venturi system can be varied by
      (1) Altering the size of the venturi's stenosis
      (2) Altering the size of the entrainment ports
   g. Back pressure on a venturi system will decrease the volume of fluid or gas entrained. This will cause the

oxygen concentration delivered by the system to increase.

G. *Poiseuille's Law*

1. Poiseuille's law originally was used in determination of viscosity of a fluid.

2. Poiseuille's law states that viscosity (n) is equal to the change in pressure (ΔP) times pi (π) times the radius to the fourth power (r^4) divided by eight times the length of the system (1) times flow ($\dot{V}$):

$$n = \frac{\Delta P \pi r^4}{8 l \dot{V}}. \tag{43}$$

3. Rearranging Eq. 42 and placing on the left side of the equation those factors that would be constant when ventilating a patient and on the right side of the equation those factors that would vary, the result is

$$\frac{n 8 l}{\pi} = \frac{\Delta P r^4}{\dot{V}}. \tag{44}$$

4. The right side of Eq. 43 indicates the relationship between pressure, flow and radius of a gas flow system.

5. If the radius were to decrease by one-half, there would be a 16-fold change in the left side of the equation.

6. In order to maintain the left side of the equation constant, a 16-fold change in pressure or flow or a combination of both would be necessary to minimize the effects of the decrease in radius.

7. Thus in order to minimize the effects of an airway diameter decrease, it would be necessary to increase the pressure gradient and/or decrease the flow in the system.

I. Normal airway resistance is equal to about 0.6–2.4 cm H_2O/L/second when measured at a standard flow rate of 0.5 L/second.

J. The airway resistance of a patient being mechanically ventilated on a square-wave flow-pattern ventilator may be estimated by dividing the peak pressure minus the plateau pressure by the flow rate:

$$\text{Airway resistance} \approx \frac{\text{peak pressure} - \text{plateau pressure}}{\text{flow}}. \tag{45}$$

K. In general, the *pressure* necessary to overcome the effects of airway resistance in a ventilator system can be decreased by *decreasing the flow rate.*

1. There would be a decrease in peak pressure but no change in plateau pressure.
2. The plateau pressure reflects compliance changes.
3. The difference between peak and plateau pressures reflects airway resistance.

BIBLIOGRAPHY

Carr, H. Y., and Weidner, R. T.: *Physics from the Ground Up* (New York: McGraw-Hill Book Co., 1971).

Cherniack, R. M., Cherniack, L., and Naimark, A.: *Respiration in Health and Disease* (2d ed.; Philadelphia: W. B. Saunders Co., 1972).

Comroe, J. H.: *Physiology of Respiration* (2d ed.; Chicago: Year Book Medical Publishers, Inc., 1974).

Dejours, P.: *Respiration* (New York: Oxford University Press, 1966).

Egan, D. F.: *Fundamentals of Respiratory Therapy* (3d ed., St. Louis: C. V. Mosby Co., 1977).

Epstein, L. I., and Kuzava, B. A.: *Basic Physics in Anesthesiology* (Chicago: Year Book Medical Publishers, Inc., 1976).

Guyton, A. C.: *Textbook of Medical Physiology* (5th ed.; Philadelphia: W. B. Saunders Co., 1976).

Murray, J. F.: *The Normal Lung* (Philadelphia: W. B. Saunders Co., 1976).

Nunn, J. F.: *Applied Respiratory Physiology with Special Reference to Anaesthesia* (London: Butterworth & Co., Ltd., 1969).

Schaim, U. R., et al.: *College Physics,* Physical Science Study Committee (New York: Raytheon Education Co., 1968).

Young, J. A., and Crocker, D.: *Principles and Practice of Respiratory Therapy* (2d ed.; Chicago: Year Book Medical Publishers, Inc., 1976).

3 / Anatomy of the Respiratory System

I. Boundaries and Functions of the Upper Airway
   - Boundaries: From the anterior nares to the true vocal cords
   - Functions
     1. Heating or cooling inspired gases to body temperature (37 C)
     2. Filtering inspired gases
     3. Humidifying inspired gases to a relative humidity of about 100% at body temperature
     4. Olfaction: Act of smelling
     5. Phonation: Production of sound
     6. Conduction passageway for ventilating gases
   A. The nose
     1. The nose is a rigid structure of cartilage and bone, the superior one-third made up of the nasal and maxilla bones, the inferior two-thirds made up of five large pieces of cartilage.
     2. The two external openings are called the nostrils, external nares or anterior nares. Their lateral borders are termed the alae.
     3. The nasal cavity is divided into two nasal fossae by the septal cartilage.
     4. Each nasal fossa is divided into three regions: vestibular, olfactory and respiratory.
        a. *Vestibular* region: An area of slight dilatation inside the nostril, bordered laterally by the alae and medially by the nasal septal cartilage.
           (1) Contained are coarse nasal hairs (vibrissae) that project anteriorly and inferiorly.
           (2) Sebaceous glands secrete sebum, a greasy substance that keeps the nasal hairs soft and pliable.
           (3) The nasal hairs are the first line of defense for the upper airway, acting as very gross filters of inspired air.
           (4) The vestibular region is lined with stratified squamous epithelium.

b. *Olfactory* region: An area in each nasal cavity defined by the superior concha laterally, nasal septal cartilage medially and roof of the nasal cavity superiorly.

   (1) Contained is the olfactory epithelium responsible for the sense of smell.

   (2) The olfactory epithelium is yellowish brown and appears as pseudostratified columnar epithelial cells. These cells are interspersed with more deeply placed olfactory cells whose sensory filament, the olfactory hairs, protrude to the epithelial surface.

   (3) Due largely to the architecture of the nasal cavity, sniffing causes inspired gases to be drawn to the olfactory region and not much farther into the respiratory tract. This provides a protective mechanism for sampling potentially noxious environmental gases.

c. *Respiratory* region: An area in each nasal cavity inferior to the olfactory region and posterior to the vestibular region. The respiratory region comprises most of the surface area of the nasal fossa.

   (1) Contained in the respiratory region of each nasal fossa are three bony plates called turbinates or conchae. The turbinates extend in a medial and inferior direction from the lateral walls of the nasal fossa.

   (2) The three turbinates (superior, middle and inferior) overhang and define the three corresponding passageways through each nasal cavity, respectively the superior, middle and inferior meati.

   (3) Because of the arrangement of the turbinates and folded mucous membrane covering the turbinates in the nose, it has a volume of about 20 cc and a remarkably large surface area of about 160 sq cm.

   (4) Turbulent flow is created through the respective meati, which serve the three primary functions of the nose: heating, humidifying and filtering inspired gases.

   (5) Heating, humidifying and filtering of inspired gases are accomplished by the turbulent flow, which provides a greater probability that each gas molecule will come in contact with the very large surface area of the vascular nasal mucous membrane. This large gas to nasal surface interface allows the following:

(a) The abundant underlying vasculature to heat inspired gases to body temperature.

(b) The moist nasal mucous membrane to give up 650–1000 ml of H_2O per day in bringing inspired gases to a relative humidity of 80% upon leaving the nose and entering the nasopharynx.

(c) Particles suspended in the inspired gas to contact the sticky mucous membrane, thus filtering out particles greater than 5 μ by inertial impaction to an efficiency of about 100%.

(6) The epithelial lining of the respiratory region of the nasal cavity is pseudostratified ciliated columnar epithelium.

(a) The cells are cylindrical and appear to be two cell layers thick due to the high lateral pressures compressing the cells. Actually the epithelium is only one cell layer thick, each columnar cell making contact with the basement membrane.

(b) Each columnar cell has 200–250 cilia on its luminal surface. Each of the cilia contains two central and nine paired peripheral fibrils. It is the sliding interaction of these fibrils that is thought to cause the beating of the cilia.

(c) Goblet cells and submucosal glands are interspersed throughout the epithelium and, along with capillary seepage, are responsible for production of mucus (100 ml per day in health).

(d) Mucus exists in two layers:
   (i) Sol layer: Fluid bottom layer housing the cilia
   (ii) Gel layer: A viscous layer overlying the cilia

(e) On the forward stroke, the cilia become rigid. Their tips touch the undersurface of the gel layer and propel it toward the oropharynx. On the backward stroke, the cilia become flaccid, fold upon themselves and slide entirely through the sol layer to their resting position without producing a retrograde motion of the gel layer.

(f) The cilia of a particular cell and adjacent cells beat in a coordinated and sequential fashion that produces a motion very similar to a wave. This allows a unidirectional flow of mucus. The cilia beat about 1000–1500 times per minute and move the mucous layer at a rate of 2 cm per minute.

  (g) Function of the mucus and pseudostratified ciliated columnar epithelium (mucociliary blanket)
     (i) To entrap inspired particles.
     (ii) To humidify inspired gas.
     (iii) To transport debris-laden mucus out of the respiratory tract.

5. The nose is responsible for one half to two thirds of the total airway resistance during nasal breathing. It therefore is not surprising that during stress (e.g., exercise or disease) a switch is made to mouth breathing.
6. The nose ends with the outlet of the nasal cavity into the nasopharynx through the internal nares (posterior nares or choanae).

B. Paranasal sinuses
  1. Sinuses are cavities of air in the bones of the cranium.
  2. The function of the sinuses is not clearly understood, but it may be twofold:
    a. To give the voice resonance (prolongation and intensification of sound).
    b. To lighten the head to some extent, the space occupied by the sinuses being filled with air rather than bone.
  3. The sinuses are absent or rudimentary at birth and grow most simultaneously with the development of the permanent teeth. Formation of the sinuses is responsible for the alteration in facial shape that occurs at this time.
  4. All of the air sinuses are lined with pseudostratified ciliated columnar epithelium and produce mucus, which drains into the nasal meati.
  5. If sinus drainage is blocked by nasograstric tubes or nasotracheal intubation, sinusitis and sinus infection often result.
  6. Groups of paranasal sinuses: Frontal, maxillary, sphenoidal and ethmoidal.
    a. The *frontal sinuses* appear as paired sinuses medial to the orbits of the eye and superior to the roof of the nasal cavity between external and internal surfaces of the

frontal bone. They drain into the anterior portion of the middle meati.
  b. The *maxillary sinuses* appear as paired sinuses lateral to each nasal cavity and inferior to the orbits of the eye in the body of the maxilla. These sinuses, the largest of all the air sinuses, drain into the middle meati.
  c. The *sphenoidal sinuses* appear as paired sinuses posterior and inferior to the roof of the nasal cavity and superior to the internal nares (choanae) in the body of the sphenoid bone. They drain into the superior meati.
  d. The *ethmoidal sinuses* are paired sinuses that exist in three groups: anterior, medial and posterior ethmoidal. They exist just lateral to the superior and middle conchae, medial to the orbits of the eyes, inferior to the frontal sinuses and superior to the maxillary sinuses in the ethmoid bone. The ethmoidal sinuses drain into the superior and middle meati.
C. Pharynx
  1. The pharynx is a hollow muscular structure lined with epithelium.
  2. Major functions
    a. To produce the vowel sounds (phonation) by changing its shape.
    b. To serve as a common passageway for ventilating gases, food and liquid.
  3. The pharynx is about 5 in. long and extends from the internal nares (choanae) inferiorly to the esophagus.
  4. Sections of the pharynx: Nasopharynx, oropharynx and laryngopharynx.
    a. The *nasopharynx* is located behind the nasal cavity and extends from the internal nares superiorly to the tip of the uvula inferiorly.
      (1) The epithelium is continuous with the epithelium of the nasal cavity and is pseudostratified ciliated columnar epithelium.
      (2) The eustachian or auditory tubes open into the nasopharynx on each of its lateral walls and communicate with the tympanic cavity or middle ear.
        (a) This allows equilibration of pressure on each side of the tympanic membrane (eardrum) with environmental pressure changes.

        (b) Nasal intubation commonly blocks the eustachian tube openings and may cause otitis media.

    (3) The pharyngeal tonsil or adenoid is located in the superior and posterior wall of the nasopharynx.

        (a) The pharyngeal tonsil consists of a large concentration of lymphoid tissue comprising the superior portion of Waldeyer's ring. This ring of lymphoid tissue surrounds and guards the entrance to the respiratory and gastrointestinal tracts.

    (4) During the process of swallowing, the uvula and soft palate move in a posterior and superior direction to protect the nasopharynx and nasal cavity from the entrance of food and/or liquid.

    (5) Major functions of nasopharynx

        (a) Gas conduction

        (b) Filtration of gases

        (c) Defense mechanism of the body (tonsils)

  b. The *oropharynx* is located behind the oral or buccal cavity and extends from the tip of the uvula superiorly to the tip of the epiglottis inferiorly.

    (1) The epithelial lining is stratified squamous epithelium.

    (2) The palatine tonsils are located lateral to the uvula on the lateral and anterior aspects of the oropharynx.

    (3) The lingual tonsil is located at the base of the tongue, superior and anterior to the vallecula (the space between the epiglottis and base of the tongue).

    (4) The two palatine tonsils, one lingual and one pharyngeal (adenoid), comprise the major components of Waldeyer's ring.

    (5) Major functions of oropharynx

        (a) Gas conduction

        (b) Food and fluid conduction

        (c) Filtration of inspired gases

        (d) Defense mechanism of the body (Waldeyer's ring)

  c. The laryngopharynx or hypopharynx extends superiorly from the tip of the epiglottis to a point inferiorly where it bifurcates into larynx and esophagus.

(1) The epithelial lining is stratified squamous epithelium.
(2) Major functions of laryngopharynx
   (a) Gas conduction
   (b) Food and fluid conduction
(3) The laryngopharynx leads anteriorly into the larynx and posteriorly into the esophagus.
(4) The larynx* is considered the connection between the upper and lower airways, the exact division being the true vocal cords.

II. Boundaries and Functions of the Lower Airway
- Boundaries: From the true vocal cords to the terminal air spaces (alveoli).
- Functions
  1. Ventilation: To and fro movement of gas (gas conduction).
  2. External respiration: Actual gas exchange between body (pulmonary capillary blood) and external environment (alveolar gas).
  3. Sphincter or glottic mechanisms
     a. Valsalva maneuver: Forced expiration against closed glottis.
     b. Müller maneuver: Forced inspiration against closed glottis.
     c. Cough mechanism.
     d. Protection of laryngeal inlet.
  4. Phonation: Production of sound.

A. The larynx
  1. The larynx is a boxlike structure made of cartilage connected by extrinsic and intrinsic muscles and ligaments. It is lined internally by a mucous membrane.
  2. Functions
     a. Gas conduction: Ventilation.
     b. Phonation: Production of sound.
     c. Sphincter or glottic mechanism.
  3. The larynx extends from the third to sixth cervical vertebrae in the anterior portion of the neck.
  4. Unpaired cartilages of the larynx: Epiglottis, thyroid and cricoid.

---

*For discussion and organizational purposes a complete description of the larynx will follow after Section II on the lower airway (please note that the superior portion of the larynx is part of the upper airway and the inferior portion of the larynx is part of the lower airway).

a. *Epiglottic cartilage*
   (1) Leaf-shaped piece of fibrocartilage.
   (2) Anteriorly attached to thyroid cartilage just inferior to thyroid notch.
   (3) Laterally attached to folds of mucous membrane called aryepiglottic folds.
   (4) On swallowing, the epiglottis is squeezed between the base of the tongue and thyroid cartilage, causing the epiglottis to pivot in a posterior and inferior direction to cover the laryngeal inlet.
b. *Thyroid cartilage*
   (1) The largest laryngeal cartilage.
   (2) The anterior aspect is called the laryngeal prominence or Adam's apple.
   (3) Directly superior to the laryngeal prominence is the thyroid notch.
   (4) The posterior and lateral aspects of this cartilage have two superior and two inferior projections, the superior and inferior cornua.
       (a) The superior cornu articulates with the hyoid bone, which serves as a support from which the lower respiratory tract is suspended.
       (b) The inferior cornu articulates with the cricoid cartilage below.
c. *Cricoid cartilage*
   (1) Shaped like a signet ring.
   (2) Forms the entire inferior aspect and most of the posterior aspect of the larynx.
   (3) On the posterior-lateral surface exist articulating surfaces for the inferior cornu of the thyroid cartilage.
   (4) On the posterior-superior surface exist articulating surfaces for the paired arytenoid cartilages.
   (5) Lies inferior to the thyroid and superior to the trachea to which it attaches.
   (6) Lies anterior to the esophagus. Therefore, external cricoid pressure may facilitate viewing of the glottis during tracheal intubation and prevent reflux from the stomach by compressing the esophagus.
5. Paired cartilages of the larynx: Arytenoid, corniculate and cuneiform.
a. *Arytenoid cartilages*

      (1) Shaped like upright pyramids.

      (2) The base of each cartilage articulates with the posterior-superior surface of the cricoid cartilage.

      (3) Each arytenoid cartilage has a ventral-medial projection from its base called the vocal process to which the vocal ligaments attach.

      (4) Arytenoid cartilages, along with the cricoid cartilage, make up the entire posterior surface of the larynx.

  b. *Corniculate cartilages*

      (1) Shaped like cones and are the smallest cartilages of the larynx.

      (2) Articulate with the arytenoid cartilages on their superior surface to which the corniculate cartilages are sometimes fused.

      (3) When the larynx is viewed from above, the corniculate cartilages appear as two small elevations on the posterior-medial aspect of the laryngeal inlet.

      (4) Housed in mucosal folds called the aryepiglottic folds.

  c. *Cuneiform cartilages*

      (1) Shaped like small, elongated clubs.

      (2) Located lateral and anterior to the corniculate cartilages.

      (3) When the larynx is viewed from above, the cuneiform cartilages appear as two small elevations just lateral and anterior to the corniculate cartilages.

      (4) Housed in the aryepiglottic folds.

      (5) The cuneiforms, along with the aryepiglottic folds, form the lateral aspect of the laryngeal inlet. The epiglottis forms the anterior aspect, the corniculates the posterior aspect of the laryngeal inlet.

6. Extrinsic ligaments of the larynx

  a. Extrinsic ligaments attach cartilages of the larynx to structures outside the larynx.

  b. The *thyrohyoid membrane* is a broad fibroelastic sheet that attaches the anterior and lateral superior aspects of the thyroid cartilage to the inferior surface of the hyoid bone (the posterior portion of the thyroid cartilage is attached to the hyoid bone by the superior cornu of the thyroid cartilage).

  c. The *hyoepiglottic ligament* is an elastic band that attaches the anterior surface of the epiglottis to the hyoid bone.

d. The *cricotracheal ligament* connects the lower portion of the cricoid cartilage to the trachea by a very broad fibrous membrane.

7. Intrinsic ligaments of the larynx

a. Intrinsic ligaments attach cartilages of the larynx to one another.

b. The *thyroepiglottic ligament* attaches the inferior aspect of the epiglottis to the thyroid cartilage on its internal surface below the thyroid notch.

c. The *aryepiglottic ligament* attaches the arytenoid cartilages to the epiglottis and acts as a point of attachment for the aryepiglottic folds.

d. The *cricothyroid ligament* attaches the anterior portion of the thyroid cartilage to the anterior portion of the cricoid cartilage. It is through this ligament that an emergency cricothyroidotomy is performed.

e. The *vocal ligament* is a thick band that stretches from the vocal process of the arytenoid cartilages across the cavity of the larynx to attach to the thyroid cartilage just inferior to the thyroepiglottic ligament. The lateral borders of the vocal ligament attach to the inverted free borders of the cricothyroid ligament.

f. The *ventricular ligament* is a thick band that stretches from the arytenoid cartilage across the cavity of the larynx to the thyroid cartilage. It exists superior and lateral to the vocal ligament.

8. Cavity of the larynx

a. The larynx is divided into three sections by the pair of ventricular folds and vocal folds.

b. The *upper section*, the vestibule of the larynx, extends from the laryngeal inlet to the level of ventricular folds.

(1) The ventricular folds are called the false vocal cords.

(2) The space between the ventricular folds is the rima vestibuli.

c. The *middle section*, the ventricle of the larynx, extends from ventricular folds to vocal cords.

(1) The vocal folds are the true vocal cords.

(2) The space between the vocal folds is the rima glottidis or glottis.

(a) The glottis is triangular, the base being posterior, the apex anterior.

(b) It is the smallest opening of the adult airway (important when selecting endotracheal tube size).

(c) The dimensions of the glottis are smaller in the female than in the male.

   (i)   Average female transverse diameter: 7–8 mm.

   (ii) Average male transverse diameter: 9–10 mm.

   (iii) Average anteroposterior diameter in the female: 17 mm.

   (iv) Average anteroposterior diameter in the male: 24 mm.

(3) The size of the rima glottidis also is variable, depending on the state of the vocal cords.

   (a) Adduction is accomplished by medial rotation and approximation of the arytenoids, thus sealing the glottis.

   (b) Abduction is accomplished by lateral rotation of the arytenoids, thus increasing the size of the glottis.

(4) The glottic or sphincter mechanism requires aryepiglottic folds, epiglottis, ventricular folds and vocal folds to act in a very coordinated fashion in sealing the laryngeal inlet.

   d. The *lower section* of the larynx extends from vocal folds to cricoid cartilage.

   e. The epithelial lining of the larynx above the true vocal cords is continuous with the laryngopharynx and is stratified squamous epithelium.

   f. The epithelial lining of the larynx below the true vocal cords is pseudostratified ciliated columnar epithelium.

B. Tracheobronchial tree and lung parenchyma

   1. The tracheobronchial tree functions in ventilation (to and fro movement of air) and is sometimes referred to as the conducting airway.

   2. The lung parenchyma functions in external respiration and is the area of the lung where actual gas exchange occurs.

   3. As the lower airway subdivides, it gives way to more and more airways (generations). Each new generation of air-

ways is assigned a number. The numbering system below begins with assigning generation #0 to the trachea. The first branching or division of the trachea constitutes the mainstem bronchi, which are assigned generation #1. Each subsequent branching of the lower airway is assigned the subsequent generation number.

C. Trachea (generation #0)

1. The trachea is a cartilaginous, membranous tube 10–13 cm in length and 2–2.5 cm in diameter.

2. The trachea extends from the cricoid cartilage at the sixth cervical vertebra to its point of bifurcation (carina) at the fifth thoracic vertebra.

3. Sixteen to twenty incomplete cartilaginous rings open posteriorly and are arranged horizontally. The open ends of the cartilage and the area between individual cartilages are joined by a combination of fibrous, elastic and smooth muscle tissue.

   a. The smooth muscle is arranged longitudinally to shorten and elongate the trachea.

   b. The smooth muscle also is arranged transversely to constrict and dilate the trachea.

4. The posterior wall of the trachea is separated from the anterior wall of the esophagus by loose connective tissue.

5. The trachea and following large airways (bronchi) contain three characteristic layers:

   a. Cartilaginous layer.

   b. Lamina propria, which contains small blood vessels, lymphatic vessels, nerve tracts, elastic fibers, smooth muscle and submucosal glands.

   c. Epithelial, or intraluminal, layer, which is separated from the lamina propria by a noncellular basement membrane.

6. The epithelial lining of the trachea is continuous with the larynx above and is pseudostratified ciliated columnar epithelium.

D. Mainstem bronchi (generation #1)

1. The trachea bifurcates into two airways, right and left mainstem bronchi at the carina.

   a. Right mainstem bronchus

      (1) Branches off the trachea at an angle of about 20 to 30 degrees with respect to the midline.

      (2) Diameter: About 1.4 cm.

      (3) Length: About 2.5 cm.

   b. Left mainstem bronchus

      (1) Branches off the trachea at an angle of 40 to 60 degrees with respect to the midline.

      (2) Diameter: About 1.0 cm.

      (3) Length: About 5 cm.

2. A portion of mainstem bronchi is extrapulmonary (exists outside the lung, in the mediastinum) with the majority of it lying in an intrapulmonary location (inside the lung proper).

3. The structural arrangement of the mainstem bronchi is the same as that of the trachea, with C-shaped pieces of cartilage, a lamina propria and pseudostratified ciliated columnar epithelium.

4. The only structural difference of the mainstem bronchi from the trachea is that the intrapulmonary section of the mainstem bronchi is covered with a sheath of connective tissue, the peribronchiolar connective tissue.

   a. The function of peribronchiolar connective tissue is to encase large nerve, lymphatic and bronchial blood vessels as they follow the branchings of the subdividing airways.

   b. The peribronchiolar connective tissue continues to follow the branching of the airways until the level of the bronchioles, where it disappears.

5. Mainstem bronchi are sometimes referred to as primary bronchi.

E. Lobar bronchi (generation #2)

1. Five lobar bronchi correspond, respectively, to the five lobes of the lung.

2. The right mainstem bronchus trifurcates into right upper, middle and lower lobar bronchi.

3. The left mainstem bronchus bifurcates into left upper and lower lobar bronchi.

4. The structural arrangement of lobar bronchi is the same as that of mainstem bronchi.

5. The epithelial lining of lobar bronchi is pseudostratified ciliated columnar epithelium.

6. Lobar bronchi are sometimes referred to as secondary bronchi.

F. Segmental bronchi (generation #3)
   1. There are 18 segmental bronchi, corresponding respectively to the 18 segments of the lung.
   2. The structural arrangement of segmental bronchi is similar to that of lobar and mainstem bronchi except that the C-shaped pieces of cartilage become less regular in shape and volume.
   3. The epithelial lining of segmental bronchi is pseudostratified ciliated columnar epithelium.
   4. Segmental bronchi are sometimes referred to as tertiary bronchi.
G. Subsegmental bronchi (generations #4–9)
   1. Diameter of subsegmental bronchi ranges from 1 mm to 6 mm.
   2. Cartilaginous rings give way to irregularly placed pieces of cartilage circumscribing the airway, the cartilaginous plaques.
   3. By the ninth generation of airways, cartilage is only scantily present.
   4. As volume and regularity of cartilage have decreased from generation #0 to generation #9, so has the number of submucosal glands and goblet cells.
   5. The epithelial lining of subsegmental bronchi is pseudostratified ciliated columnar epithelium.
H. Bronchioles (generations #10–15)
   1. Diameter is characteristically 1 mm.
   2. Cartilage is totally absent.
   3. Peribronchiolar connective tissue is absent, the lamina propria of these airways being directly embedded in surrounding lung parenchyma.
   4. Airway patency is dependent not on the structural rigidity of surrounding cartilage, but on fibrous, elastic and smooth muscle tissue.
   5. The epithelial lining of bronchioles is pseudostratified ciliated cuboidal epithelium.
      a. This epithelium is functionally the same as pseudostratified ciliated columnar epithelium.
      b. It differs from pseudostratified ciliated columnar epithelium in three ways:
         (1) It is thinner, being constructed of cuboidal cells versus columnar cells.
         (2) The number of goblet cells and submucosal glands

gradually decreases, being almost nonexistent by generation #15.

(3) The number of cilia also is decreased and all but gone by the end of generation #15.

I. Terminal bronchioles (generation #16)

1. Average diameter is 0.5 mm.

2. Goblet cells and submucosal glands disappear, although mucus is found in these airways.

3. Cilia are absent from the epithelium of terminal bronchioles. This epithelium serves as a transition from the cuboidal epithelium of generation #15 to the squamous epithelium of generation #17.

4. Clara cells are located in the terminal bronchioles.

    a. Plump columnar cells that bulge into the lumen of terminal bronchioles

    b. Probably responsible for mucus and/or surfactant found in terminal bronchioles

5. Terminal bronchioles mark the end of the conducting airways; all airway generations distal to the terminal bronchioles are considered part of the lung parenchyma.

J. Respiratory bronchioles (generations #17–19)

1. Average diameter is 0.5 mm.

2. Alveoli arise from the external surface of the respiratory bronchioles, where a very small portion of external respiration takes place.

3. The epithelial lining of respiratory bronchioles is a very low cuboidal epithelium interspersed with actual alveoli (simple squamous epithelium).

K. Alveolar ducts (generations #20–24)

1. Alveolar ducts arise from respiratory bronchioles.

2. The only difference between alveolar ducts and respiratory bronchioles is that the walls of the alveolar ducts are totally made up of alveoli.

3. About one half of the total number of alveoli arise from alveolar ducts.

4. Alveolar ducts give way to alveolar sacs.

L. Alveolar sacs (generation #25)

1. Alveolar sacs are the last generation of airways and are blind passageways.

2. These appear functionally the same as alveolar ducts but differ in that they form grapelike clusters having common walls with other alveoli.

      3. The remaining half of alveoli rise from alveolar sacs.

M. Alveoli

    1. The alveoli are terminal air spaces that contain numerous capillaries in their septa, which serve as sites for gas exchange.

    2. The average number of total alveoli contained in both lungs combined is 300,000,000, but varies directly with the height of the individual.

    3. The total cross-sectional area provided by the alveolar surface is about 80 sq m.

    4. The total cross-sectional area provided by the pulmonary capillaries is 70 sq m, thus constituting an alveolar gas, pulmonary blood interface of 70 sq m (the size of a tennis court).

N. Alveolar capillary membrane

    1. The alveolar capillary membrane has four components: surfactant layer, alveolar epithelium, interstitial space and capillary endothelium.

       a. The surfactant is composed of a phospholipid attached to a lecithin molecule.

          (1) Surfactant lines the internal alveolar surface.

          (2) It reduces surface tension, facilitating inspiration and expiration.

       b. Alveolar epithelium (simple squamous epithelium) is a continuous layer of tissue made up of Type I and II cells lying on a basement membrane.

          (1) Type I cells, or squamous pneumocytes: Very flat, thin simple squames making up 95% of alveolar surface.

          (2) Type II cells, or granular pneumocytes: Plump, highly metabolic cells credited with surfactant production and alveolar repair.

          (3) Type III cells, or alveolar macrophages: Free, wandering phagocytic cells, which ingest foreign material on the alveolar surface.

       c. The interstitial space is the area that separates the basement membrane of alveolar epithelium from the basement membrane of capillary endothelium.

          (1) It contains interstitial fluid.

          (2) This space may be so small, especially where diffusion is to take place, that the basement membranes appear fused.

  d. Capillary endothelium is a continuous layer of tissue made up of flat, interlocking squames supported on a basement membrane.

  2. Thickness of the alveolar capillary membrane varies from 0.35μ to 1μ.

III. The Lung

  A. The lung is situated in the thoracic cavity separated by a structure (mediastinum) containing the heart, great vessels, esophagus and trachea.

  1. Each thoracic cavity is lined with a very fine serous membrane, the parietal pleura, which also covers the dome of each hemidiaphragm.

  2. The lung and each of its lobes are encased in a similar serous membrane called the visceral pleura.

  3. A potential space (intrapleural space) between the two pleura contains a small amount of fluid called pleural fluid.

  a. Pleural fluid allows cohesion of visceral and parietal pleura.

  b. Pleural fluid allows the two pleura to slide over each other with reduced frictional resistance.

  B. The lung is a conical-shaped organ with four surfaces: apex, base, medial surface and costal surface.

  1. The apices are rounded superior sections of the lung. They extend 1–2 inches above the clavicles.

  2. The bases are concave inferior surfaces of the lung. They rest on the hemidiaphragm. The right base lies higher in the thorax than does the left to accommodate the large, underlying liver.

  3. The medial surface of each lung exhibits a deep concavity to accept the heart and great vessels. This concavity is called the cardiac impression. The left cardiac impression is deeper than the right because the heart projects itself to the left of the midline.

  4. The costal surface constitutes most of the lung surface in contact with the pleura lining the thoracic cavity.

  C. The root of the lung enters the lung proper at the hilum.

  1. The root of the lung consists of a mainstem bronchus, a pulmonary artery, two pulmonary veins, major lymph vessels and nerve tracts.

  2. The hilum is the area where the root enters the lung. There the mediastinal and visceral pleura become continuous, forming the pulmonary ligament. This arrangement

keeps the pleural cavity sealed and allows the root to enter the sealed lung.
D. The right lung is divided into three lobes by the horizontal and oblique fissures.
  1. The oblique fissure isolates the right lower lobe from the right middle and right upper lobe.
  2. The horizontal fissure divides the right upper lobe from the right middle lobe.
  3. Externally the oblique fissure courses through the following landmarks:
     a. Junction of sixth rib and midclavicular line
     b. Junction of fifth rib and midaxillary line
     c. Spinous process of third thoracic vertebra
  4. Externally the horizontal fissure courses through the following landmarks:
     a. Junction of fifth rib and midaxillary line
     b. Follows the medial course of fourth rib
E. The left lung is divided into two lobes by the oblique fissure.
  1. The oblique fissure divides the left upper lobe from the left lower lobe.
  2. Externally the left oblique fissure courses through the same landmarks as does the right oblique fissure.
F. The lobes of the lung are further subdivided into segments.
  1. Right upper lobe
     a. Anterior segment
     b. Apical segment
     c. Posterior segment
  2. Right middle lobe
     a. Lateral segment
     b. Medial segment
  3. Right lower lobe
     a. Superior segment
     b. Anterior basal segment
     c. Lateral basal segment
     d. Medial basal segment
     e. Posterior basal segment
  4. Left upper lobe
     a. Apical-posterior segment
     b. Anterior segment
     c. Superior segment⎤Lingula (anatomically corresponds
     d. Inferior segment ⎦   to right middle lobe)

    5. Left lower lobe
       a. Superior segment
       b. Anteromedial basal segment
       c. Lateral basal segment
       d. Posterior basal segment
    6. Knowledge of bronchopulmonary segmentation becomes important when postural drainage, auscultation, x-ray findings and bronchoscopy are considered.

G. The segments are further subdivided into secondary lobules.
    1. *Secondary lobules* consist of a 15th order airway (bronchiole) associated with three to five terminal bronchioles and the distal respiratory bronchioles, alveolar ducts and alveolar sacs.
    2. The secondary lobule is the smallest self-contained unit of the lung that is surrounded by connective tissue.
    3. Secondary lobules appear as polyhedral masses observable on the lung surface and between fissures as dark intersecting lines.
    4. Secondary lobules have their own discrete single pulmonary arteriole, venule, lymphatic and nerve supply.
    5. Secondary lobules are the building blocks of segments and are discernible on chest x-ray.
    6. Each secondary lobule comprises 30 to 50 primary lobules and measures 1–2.5 cm in diameter.
       a. Primary lobules consist of a 19th order respiratory bronchiole and every generation distal to it.
       b. Primary lobules are not self-contained in connective tissue.
       c. There are about 23 million primary lobules in the lung.
    7. Secondary lobules may be important in isolating and maintaining disease entities locally. They also may be responsible for local matching of ventilation to perfusion.

H. Bronchiolar and alveolar intercommunicating channels
    1. The canals of Lambert may be important structures implicated in collateral ventilation of bronchioles.
    2. The pores of Kohn are interalveolar pores, which allow collateral ventilation of alveoli. Their diameter varies from $3\,\mu$ to $13\,\mu$.

IV. Bony Thorax
A. It is a bony and cartilaginous frame within which lie the principal organs of circulation and respiration.

B. It is conical, narrow above and broad below.
C. Posteriorly the thorax includes the 12 thoracic vertebrae and the posterior portion of the ribs.
D. Laterally the thorax is convex and formed by the ribs.
E. Anteriorly it is composed of the sternum, anterior ends of the ribs and the costal cartilage.
F. The superior opening into the thorax – defined by the manubrium, first rib and first thoracic vertebra – is called the thoracic inlet or operculum.
G. The inferior opening out of the thorax – defined by the 12th rib, costal cartilage of ribs (7 through 10) and 12th thoracic vertebra – is called the thoracic outlet.
H. Functions of the bony thorax are to protect underlying organs, to aid in ventilation and to provide a point of attachment for various bones and muscles.
I. Sternum
    1. The sternum is about 17 cm long.
    2. Divided into 3 sections
        a. Manubrium: Superior portion
        b. Body: Middle portion
        c. Xiphoid process: Inferior portion
    3. The manubrium articulates with the clavicle and the first and second ribs.
    4. The junction of the manubrium and the body is called the angle of Louis. The trachea bifurcates beneath this junction.
    5. The body of the sternum articulates with ribs 2 through 7.
    6. The xiphoid process articulates with the 7th rib.
J. Ribs
    1. Twelve elastic arches of bone, posteriorly connected to vertebral column.
    2. Types of ribs: True, false and floating.
    3. True ribs
        a. Rib pairs 1 through 7.
        b. Called vertebrosternal ribs because they connect to sternum via costal cartilage and vertebrae of spinal column.
    4. False ribs
        a. Rib pairs 8 through 10.
        b. Called vertebrocostal ribs because they connect to costal cartilage of superior rib and vertebrae of spinal column.

5. Floating ribs
   a. Rib pairs 11 and 12.
   b. Have no anterior attachment, lying free in abdominal musculature.
6. The space between the ribs is called the intercostal space.
   a. Wider anteriorly than posteriorly.
   b. Wider superiorly than inferiorly.
7. All 12 pairs of ribs are positioned in an inferior direction.
   a. Contraction of the intercostal muscles elevates the ribs from their natural inclined position.
      (1) A superior-inferior motion of the ribs causes an increase in the transverse diameter of the thorax and is called the bucket-handle effect.
      (2) An anterior-posterior motion of the ribs causes an increase in the anteroposterior diameter of the thorax and is called the pump-handle effect.

V. Muscles of Inspiration
   A. The diaphragm and external intercostal muscles are those normally used for resting inspiration.
      1. Diaphragm: Dome-shaped muscle that separates thoracic from abdominal cavity.
         a. It is the major muscle of ventilation.
         b. Origin: Thoracic outlet.
         c. Insertion: Central tendon.
         d. Action: Increases vertical diameter of thorax.
         e. Innervation: Cervical spinal motor nerves 3, 4 and 5 (phrenic nerve).
      2. External intercostals
         a. Origin: Inferior border of superior rib.
         b. Insertion: Superior border of inferior rib.
         c. Action: Elevate ribs, increasing anterior-posterior and transverse diameters of thorax (pump- and bucket-handle effects).
         d. Innervation: Thoracic spinal motor nerves 1 through 11.
         e. Along with internal intercostals, this muscle group prevents the intercostal space from bulging and recessing with normal ventilatory efforts.
   B. Accessory muscles of inspiration
      1. Each tends to perform one of two actions; either raising the thorax or stabilizing the thorax so that other muscles can effectively raise the thorax.
         a. Sternocleidomastoid

     b. Scalenes
       (1) Anterior
       (2) Middle
       (3) Posterior
     c. Pectoralis major
     d. Pectoralis minor
     e. Trapezius
     f. Serratus anterior
     g. Levatores costarum
     h. Serratus posterior
     i. Sacrospinalis

  2. It should be noted that use of accessory muscles for resting inspiration is abnormal and that accessory muscle use should occur only with deep or forced inspiration.

VI. Accessory Muscles of Expiration

  A. There are no muscles of quiet resting expiration. Expiration is purely a passive process brought about by the normal elastic tendencies of the lung coupled with cessation of inspiratory muscle contraction. Therefore, any muscles used for expiration are termed accessory muscles of expiration.

  B. Any muscle usage for quiet resting expiration is abnormal.

  C. Accessory muscles of expiration are used only for forced expiration, making expiration an active process.

  D. The accessory muscles of expiration are either of the back, thorax or abdomen and tend either to pull the thorax down or to support the thorax so that other muscle groups can effectively pull down on the thorax.

    1. Latissimus dorsi
    2. Internal intercostals
    3. Rectus abdominis
    4. External oblique
    5. Internal oblique
    6. Transverse abdominis

BIBLIOGRAPHY

Anthony, C. P., and Kolthoff, N. J.: *Textbook of Anatomy and Physiology* (8th ed.; St. Louis: C..V. Mosby Co., 1971).

Comroe, J. H.: *Physiology of Respiration* (2d ed.; Chicago: Year Book Medical Publishers, Inc., 1974).

Crowley, L. V.: *Introductory Concepts in Anatomy and Physiology* (Chicago: Year Book Medical Publishers, Inc., 1976).

Egan, D. F.: *Fundamentals of Respiratory Therapy* (3d ed.; St. Louis: C. V. Mosby Co., 1977).

Fraser, R. G., and Paré, J. A. P.: *Organ Physiology: Structure and Function of the Lung* (Philadelphia: W. B. Saunders Co., 1977).

Gray, H., and Goss, C. M.: *Gray's Anatomy of the Human Body* (29th ed.; Philadelphia: Lea & Febiger, 1973).

Guyton, A. C.: *Textbook of Medical Physiology* (5th ed.; Philadelphia: W. B. Saunders Co., 1976).

Jacob, S. W., and Francone, C. A.: *Structure and Function in Man* (3d ed.; Philadelphia: W. B. Saunders Co., 1974).

McLaughlin, A. J.: *Essentials of Physiology for Advanced Respiratory Therapy* (St. Louis: C. V. Mosby Co., 1977).

Murray, J. F.: *The Normal Lung* (Philadelphia: W. B. Saunders Co., 1976).

Ruch, T. C., and Patton, H. D.: *Physiology and Biophysics* (20th ed.; Philadelphia: W. B. Saunders Co., 1974).

Shapiro, B. A., Harrison, R. A., and Trout, C. A.: *Clinical Application of Respiratory Care* (Chicago: Year Book Medical Publishers, Inc., 1975).

Shibel, E. M., and Moser, K. M.: *Respiratory Emergencies* (St. Louis: C. V. Mosby Co., 1977).

Slonim, N. B., and Hamilton, L. H.: *Respiratory Physiology* (2d ed.; St. Louis: C. V. Mosby Co., 1971).

Wylie, W. D., and Churchill-Davidson, H. C.: *A Practice of Anesthesia* (2d ed.; Chicago: Year Book Medical Publishers, Inc., 1966).

4 / Anatomy and Physiology of the Nervous System

I. Structure of the Nerve Fiber
  A. Each nerve fiber has three components.
    1. Cell body or soma: primary metabolic area.
    2. Dendrites (branchlike structures): Carry impulses to cell body.
    3. Axons: Carry impulses from cell body to other nerves, muscles or organs.
II. Classification of Neurons
  A. Each neuron is classified by direction of impulse transmission.
    1. Sensory (afferent) neurons: Transmit nerve impulses to spinal cord or brain.
    2. Motor (efferent) neurons: Transmit nerve impulses from brain or spinal cord to muscle or gland (effector organ).
    3. Interneurons (internuncial): Conduct impulses from sensory to motor neurons entirely within central nervous system (CNS).
III. Nerve Cell Membrane Potential
  A. In the resting state, the inner surface of the cell membrane is negative as compared to the positive outer surface. This sets up an electric potential across the cell membrane (normal polarity).
    1. Intracellular: The primary cation, potassium (K^+), is readily diffusible across the cell membrane.
    2. Extracellular: The primary cation, sodium (Na^+), is poorly diffusible across the cell membrane.
    3. High extracellular Na^+ and low extracellular K^+ levels, along with high intracellular K^+ and low intracellular Na^+ levels, are maintained in the resting state by the *Na pump* (active transport).
    4. Continual K^+ diffusion to the outside of the membrane sets up a negative intracellular membrane charge and a positive extracellular membrane charge.

IV. Action Potential
  A. The action potential is any factor that increases the nerve cell membrane's permeability to sodium ions (depolarization).
  B. Depolarization will result in a rapid change in membrane potential.
  C. Causes of action potential
    1. Electric stimulation.
    2. Chemicals.
    3. Mechanical damage to membrane.
    4. Heat or cold.
    5. Decreased serum calcium (Ca^{+2}), which increases the tendency for development of an action potential (low calcium tetany).
  V. Nerve Impulse Propagation
  A. The nerve impulse is a self-propagating wave of electric charge that travels along the surface of the neuron membrane.
  B. Depolarization: Stage 1 of the action potential, in which an impulse travels along nerve fibers.
    1. Sodium ions rush to inside of the cell membrane.
    2. A positive intracellular membrane charge is set up with a negative extracellular membrane charge.
    3. This is a complete reversal of the membrane potential.
  C. Repolarization: Stage 2 of the action potential, in which membrane returns to normal resting membrane potential state.
    1. Immediately after the impulse passes a point on the membrane, the membrane's permeability to Na^+ is again decreased.
    2. Na^+ ions are actively removed by the Na pump.
    3. The resting membrane potential is re-established.
 VI. Nerve Synapse
  A. The nerve synapse is the junction between one neuron (motor, interneuron or sensory) and the next. It is an actual space between nerve fibers.
  B. Transmission of an impulse from the axon of one nerve to a dendrite, soma or effector organ occurs across the synapse. Distance across the synapse is about 200 Å.
  C. Presynaptic terminals are located on the axon and contain vesicles that store and secrete a transmitter substance into the synapse. The transmitter substance excites the den-

drite or soma of the next nerve, stimulating an action potential.
1. Primary transmitter substances
    a. Acetylcholine
    b. Norepinephrine
D. Postsynaptic terminals are located on dendrite, soma, or effector organ. After being stimulated, these terminals secrete a substance into the synapse to metabolize the transmitter substance.
    1. Transmitter substance acetylcholine is metabolized by cholinesterase (acetylcholinesterase).
    2. Transmitter substance norepinephrine is metabolized by monamine oxidase or catechol-O-methyltransferase.
VII. Alteration of Nerve Impulse Transmission
    A. Acidosis decreases transmission across synapse.
    B. Alkalosis increases transmission across synapse.
VIII. Neuromuscular Junction
    A. This junction is the site of transmission of impulses from nerves to skeletal muscle fibers.
    B. The axon of the nerve branches at its end to form a structure called the motor end plate, which invaginates in muscle fiber but does not penetrate muscle membrane.
    C. The motor end plate's terminal aspects are referred to as sole feet.
    D. Sole feet provide a large area of "contact" on the muscle surface. It is from the sole feet that the transmitter substance acetylcholine is secreted.
    E. After stimulation by an impulse, cholinesterase is secreted by muscle to metabolize acetylcholine.
IX. Reflex Arc or Reflex Action
    A. The reflex arc is the functional process of the nervous system. Most neuromuscular and neuroglandular mechanisms are controlled by it.
    B. The reflex arc consists of a series of neurons in which impulses are transmitted from a receptor or sense organ to the CNS, and then to a motor neuron to elicit a response.
    C. Most simple reflexes consist of an impulse from a sensory neuron being transmitted (normally in the spinal cord) to a motor neuron.
    D. Complex reflexes may comprise many internuncial neurons.
    E. Reflex actions are involuntary, specific, predictable and adaptive.

X. Organization of the Nervous System
  A. Composition of nervous system: brain, spinal cord, ganglia (an aggregation of nerve cell bodies) and nerves, which regulate and coordinate bodily activities.
  B. Divisions of nervous system
    1. Central nervous system (CNS): brain and spinal cord, which acts as a switchboard, receiving and sending impulses to all areas of the body.
    2. Peripheral nervous system:
      a. Motor and sensory nerves enter and leave the CNS (somatic system). These nerves control all voluntary bodily functions.
      b. Autonomic nervous system (ANS): controls unconscious involuntary bodily functions innervating all visceral organs. Autonomic impulses are transmitted through two major subdivisions:
        (1) Parasympathetic (craniosacral) nervous system
        (2) Sympathetic (thoracolumbar) nervous system
XI. Autonomic Nervous System (ANS)
  A. Activated and controlled primarily by
    1. Spinal cord
    2. Brain stem
    3. Hypothalamus
  B. Activated secondarily by
    1. Cerebral cortex
    2. Visceral reflexes
  C. Sympathetic and parasympathetic subdivisions of the ANS.
    1. Sympathetic nervous system (SNS): Nerves of the SNS originate from the spinal cord at levels T1 (thoracic) through L2 (lumbar).
      a. Nerve fibers that transmit SNS impulses
        (1) Preganglionic fibers
        (2) Postganglionic fibers
      b. The SNS fibers synapse primarily at ganglia located along the spinal cord (sympathetic chain). The ganglia of the chain are in turn connected to each other.
      c. The SNS fibers may synapse at peripheral ganglia (celiac ganglion and hypogastric plexus), bypassing the sympathetic chain.
      d. Transmitter substances
        (1) Preganglionic fiber: Acetylcholine.
        (2) Postganglionic fiber: Norepinephrine.

   e. Transmitter substance metabolism
      (1) Acetylcholine: Metabolized by cholinesterase.
      (2) Norepinephrine: Metabolized by monamine oxi-
          dase or catechol-O-methyltransferase, or reab-
          sorbed into the axon.
   2. Parasympathetic nervous system (PNS): Nerves of the
      PNS originate from sacral nerves 1 through 4 and crani-
      al nerves III, VII, IX and X. Eighty percent (80%) of all
      PNS impulses originate from *X cranial (vagus) nerve.*
      a. Nerve fibers that transmit impulses in the PNS
         (1) Preganglionic fiber
         (2) Postganglionic fiber
      b. These fibers synapse at the ganglia of the PNS, which
         are located very close to the organs they innervate.
      c. The transmitter substance for both pre- and postgan-
         glionic fibers is acetylcholine (metabolized by cholin-
         esterase).
   D. Adrenal medulla: Secretes epinephrine (75% by volume)
      and norepinephrine (25% by volume) into the bloodstream,
      resulting in stimulation of the SNS.
      1. Innervation is via specific preganglionic fibers of the SNS.
      2. Adrenal secretions maintain normal tone of the SNS.
   E. Effects of SNS and PNS
      1. Adrenergic effect: An effect activated or transmitted by
         epinephrine.
      2. Cholinergic effect: An effect activated or transmitted by
         acetylcholine.
      3. Effects on various organ systems
         a. Bronchi
            SNS: Relaxes smooth muscles (bronchodilatation)
            PNS: Stimulates glands, contracts smooth muscles
                 (bronchoconstriction)
         b. Blood vessels
            SNS: Strong vasoconstriction or mild vasodilatation
            PNS: Vasodilatation
         c. Heart
            SNS: Increases heart rate (+ chronotropic effect) and
                 force of contraction (+ inotropic effect)
            PNS: Decreases heart rate and force of contraction
         d. Intestine
            SNS: Constricts sphincters of gastrointestinal tract,

decreases glandular secretion of gastrointestinal tract and decreases general motility

PNS: Relaxes sphincters of gastrointestinal tract, increases glandular secretions and increases general motility

e. Salivary gland

SNS: Produces viscid secretions

PNS: Produces profuse watery secretions

f. Eye

SNS: Relaxes ciliary muscle and dilates pupil

PNS: Contracts ciliary muscle and constricts pupil

BIBLIOGRAPHY

Carrier, O.: *Pharmacology of the Peripheral Autonomic Nervous System* (Chicago: Year Book Medical Publishers, Inc., 1972).

Egan, D. F.: *Fundamentals of Respiratory Therapy* (3d ed.; St. Louis: C. V. Mosby Co., 1977).

Ganong, W. F.: *Review of Medical Physiology* (6th ed.; Los Altos, Calif.: Lange Medical Publications, 1973).

Goodman, L. S., and Gilman, A. (eds.): *The Pharmacological Basis of Therapeutics* (5th ed.; Macmillan Publishing Co., Inc., 1975).

Guyton, A. C.: *Textbook of Medical Pharmacology* (5th ed.; Philadelphia: W. B. Saunders Co., 1976).

5 / Neurologic Control of Ventilation

I. Medulla Oblongata
   A. The medulla oblongata acts as an overall integrating center for all afferent impulses.
   B. Afferent impulses are interpreted and efferent impulses are initiated in the medulla oblongata.
   C. The medullary respiratory center maintains the normal rhythmic pattern of ventilation.
   D. Two fairly distinct areas in the medullary center contain respiratory neurons.
      1. Dorsal respiratory group
         a. Functions as initial processing center of afferent impulses.
         b. Originates inspiratory efferent impulses, which travel to ventral respiratory neurons and spinal cord.
      2. Ventral respiratory group
         a. Functions primarily by sending efferent impulses to all expiratory motor neurons.
         b. Originates some inspiratory efferent impulses.
   E. Areas from which afferent impulses are sent to medulla oblongata
      1. Cerebral cortex
      2. Pons
      3. Upper airway reflexes
      4. Vagus (X cranial) nerve
      5. Peripheral chemoreceptors
      6. Central chemoreceptors
      7. Glossopharyngeal (IX cranial) nerve
      8. Miscellaneous reflexes
II. Cerebral Cortex
   A. Initiates all conscious respiratory control.
   B. Mediates ventilatory changes as a result of pain, anxiety or other emotional stimuli.
   C. Governs ventilatory control during speech.
III. The Pons
   A. Two distinct centers in the pons contain afferent respiratory neurons.

    1. Pneumotaxic center
      a. Located in upper pons.
      b. Afferent impulses from pneumotaxic center "fine tune" ventilatory rhythmicity by inhibiting length of inspiration.
      c. Rhythmic ventilation may exist even when the pneumotaxic center is impaired.
      d. If the pneumotaxic center is destroyed, apneustic ventilation (long, sustained inspirations) occurs.
    2. Apneustic center
      a. Located in lower pons.
      b. Afferent impulses from apneustic center cause a sustained inspiratory pattern.
      c. Normal rhythmic ventilation can exist without the apneustic center.
      d. If the apneustic and pneumotaxic centers are destroyed, a rapid, irregular, gasping respiratory pattern occurs.
IV. Upper Airway Reflexes
  A. Nose
    1. Stimulation of nasal mucosa may cause exhalation.
    2. Exhalation is frequently in the form of a sneeze.
    3. Apnea and bradycardia also may result from nasal stimulation.
  B. Nasopharynx
    1. Stimulation may cause the sniff or aspiration reflex.
    2. A rapid inspiration is initiated to move the irritant from nasopharynx to oropharynx.
    3. Stimulation may cause bronchodilatation and hypertension.
  C. Larynx
    1. Stimulation may result in afferent impulses, causing
      a. Apnea
      b. Slow, deep breathing
      c. Coughing
      d. Hypertension
      e. Bronchoconstriction
  D. Trachea
    1. Stimulation may result in afferent impulses, causing
      a. Coughing
      b. Bronchoconstriction
      c. Hypertension

V. Vagus Nerve
  A. Afferent impulses via the vagus nerve originate from two areas.
    1. Baroreceptors
      a. Located in aortic arch.
      b. Stimulated by variations in blood pressure.
      c. Afferent impulses from baroreceptors cause alteration of vascular tone in order to maintain normal blood pressure levels.
      d. Ventilatory response is minimal.
        (1) Hyperventilation may be caused by hypotension.
        (2) Hypoventilation may be caused by hypertension.
    2. Pulmonary reflexes
      a. Pulmonary stretch receptors
        (1) Located in smooth muscle of conducting airways.
        (2) Stimulated by lung inflation, deflation and increased transpulmonary pressures.
        (3) Slowly adaptive to changes in inflating pressure.
        (4) Stimulation of these receptors may cause
          (a) Termination of inspiration or expiration
          (b) Bronchodilatation
          (c) Tachycardia
          (d) Decreased peripheral vascular resistance
      b. Irritant receptors
        (1) Located in epithelium of trachea, bronchi, larynx, nose and pharynx
        (2) Rapidly adaptive
        (3) Stimulated by
          (a) Inspired irritants
          (b) Mechanical factors
          (c) Anaphylaxis
          (d) Pneumothorax
          (e) Pulmonary congestion
        (4) Possible results of stimulation
          (a) Bronchoconstriction
          (b) Hyperpnea
          (c) Constriction of larynx (laryngospasm)
          (d) Closure of glottis
          (e) Cough
      c. Type J (juxtapulmonary-capillary) receptors
        (1) Located in walls of alveoli
        (2) Stimulated by

        (a) Increased interstitial fluid volume

        (b) Chemical irritants

        (c) Microembolism

    (3) Possible effects of stimulation

        (a) Rapid, shallow breathing

        (b) Severe expiratory constriction of larynx

        (c) Hypoventilation and bradycardia

        (d) Spinal reflex inhibition

VI. Peripheral Chemoreceptors

  A. Chemoreceptor cells can differentiate between concentrations or pressures of various substances.

    1. *Carotid bodies*

      a. Located at the bifurcation of the common carotid artery

      b. Innervated by the glossopharyngeal (IX cranial) nerve

      c. Primarily respond to hypoxemia

    2. *Aortic bodies*

      a. Located in the arch of the aorta

      b. Innervated by the vagus (X cranial) nerve

      c. Minor role in regulating ventilation

  B. Peripheral chemoreceptors stimulated by

    1. Decreased PO_2 levels

    2. Change in arterial pH

    3. Synergistic response to hypoxemia and acidosis

  C. Effect of altered PO_2

    1. Initial stimulation occurs at a PO_2 of 500 mm Hg and gradually increases as PO_2 decreases.

    2. Maximum stimulation when arterial PO_2 is between 40 and 60 mm Hg

    3. Gradual decrease in stimulation when arterial PO_2 is less than 30 mm Hg

    4. Additional sources of stimulation

      a. Decreased blood flow

      b. Increased temperature

    5. Conditions having no stimulating effect

      a. Carbon monoxide poisoning

      b. Anemia

  D. Effects of PCO_2 and H^+ concentrations

    1. Stimulation usually is relatively linear over a PCO_2 range of 20–60 mm Hg and an $[H^+]$ range of about 20–60 nM/L (pH 7.50–7.22).

    2. Rapid stimulation of peripheral chemoreceptors by $[H^+]$

and CO_2 but magnitude of response to stimulation is usually significantly less than that from central chemoreceptors.

   E. Slowly adaptive with time to altered PO_2, PCO_2 and $[H^+]$.

VII. Central Chemoreceptors
   A. A poorly defined group of cells located near ventrolateral surface of medulla oblongata.
   B. These cells are in contact with cerebral spinal fluid and arterial blood.
   C. Actual stimulation is caused by $[H^+]$ of cerebral spinal fluid.
   D. Composition of cerebral spinal fluid
      1. Electrolytes similar in content to those in plasma
      2. Low protein content: $15-45$ mg/100 ml
      3. PCO_2: 50.2 ± 2.6 mm Hg
      4. pH: 7.336 ± 0.012
      5. HCO_3^-: 21.5 ± 1.2 mEq/L
   E. Diffusion across blood-brain barrier
      1. The only readily diffusible substance is carbon dioxide.
      2. HCO_3^- and H^+ also move across the membrane, but extremely slowly. Active transport mechanisms are believed involved in movement of these two substances.
   F. Mechanism of stimulation
      1. Changes in arterial PCO_2 will alter diffusion of carbon dioxide across the blood-brain barrier, causing a change in PCO_2 of cerebral spinal fluid.
      2. The altered PCO_2 level will effect a change in cerebral spinal fluid $[H^+]$.
      3. The altered $[H^+]$ will thus stimulate or inhibit ventilation.
      4. Increased PCO_2 (increased H^+) stimulates ventilation, while decreased PCO_2 (decreased H^+) inhibits ventilation.
   G. Factors influencing cerebral spinal fluid carbon dioxide levels
      1. Cerebral blood flow
      2. CO_2 production
      3. CO_2 content of venous blood
      4. CO_2 content of arterial blood
      5. Alveolar ventilation

VIII. Efferent Impulses from Medulla Oblongata
   A. All of these impulses are directed via the spinal cord to the various muscles of ventilation.

B. Skeletal muscle is composed of two types of contractive fiber.
  1. Extrafusal fibers (main muscle): Cause of actual muscular contraction.
  2. Fusimotor fibers (muscle spindle fibers): Organs of proprioception that determine extent of muscle contraction necessary to perform a certain work load.
     a. Extent of contraction of the main muscle is controlled by a feedback mechanism via muscle spindle fibers. These fibers assess the level of contraction of the main muscle and send afferent impulses to the spinal cord, coordinating the extent of the main muscle's contraction.

IX. Medullary Adjustments in Compensated Respiratory Acidosis
  A. An increase in arterial P_{CO_2} causes an increase in cerebral spinal fluid P_{CO_2} levels.
  B. The increased P_{CO_2} levels cause a decrease in cerebral spinal fluid pH.
  C. This decrease causes an increased stimulus to ventilate.
  D. If the mechanisms that caused the increased arterial P_{CO_2} (chronic pulmonary disease, CNS depression) persist for a period of time, cerebral spinal fluid HCO_3^- ion levels will increase, causing cerebral spinal fluid pH to normalize.
  E. Results of normalization of cerebral spinal fluid pH at a new (increased) P_{CO_2} level:
     1. Decreased central chemoreceptor drive to ventilate.
     2. Decreased sensitivity to CO_2 changes.

X. Medullary Adjustments in Compensated Respiratory Alkalosis
  A. Decrease in arterial P_{CO_2} causes a decrease in cerebral spinal fluid P_{CO_2} levels.
  B. Decreased P_{CO_2} levels will result in increased cerebral spinal fluid pH.
  C. This will decrease the stimulus to ventilate.
  D. If the mechanisms that caused the decreased arterial P_{CO_2} (i.e., hypoxemia) persist for a period of time, cerebral spinal fluid HCO_3^- ion levels will decrease, causing cerebral spinal fluid pH to normalize.
  E. Results of normalization of cerebral spinal fluid pH at a new (decreased) P_{CO_2} level
     1. Increased central chemoreceptor drive to ventilate
     2. Increased sensitivity to CO_2 changes

XI. Medullary Adjustments in Compensated Nonrespiratory Acidosis
   A. Decreased plasma pH causes stimulation of peripheral chemoreceptors, increasing ventilation. This will cause a decrease in arterial P_{CO_2}.
   B. The resulting decreased arterial P_{CO_2} will cause inhibition of ventilation via central chemoreceptors.
   C. Thus ventilation via the central chemoreceptors is inhibited and ventilation via the peripheral chemoreceptors is stimulated.
   D. Since the effect on peripheral chemoreceptors is the predominant stimulus, there will be a step-wise readjustment (decrease) of cerebral spinal fluid HCO_3^- levels. This allows normalization of cerebral spinal fluid pH and a sustained increase in the drive to ventilate in order to compensate for nonrespiratory acidosis.
XII. Medullary Adjustments in Compensated Nonrespiratory Alkalosis
   A. Increased plasma pH causes only minor inhibition of peripheral chemoreceptors.
   B. The resulting increased arterial P_{CO_2} will cause increased ventilation via central chemoreceptors.
   C. Clinically only minor increases in arterial P_{CO_2} usually are seen in compensation for nonrespiratory alkalosis. The mechanisms involved in central and peripheral maintenance of normal P_{CO_2} prevent significant P_{CO_2} increases for nonrespiratory compensation. In these situations P_{CO_2} rarely increases over 50 mm Hg.

BIBLIOGRAPHY

Berger, A. J., Mitchell, R. A., and Severinghaus, J. W.: Regulation of respiration, N. Engl. J. Med. 297:92, 1977.

Cherniack, R. M., Cherniack, L., and Naimark, A.: *Respiration in Health and Disease* (2d ed.; Philadelphia: W. B. Saunders Co., 1972).

Comroe, J. H.: *Physiology of Respiration* (2d ed.; Chicago: Year Book Medical Publishers, Inc., 1974).

Dejours, P.: *Respiration* (New York: Oxford University Press, 1966).

Egan, D. F.: *Fundamentals of Respiratory Therapy* (3d ed.; St. Louis: C. V. Mosby Co., 1977).

Guyton, A. C.: *Textbook of Medical Physiology* (5th ed.; Philadelphia: W. B. Saunders Co., 1976).

Mitchell, R. A., and Berger, A. J.: Neural regulation of respiration, Am. Rev. Respir. Dis. 111:206, 1975.

Murray, J. F.: *The Normal Lung* (Philadelphia: W. B. Saunders Co., 1976).

West, J. B.: *Respiratory Physiology: The Essentials* (Baltimore: Williams & Wilkins Co., 1974).

6 / Pulmonary Mechanics

I. Forces Opposing Ventilation
  A. Elastic resistance to ventilation: Forces necessary to over-
     come elastic properties of lung-thorax system.
     1. Major component of elastic resistance: Compliance of
        lung-thorax system
        a. Compliance: Ease with which a structure can be dis-
           torted.
        b. Normally compliance is determined by dividing the
           unit volume change of the lung by the unit pressure
           change necessary to cause that volume change.

$$C = \frac{\Delta V}{\Delta P} \tag{1}$$

        c. The elastic recoil of the lung tends to cause pulmonary
           collapse, whereas the elastic recoil of the thorax tends
           to cause expansion of the thorax.
        d. Total compliance is a result of the combined effects of
           lung and thorax elastance.
        e. Causes of decrease in total compliance
           (1) Pneumonitis
           (2) Pulmonary consolidation
           (3) Pulmonary edema
           (4) Pneumothorax
           (5) Abdominal distention
           (6) Adult respiratory distress syndrome (ARDS)
           (7) Pulmonary fibrosis
           (8) Thoracic deformities
           (9) Complete airway obstruction
        f. Total compliance may be increased by any factor that
           causes a loss of elastic lung tissue.
           (1) Alveolar septal destruction
           (2) Alveolar distention
           Note: See Chapter 2 for a more detailed discussion.
     2. The secondary component of elastic resistance: Surface
        tension of fluid lining respiratory tract
        a. Surface tension: Force tending to cause a fluid to occu-

py the smallest volume possible. In occupying the smallest volume, a system may fall below its critical volume and collapse.

b. In the respiratory tract, surface tension tends to collapse alveoli.

c. Pressure as a result of surface tension is determined by using LaPlace's law as applied to a drop:

$$P = \frac{2\ ST}{r}. \tag{2}$$

d. The ideal LaPlace pressure-radius relationship is altered in the respiratory tract by pulmonary surfactant.

e. Pulmonary surfactant allows surface tension pressure to be lowest at residual volume (RV) level and to increase as inspired volume increases.

Note: See Chapter 2 for more detailed discussion.

B. Nonelastic resistance to ventilation: Forces necessary to overcome frictional resistance to gas flow and tissue displacement.

1. Major component (about 85%) of nonelastic resistance: Airway resistance

a. Airway resistance is a result of movement of molecules of inspired gas over the surface of the airway.

b. Airway resistance in laminar flow situations is equal to

$$R = \frac{\Delta P}{\dot{V}} \tag{3}$$

whereas in turbulent flow situations the relationship is

$$R = \frac{\Delta P}{\dot{V}^2}. \tag{4}$$

c. More than 60% of normal airway resistance is a result of turbulent gas flow through the nose, pharynx and larynx.

d. Resistance to gas flow decreases as gas moves into smaller generations of the airway. Since cross-sectional area of the respiratory tract increases dramatically with increasing generations, flow through any single airway becomes progressively smaller and the pressure necessary to maintain that flow becomes smaller.

e. At the level of the respiratory bronchioles, flow is al-

most absent and gas movement basically is a result of
diffusion.

    f. Airway resistance is always increased when the lumen
of the airway is decreased. Airway lumen may decrease
as a result of

      (1) Bronchospasm

      (2) Mucosal edema

      (3) Partial airway obstruction (retained secretions)

      Note: See Chapter 2 for more detailed discussion.

  2. The secondary component (about 15%) of nonelastic resistance: Tissue viscous resistance, or the force necessary to
move the nonelastic structures of the lung-thorax system
(i.e., the pleurae sliding across each other)

II. Functional Residual Capacity

  A. As stated previously, the thorax tends to expand, whereas the
lung tends to collapse. At the functional residual capacity
(FRC) level the vector forces of pulmonary and thoracic
elastance are equal in magnitude and opposite in direction.

  B. The FRC is the most stable of all lung volumes and capacities
because it is the level that is assumed when complete relaxation of ventilatory muscles occurs.

Fig 6–1.—Intrapleural (intrathoracic) pressure curve during normal spontaneous ventilation. Note that normal resting expiratory pressure is about −5
cm H_2O and decreases to −9 cm H_2O during inspiration.

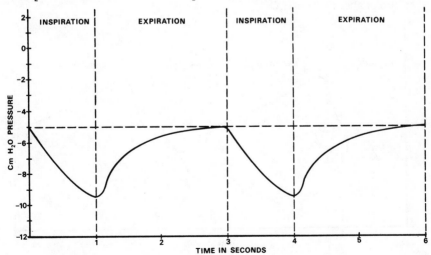

C. If elastance of thorax and/or lung were to increase or decrease, the volume of FRC would be altered.

III. Intrapleural (Intrathoracic) and Intrapulmonary Pressure

A. As a result of opposing vector forces of pulmonary and thoracic elastance, a subatmospheric intrapleural pressure normally is maintained (Fig 6–1).

B. This subatmospheric intrapleural pressure is equal to the intrathoracic pressure.

C. At the FRC level, intrapleural pressure is maintained at about -5 cm H_2O (compared to atmospheric). The -5 cm H_2O intrapleural pressure sets up a pressure gradient between the pleural space and the lung (transpulmonary pressure).

D. During normal inspiration, intrapleural pressure drops to -9 cm H_2O, increasing the transpulmonary pressure gradient. During exhalation, intrapleural pressure returns to -5 cm H_2O.

E. Intrapleural pressure is maintained at a subatmospheric level during normal quiet resting ventilation.

F. At FRC level, intrapulmonary pressure is in equilibrium with the atmosphere (Fig 6–2).

G. During inspiration the increased transpulmonary pressure gradient creates subatmospheric intrapulmonary pressures.

Fig 6–2.—Intrapulmonary pressure during normal spontaneous ventilation has a peak inspiratory pressure of about -3 cm H_2O and peak expiratory pressure of about $+3$ cm H_2O.

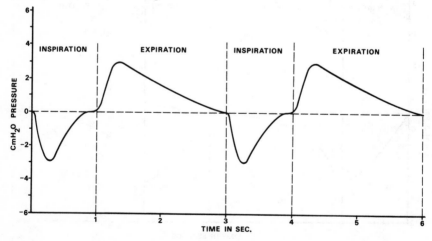

This subatmospheric pressure sets up a pressure gradient with the atmosphere and causes gas to move into the airway.

H. During normal active inspiration, intrapulmonary pressure drops to about -3 cm H_2O.

I. At the end of a normal inspiration, intrapulmonary pressure returns to baseline (atmospheric pressure).

J. During normal quiet exhalation, intrapulmonary pressure increases to about $+3$ cm H_2O.

K. At the end of a normal exhalation, intrapulmonary pressure returns to baseline atmospheric pressure. A pause then exists when there is no gas movement before the next inspiration.

IV. Inspiratory Mechanics

A. Inspiration occurs when contraction of diaphragm and external intercostals causes a decrease in intrapleural pressure. This is reflected to the alveoli, creating a pressure gradient with the atmosphere.

B. The magnitude of contraction of inspiratory muscles is determined by amount of force needed to overcome
1. Compliance of lung-thorax system
2. Surface tension
3. Airway resistance
4. Tissue viscous resistance

C. Essentially, the pressure needed to determine a specific tidal volume is based mainly on (1) compliance of the system and (2) airway resistance.

D. Both compliance and airway resistance may be altered in disease states.

E. With an increase in total compliance, there is a corresponding decrease in elastance. This tends to increase the ease of inspiration but also increases the difficulty in expiration. In this situation a slow, deep ventilatory pattern may be assumed to minimize work of breathing.

F. With a decrease in total compliance, there is a corresponding increase in elastance. This tends to decrease ease of inspiration. In this situation a rapid, shallow ventilatory pattern may be assumed to minimize work of breathing.

G. Increases in pulmonary surface tension may be a result of decreased pulmonary surfactant levels. This tends to increase significantly the work of ventilation as a result of the alveoli collapsing on exhalation as well as being less compliant on inspiration.

H. The effects of an increase in airway resistance can be minimized by a slow inspiratory pattern. This will reduce inspiratory flow rates, turbulence at the site of obstruction and the pressure gradient necessary to overcome resistance.

V. Ventilation/Perfusion Relationships
  A. Distribution of ventilation is unequal throughout the lung as a result of three factors.
    1. Variation in compliance and airway resistance from bases to apices
      a. If the compliance of part of the lung is multiplied by resistance of that part of the lung, a time constant is determined:

$$\text{Compliance} \times \text{resistance} = \text{time constant.} \qquad (4)$$

      b. The time constant of a lung unit determines the amount of time it would take for that unit to fill.
    2. Regional variation in transpulmonary pressure throughout respiratory tract
      a. In the vertical position, the transpulmonary pressure gradient is greater in the apices than in the bases. The reason for this variation is unclear but the following probably affect the gradient:
        (1) Weight of lung
        (2) Effect of gravity on total system, forcing blood flow to dependent areas
        (3) Support of lung at the hilum
      b. Transpulmonary pressure differences cause alveoli in the apices to contain a greater volume at FRC level than do alveoli in the bases.
      c. Differences in alveolar size decrease as inspiration nears total lung capacity (TLC).
    3. The results of differing pulmonary time constants and transpulmonary pressure gradients on ventilation from FRC level
      a. Alveoli in the apices fill slowly and empty slowly (slow alveoli).
      b. Alveoli in the bases fill rapidly and empty rapidly (fast alveoli).
      c. In normal tidal exchange most of the ventilation goes to the bases. Figure 6–3 illustrates the compliance curve of the total lung. The position of the apices on the curve during tidal exchange is on the flatter aspect of the curve, whereas the bases are positioned on the

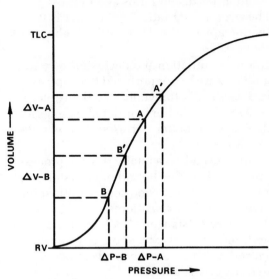

Fig 6–3. — Compliance curve of total lung at functional residual capacity (FRC). *A* to *A'* indicates volume change in the apices during tidal exchange; *B* to *B'* indicates volume change in the bases during tidal exchange. The change in volume of *B (ΔV – B)* is greater than the change in volume of *A (ΔV – A)* for the same pressure change *(ΔP – B is equal to P – A)*.

steeper aspect of the curve. Points *B* to *B'* indicate the volume change during normal ventilation in the bases; points *A* to *A'* indicate the volume change during normal ventilation of the apices. There is a considerably larger volume change in the bases than in the apices per unit pressure change.

B. Distribution of pulmonary blood flow normally is greater in the bases than in the apices as a result of three factors.

   1. Perfusion of any aspect of the lung depends on the relationship between pulmonary hydrostatic pressure and the transpulmonary pressure gradient.

   2. Since the pulmonary vascular system is a low pressure system, in the erect individual the apices of the lung receive virtually no blood flow, whereas the bases are engorged with blood.

   3. In general, the most gravity-dependent aspect of the lung receives most of the blood flow, whereas the least gravity-dependent areas receive very little blood flow.

C. Ventilation/perfusion ratios ($\dot{V}/\dot{Q}$ ratios)
 1. The overall $\dot{V}/\dot{Q}$ ratio for the lung is 0.8.
 2. In the apices the $\dot{V}/\dot{Q}$ ratio is about 3.3, in the bases about 0.6.
 3. Normal ventilation and perfusion
  a. Bases are better perfused than apices.
  b. Bases are better ventilated than apices.
  c. Apices are better ventilated than perfused.
  d. Bases are better perfused than ventilated.

VI. Expiratory Mechanics
 A. Exhalation usually is a totally passive process.
 B. Elastic recoil of the lung-thorax system and the increased pulmonary surface tension seen with inspiration assist in the passive process of exhalation.
 C. If pulmonary elastance is decreased, exhalation may be prolonged, and a forced exhalation may be necessary.
 D. Increased airway resistance also increases the amount of effort during exhalation.

VII. Diffusion
 A. Henry's and Graham's laws demonstrate that carbon dioxide diffuses about 19 times faster than oxygen (see Chap. 2).
  1. This relationship holds true where all factors affecting diffusion are equally applied to carbon dioxide and oxygen (e.g., diffusion gradient, temperature, cross-sectional area).
 B. At the alveolar capillary membrane there is a significant difference in pressure gradients for carbon dioxide and oxygen.
  1. Oxygen pressure gradient 60 mm Hg
  2. Carbon dioxide pressure gradient 6 mm Hg
 C. As a result of these different pressure gradients, oxygen diffuses slightly faster than carbon dioxide across the alveolar capillary membrane.
 D. Any factor that affects diffusibility at the alveolar capillary membrane impairs oxygen diffusibility more so than carbon dioxide.
 E. Pulmonary disease causes decreased PaO_2 much sooner than it affects $PaCO_2$. This is a result of:
  1. Oxygen and carbon dioxide's relative diffusibilities
  2. Shunting, reducing PaO_2 significantly more than $PaCO_2$

BIBLIOGRAPHY

Bendixen, H. H., et al.: *Respiratory Care* (St. Louis: C. V. Mosby Co., 1965).

Cherniack, R. M., Cherniack, L., and Naimark, A.: *Respiration in Health and Disease* (2d ed.; Philadelphia: W. B. Saunders Co., 1972).

Comroe, J. H.: *Physiology of Respiration* (2d ed.; Chicago: Year Book Medical Publishers, Inc., 1974).

Dejours, P.: *Respiration* (New York: Oxford University Press, 1966).

Murray, J. F.: *The Normal Lung* (Philadelphia: W. B. Saunders Co., 1976).

Nunn, J. F.: *Applied Respiratory Physiology with Special Reference to Anaesthesia* (London: Butterworth & Co., Ltd., 1969).

Shapiro, B. A., Harrison, R. A., and Trout, C. A.: *Clinical Application of Respiratory Care* (Chicago: Year Book Medical Publishers, Inc., 1975).

West, J. B.: *Respiratory Physiology: The Essentials* (Baltimore: William & Wilkins Co., 1974).

West, J. B.: *Ventilation/Blood Flow and Gas Exchange* (3d ed.; Oxford: Blackwell Scientific Publications, 1977).

7 / Anatomy of the Cardiovascular System

I. Blood
  A. A heterogeneous substance composed of a fluid (plasma) and a cellular component
  B. Plasma: Whole blood minus the cellular component.
    1. It is a pale yellow (strawlike) color.
    2. Plasma, along with interstitial and intracellular fluid, makes up the three major body fluids.
    3. Major constituents are water and chemical compounds (solutes).
      a. Water, the solvent, constitutes 90–91% of plasma.
      b. The major solutes constitute 9–10% of plasma:

Proteins	*Normal Ranges*
Albumin	4–5.5 gm/100 ml
Globulin	2–3 gm/100 ml
Fibrinogen	200–400 mg/100 ml
Prothrombin	
Foodstuffs	*Normal Ranges*
Glucose	65–110 mg/100 ml
Lipids	350–800 mg/100 ml
Amino acids	
Electrolytes	*Normal Ranges*
Sodium (Na^+)	136–142 mEq/L
Chloride (Cl^-)	100–110 mEq/L
Bicarbonate (HCO_3^-)	24–30 mEq/L
Potassium (K^+)	4–5.4 mEq/L
Calcium (Ca^{+2})	4.8–5.2 mEq/L
Magnesium (Mg^{+2})	1.4–2.2 mEq/L
Phosphate (HPO_4^{-2})	
Sulfate (SO_4^{-2})	
Organic acids	

    4. Plasma minus clotting factors is called blood serum.
  C. Cellular components: Red blood cells, white blood cells and platelets

1. Red blood cells (erythrocytes): Biconcave discs with a diameter of $7-8\,\mu$ and a thickness of about $2\,\mu$.
   a. Mature red blood cells have no nucleus.
   b. Red blood cells are surrounded by a semipermeable membrane.
      (1) Placed in a hypotonic solution (less than 0.9% NaCl), they will swell and can rupture (hemolysis).
      (2) Placed in a hypertonic solution (greater than 0.9% NaCl), they will shrivel (crenation).
   c. Red blood cells are relatively flexible and are able to accommodate changes in shape without rupturing. This becomes important when they pass through tight spots in the circulation (e.g., capillaries or sinusoids).
   d. Red blood cells are produced in myeloid tissue (red bone marrow) — a process termed erythropoeisis.
   e. The normal number of red blood cells is higher in males than in females.
      (1) Female: 4.1–5.1 million RBC/cu mm.
      (2) Male: 4.8–6.0 million RBC/cu mm.
   f. Reticulocytes are newly released red blood cells that retain a small portion of the hemoglobin-forming endoplasmic reticulum.
      (1) In 2 to 3 days, formation of hemoglobin will be complete. At this point, the endoplasmic reticulum disappears and the cell is a mature erythrocyte.
      (2) The percentage of total red blood cells that are reticulocytes indicates the rate of erythropoeisis.
      (3) The normal range (percentage) of reticulocytes is 0.5–1.5% of the total number of red blood cells.
         (a) Greater than 1.5% usually indicates increased erythropoeisis.
         (b) Less than 0.5% usually indicates decreased erythropoeisis.
   g. Hemoglobin is the major solute contained within the red blood cell.
      (1) The normal amount of hemoglobin contained in the blood is higher in males than females:
         (a) Female: 12–14 gm Hb/100 ml of blood
         (b) Male: 13–16 gm Hb/100 ml of blood
   h. The hematocrit is the volume percentage of red blood cells in whole blood, i.e., a hematocrit equal to 45 means that 45% of whole blood is red blood cells by volume.

      (1) The normal hematocrit is higher in males than females:
         (a) Female: 37–47
         (b) Male: 40–54
   i. Normally hemoglobin levels are equal to about one third of the hematocrit.
2. Types of white blood cells (leukocytes): Polymorphonuclear neutrophils, eosinophils and basophils and mononuclear monocytes and lymphocytes.
   a. Polymorphonuclear leukocytes
      (1) Are formed in myeloid tissue.
      (2) Have a multilobed nucleus.
      (3) Are collectively called "polys."
      (4) Appear histologically to possess granulated cytoplasm and are collectively termed granulocytes.
      (5) All can perform phagocytosis.
      (6) Polymorphonuclear neutrophils
         (a) Have a diameter of about 10μ.
         (b) Have a nucleus that contains one to five lobes.
         (c) Are highly phagocytic.
         (d) Comprise 50–75% of the total number of leukocytes.
      (7) Polymorphonuclear eosinophils
         (a) Readily absorb an acid stain.
         (b) Have a bilobed nucleus.
         (c) Are implicated in parasitic as well as allergic processes.
         (d) Comprise 2–4% of the total number of leukocytes.
         (e) Have a diameter of about 10μ.
      (8) Polymorphonuclear basophils
         (a) Readily absorb a basic stain.
         (b) Have a three- or four-lobed nucleus.
         (c) Contain heparin, which may serve to prevent coagulation of blood at sites of inflammation.
         (d) Comprise less than 0.5% of the total number of leukocytes.
         (e) Have a diameter of about 10μ.
   b. Mononuclear leukocytes
      (1) Are formed in lymphoid tissue.
      (2) Mononuclear monocytes
         (a) Have a diameter of $10 – 15 \mu$.

  (b) Have a crescent-shaped nucleus.
  (c) Have cytoplasm containing very fine granules.
  (d) Are highly phagocytic cells.
  (e) Comprise 3–8% of the total number of leukocytes.
(3) Mononuclear lymphocytes
  (a) Have a diameter of about 6–9 μ.
  (b) Have a round nucleus.
  (c) Have cytoplasm that appears clear.
  (d) Form antibodies that remain intracellular
  (cellular antibodies) or form antibodies that are
  released into the bloodstream (circulating antibodies).
  (e) Comprise 20–40% of the total number of leukocytes.
  c. Total white blood cell count has the normal range of
  5,000 to 10,000 white blood cells/cu mm.
  d. A differential count identifies the percentage of the
  total white blood cell count that each white blood cell
  type comprises. (Note normal range [%] in each of the
  white blood cell types previously described.)
  e. Megakaryocyte: a special type of blood cell
  (1) Formed in myeloid tissue.
  (2) Fragments into small irregular pieces of proto-
  plasm called thrombocytes or platelets
  (a) Are 2–4 μ in diameter.
  (b) Have no nucleus.
  (c) Have a granular cytoplasm.
  (d) Normal platelet count 200,000 to 350,000/
  cu mm.
  (e) Function in clot formation (hemostasis).
  D. Total blood volume of an individual
  1. This is equal to about 70–72 ml of blood per kilogram of
  body weight.
  2. This relationship varies inversely with the amount of
  excess body fat, i.e., an obese individual has less blood
  volume per kilogram than does a slender individual.
II. The blood vessels
  A. The blood vessels consist of a closed system of connected arteries, arterioles, capillaries, venules and veins.
  B. *Arteries* contain three characteristic layers: tunica intima, tunica media and tunica adventitia.

    1. Tunica adventitia (external layer)
       a. Consists of connective tissue surrounding a network of collagenous and elastic fibers.
       b. Supports and protects the blood vessels.
       c. Contains vasa vasorum, very fine vessels that serve the tunica adventitia with its blood supply.
       d. Contains lymphatic vessels and nerve fibers.
    2. Tunica media (middle layer)
       a. Thickest layer of the artery.
       b. Composed of circularly arranged smooth muscle and elastic fibers.
       c. Nerve fibers contained in tunica adventitia terminate in the smooth muscle layer of the tunica media.
    3. Tunica intima (internal layer)
       a. Thinnest layer of the artery.
       b. Consists of flat layer of simple squamous cells called the endothelium:
          (1) The endothelium is supported by a fine layer of connective tissue.
          (2) The connective tissue is surrounded by a longitudinally placed network of elastic fibers.
       c. Common to all blood vessels, the endothelium even being continuous with the endocardium of the heart.
  C. Large arteries: Termed "elastic arteries" because the tunica media has less smooth muscle and more elastic fibers.
  D. Medium-sized arteries: Sometimes called "nutrient arteries" because they control flow of blood to various areas of the body. Their ability to regulate blood flow lies in a tunica media, which is almost entirely composed of smooth muscle.
  E. *Arterioles* (small arteries)
    1. The arterioles have a thin tunica intima and adventitia but have a thick, smooth muscle layer in the tunica media.
    2. The arterioles range in diameter from 20μ to 50μ.
    3. The tunica media is extensively innervated by postsynaptic sympathetic nerve fibers.
    4. Due to the extensive innervation and abundance of smooth muscle, the arterioles control regional blood flow to the capillary beds.
    5. The arterioles are frequently called the "resistance vessels." By vasomotion, they control the rate of arterial run-

off (the rate at which blood leaves the arterial tree) and thereby arterial blood volume.

   6. The arterioles terminate in either metarterioles or capillaries.

      a. Metarterioles range in diameter from 10μ to 20μ.

      b. Metarterioles can bypass a capillary bed entirely by shunting blood directly to the venules.

      c. Metarterioles can also allow blood to pass from arterioles to capillaries.

F. *Capillaries*

   1. Consist only of tunica intima.

   2. Vary in diameter from 5μ to 10μ.

   3. Where capillaries originate from arterioles or metarterioles, there frequently is a small band of smooth muscle called the precapillary sphincter.

      a. This sphincter controls blood flow through the distal capillary.

      b. It is responsive (vasoactive) to local P_{CO_2}, P_{O_2}, pH and temperature.

   4. Capillaries frequently are called "exchange vessels," because they are the site of gas, fluid, nutrient and waste exchange.

      a. An intracellular cleft lies between the individual squames comprising the endothelium.

         (1) They are about $50-60$ Å wide.

         (2) They act as pores through which substances can move into and out of the capillaries.

      b. The basement membrane usually is continuous in the capillaries and may limit movement of substances into and out of the capillaries.

G. *Veins* consist of a tunica intima, media and adventitia but each layer is thinner than its counterpart in the arteries.

   1. Tunica adventitia

      a. One to five times as thick as tunica media.

      b. Made up of connective, elastic and smooth muscle tissue.

   2. Tunica media

      a. Made up of circularly arranged smooth muscle, collagenous and elastic tissue.

      b. Innervated with postsynaptic fibers of sympathetic nervous system.

          (1) Veins are not as extensively innervated as arteries.

          (2) By venodilatation or venoconstriction, veins can alter venous blood volume and "venous return."

     3. Tunica intima

       a. Consists of endothelial cells supported by delicate elastic fibers and connective tissue.

  H. In general, all vessels of the venous system have smaller amounts of elastic and smooth muscle tissue than do their arterial counterparts.

  I. *Venules* (small veins) have the three characteristic layers, but they are very thin and almost indistinguishable.

  J. Veins are called "capacitance vessels" or "reservoir vessels" because 70–75% of the blood volume exists in the venous system.

  K. Veins contained in the periphery of the body contain one-way valves.

     1. Valves are formed by duplication of endothelial lining of veins.

     2. Valves are semilunar and prevent retrograde flow of blood.

     3. Valves are found in veins greater than 2 mm in diameter and exist in areas subjected to muscular pressure, e.g., arms and legs.

     4. Valves are absent in veins smaller than 1 mm in diameter and in areas such as the abdominal and thoracic cavities.

III. The lymphatic vessels

  A. These vessels are a type of circulatory system that collects fluid and other material in the interstitial space and returns them to the venous vasculature.

  B. Lymphatic vessels originate as blind end vessels called lymphatic capillaries.

     1. They have no basement membrane and consist only of loosely fitting endothelial cells.

     2. They are invested in every tissue of the body except for cartilage, bone, epithelium and the CNS.

  C. Lymphatic capillaries drain into larger lymphatic vessels, which take on three characteristic layers similar to those of the veins.

     1. Larger lymphatic channels contain smooth muscle, elastic, fibrous and connective tissue.

     2. These vessels resemble the veins except that the three layers composing the lymphatics are much thinner.

   3. One-way semilunar valves are found about every milli-
      meter and are more frequent in the lymphatics than in the
      veins.
D. The larger lymphatic vessels drain into lymph nodes.
   1. Lymph nodes are found in neck, axilla, groin, thorax,
      breast, arms and mouth.
   2. Lymph nodes are bean or oval shaped.
   3. Lymph moves into the lymph nodes via afferent lymphat-
      ic channels.
      a. The lymph is exposed to phagocytic reticular endo-
         thelial cells lining the sinus of the nodes.
      b. The lymph is filtered and exits from the lymph node
         via efferent lymphatic channels.
E. The large efferent lymphatic vessels join one of two major
   lymphatic ducts.
   1. Right lymphatic duct
      a. Drains right upper quadrant of the trunk.
      b. Drains right side of head and neck.
      c. Drains filtered lymph into right subclavian vein.
   2. Thoracic duct
      a. Drains remainder of the body.
      b. Largest lymphatic vessel but smaller than either vena
         cava.
         (1) The duct is 15–18 in. long.
         (2) It originates in lumbar region of abdominal cavity
             and ascends to the neck.
      c. Drains filtered lymph into left subclavian vein.
IV. The heart
A. The heart is a muscular pump that maintains circulation of the
   blood through the vessels to all parts of the body.
B. The heart is located between the lungs in the mediastinum.
C. The apex is the inferior portion of the heart and is directed
   inferiorly, anteriorly and to the left, with most of it left of the
   midline.
D. The base is the superior aspect of the heart.
E. The heart is about the size of the clenched fist.
F. The heart is encased by a loose nondistensible sac called the
   pericardium.
G. Layers of pericardium
   1. *Fibrous pericardium*
      a. Outermost layer of pericardium.
      b. Attaches to great vessels (major vessels entering and

exiting from the heart) of the heart and loosely encases the heart proper.

    c. Made of white fibrous tissue that protects and anchors the heart to some extent.

    d. Externally attached to sternum, vertebral column, central tendon and left hemidiaphragm.

  2. *Parietal serous pericardium*

    a. Lines the fibrous pericardium, to which it is closely adherent.

    b. A moist serous membrane that forms a smooth surface to reduce frictional resistances.

    c. Produces a small volume of serous fluid called pericardial fluid.

    d. Becomes continuous with the visceral serous pericardium.

  3. *Visceral serous pericardium*

    a. Directly adherent to the heart.

    b. Commonly called epicardium of the heart.

    c. A serous membrane which produces serous pericardial fluid.

    d. The small space between visceral and parietal serous pericardial layers is called the pericardial space.

  4. The fact that the visceral and parietal serous pericardial layers are smooth membranes with a small volume of lubricating pericardial fluid between them allows the heart to move freely in the pericardial sac opposed by reduced frictional forces.

H. The heart wall has three distinctive layers.

  1. *Epicardium* or visceral serous pericardium

    a. Most superficial layer.

    b. A transparent serous sheet lying on a delicate network of connective tissue.

    c. Contains fat, coronary blood vessels and coronary nerves, which are observable on cardiac surface.

  2. *Myocardium*

    a. Located just deep to the epicardium and is the middle layer of heart wall.

    b. Composed almost exclusively of cardiac muscle with exception of coronary blood vessels.

    c. Thickest of three cardiac layers.

  3. *Endocardium*

    a. Deepest cardiac layer and is the internal lining of the heart.

      b. Smooth layer of squamous epithelium.

      c. Continuous with endothelial lining of all blood vessels.

      d. Duplication of this layer in the heart forms the cardiac valves.

I. The heart has four chambers.

    1. The two superior chambers, or atria.

    2. The two inferior chambers, or ventricles.

    3. Externally the two atria are separated from the two ventricles by a groove that circumscribes the heart, the coronary sulcus.

    4. Externally the two atria are separated from each other by the roots of both the aorta and pulmonary artery.

    5. Externally the two ventricles are separated from each other by a groove, the interventricular sulcus.

    6. Internally the two atria are separated from each other by a wall, the interatrial septum.

      a. The fossa ovalis, a depression in the atrial septal wall, is the remnant of the fetal foramen ovale.

    7. Internally the two ventricles are separated from each other by a fibrous and muscular interventricular septum. It is continuous with the interatrial septum through its fibrous portion.

    8. Internally the atria are separated from the ventricles by a structure known as the fibroskeleton of the heart.

      a. The fibroskeleton consists of fibrous rings (which surround the atrioventricular cardiac valves, pulmonic and aortic semilunar valves), fibrous interventricular septum, right and left trigone and tendon of conus.

        (1) The right fibrous trigone consists of fibrous tissue, which connects the two atrioventricular rings, fibrous interventricular septum and ring of the aortic semilunar valve.

        (2) The left fibrous trigone consists of fibrous tissue, which connects the fibrous ring of the left atrioventricular valve with the aortic semilunar valve.

        (3) The tendon of conus is fibrous tissue, which connects the fibrous ring of the pulmonic semilunar valve with the ring surrounding the aortic semilunar valve.

      b. Functions of fibroskeleton

        (1) It houses the four cardiac valves.

      (2) It serves as the origin and insertion of atrial and ventricular bands of muscle.

      (3) It electrically isolates atrial muscle bundles from ventricular muscle bundles.

         (a) The fibroskeleton is bridged only by the common bundle branch of the electrical conduction system of the heart called the bundle of His.

         (b) This arrangement allows repolarization and depolarization of the atria separate from the ventricles.

9. The *right atrium* is positioned atop the right ventricle.

   a. It is anterior to the left atrium because the heart is rotated to the left.

      (1) Thus, the bulk of the anterior surface of the heart is composed of the right heart (right atrium and ventricle).

      (2) Most of the posterior surface of the heart is composed of the left heart (left atrium and ventricle).

   b. The right atrium is larger than the left atrium and has a thinner wall.

      (1) The right atrial wall is about 2 mm thick.

      (2) The atrial musculature is divided into deep atrial muscle, which encircles each atrium individually, and superficial atrial muscle, which encircles both atria.

      (3) The deep and superficial muscle fibers run perpendicularly to one another and originate and insert on the fibroskeleton of the heart.

      (4) Contraction of the two major groups of atrial muscle fibers tends to decrease the size of the respective atria in all dimensions.

   c. The cavity of the right atrium consists of two parts:

      (1) The major cavity of the right atrium, or sinus venarum.

      (2) The smaller cavity, which appears externally as a pouch, called the right auricle. (*Note:* Auricle is a term formerly used to denote the entire atrium.)

   d. The right atrium accepts venous blood from the following veins:

      (1) The superior vena cava, which opens into the su-

perior and posterior portions of the major cavity of the right atrium.

(2) The inferior vena cava, which opens into the most inferior portion of the right atrium very near the interatrial septal wall.

(3) The coronary sinus, which opens into the right atrium between the tricuspid valve and the opening of the inferior vena cava.

10. The *left atrium* is positioned atop the left ventricle.
    a. The left atrium is smaller than the right atrium and has a thicker wall.
       (1) The left atrial wall is about 3 mm thick.
       (2) The left atrial muscle fibers are divided into deep and superficial muscle groups and have an arrangement similar to that of the right atrium.
    b. The cavity of the left atrium consists of two parts:
       (1) The major cavity of the left atrium.
       (2) The left auricle, which appears externally as a pouchlike structure.
    c. The left atrium accepts arterial blood from the four pulmonary veins, which open into its superior and posterior aspects.

11. Right ventricle
    a. It constitutes most of the anterior surface of the heart.
    b. The right ventricular wall is one-third the thickness of the left ventricular wall.
    c. The ventricular musculature classically is separated into deep and superficial muscle groups.
       (1) Both deep and superficial muscle groups appear to originate on the fibroskeleton of the heart.
       (2) Superficial fibers follow a clockwise spiral course to the apex of the heart. At the apex, these fibers turn inward and follow a spiraled course upward counterclockwise toward the base of the heart to insert on the fibroskeleton.
       (3) Deep fibers follow a similar course to the superficial ventricular fibers, with three exceptions:
          (a) The spiraled course of the deep fibers is in a direction opposite to that of the superficial fibers.
          (b) Deep fibers may not follow a course all the way to the apex of the heart before starting to ascend.

(c) Deep fibers may insert themselves in the cardiac fibroskeleton, papillary muscles or trabeculae carneae.

    (i) Papillary muscles are fingerlike projections of cardiac muscle located in the cavity of each ventricle.

    (ii) Trabeculae carneae are irregular bundles of muscle that form ridges along the internal wall of the ventricular cavity.

(4) Contraction of ventricular muscle fibers tends to decrease the internal anteroposterior and transverse diameter significantly, but leaves the vertical diameter virtually unchanged.

d. The right ventricle receives venous blood from the right atrium through an opening called the right atrioventricular orifice.

    (1) This orifice is surrounded by a fibrous ring that is a part of the cardiac fibroskeleton.

    (2) The right atrioventricular orifice is about 4 cm in diameter.

    (3) The right atrioventricular orifice contains the tricuspid valve.

        (a) The tricuspid valve contains three cusps, each fused at their origin in the atrioventricular ring.

        (b) The cusps are formed by a duplication of the endocardial layer of the heart and are supported with fibrous tissue.

        (c) The three cusps collectively have a funnel shape that projects into the cavity of the right ventricle.

        (d) The free borders (inferior border) of each cusp have an attached fibrous cordlike structure, the chordae tendineae.

        (e) The chordae tendineae are in turn attached to the intraventricular papillary muscles.

        (f) The chordae tendineae commonly cross, passing from one of the cusps to a group of papillary muscles on the opposite side of the ventricle.

e. The cavity of the right ventricle is lined with muscular ridges (trabeculae carneae) and papillary muscle covered by endocardium.

    (1) The cavity of the right ventricle has a bellows or U shape.

       (2) The muscular arrangement and shape of the right ventricle is well suited to its function of pumping blood under low pressure.

  f. Blood exits from the cavity of the right ventricle by passing through an opening called the orifice of the pulmonary trunk (pulmonary artery).

       (1) This orifice is surrounded by a fibrous ring, a component of the cardiac fibroskeleton.

       (2) The pulmonary orifice is located in the superior, anterior and medial section of the right ventricle.

       (3) The pulmonary orifice contains the pulmonic semilunar valve.

          (a) The pulmonic semilunar valve is composed of three half-moon-shaped cusps.

          (b) This valve resembles the type found in the large veins of the periphery.

          (c) This valve, like the atrioventricular valves, is formed by duplication of the endocardial layer and is supported by fibrous tissue.

12. Left ventricle

  a. It constitutes most of the posterior surface of the heart.

  b. The left ventricular wall is three times the thickness of the right ventricular wall.

  c. Left ventricular muscle fibers are part of the continuum of muscle circumscribing both ventricles and cannot be anatomically separated from right ventricular fibers. (*Note:* The arrangement of the ventricular muscle fibers is described in the foregoing section on the right ventricle.)

  d. The left ventricle receives arterial blood from the left atrium through the left atrioventricular orifice.

       (1) This orifice is surrounded by a fibrous ring, which is one of the components of the cardiac fibroskeleton.

       (2) Contained in the left atrioventricular orifice is the bicuspid or mitral valve.

          (a) The mitral valve is composed of two cusps.

          (b) The anatomical structure is very similar to that of the previously discussed tricuspid valve except that the chordae tendineae are thicker and stronger in the left ventricle.

  e. The cavity of the left ventricle is lined with muscular ridges (trabeculae carneae), which appear in a more numerous and dense arrangement than in the right ventricle. Papillary muscles with the corresponding thick chordae tendineae, along with the trabeculae carneae, are covered by the endocardial layer.

    (1) The cavity of the left ventricle is conical.

    (2) The arrangement of the left ventricular musculature coupled with its conical shape lends well to its function of pumping blood under high pressure.

  f. Blood exits from the cavity of the left ventricle by passing through the aortic opening.

    (1) This opening is surrounded by a fibrous ring, a component of the cardiac fibroskeleton.

    (2) The aortic opening exists in the superior, posterior and medial section of the left ventricle.

    (3) The aortic opening contains the aortic semilunar valve.

      (a) The aortic semilunar valve is anatomically similar to the pulmonic semilunar valve, except that the aortic cusps are stronger, larger and thicker.

BIBLIOGRAPHY

Anthony, C. P., and Kolthoff, N. J.: *Textbook of Anatomy and Physiology* (8th ed.; St. Louis: C. V. Mosby Co., 1971).

Ayres, S. M., Giannelli, S., Jr., and Mueller, H. S.: *Care of the Critically Ill* (2d ed.; New York: Appleton-Century-Crofts, 1974).

Crowley, L. V.: *Introductory Concepts in Anatomy and Physiology* (Chicago: Year Book Medical Publishers, Inc., 1976).

Gray, H., and Goss, C. M.: *Gray's Anatomy of the Human Body* (29th ed.; Philadelphia: Lea & Febiger, 1973).

Guyton, A. C.: *Textbook of Medical Physiology* (5th ed.; Philadelphia: Lea & Febiger, 1976).

Jacob, S. W., and Francone, C. A.: *Structure and Function in Man* (3d ed.; Philadelphia: W. B. Saunders Co., 1974).

Little, R. C.: *Physiology of the Heart and Circulation* (Chicago: Year Book Medical Publishers, Inc., 1977).

McLaughlin, A. J.: *Essentials of Physiology for Advanced Respiratory Therapy* (St. Louis: C. V. Mosby Co., 1977).

Ruch, T. C., and Patton, H. D.: *Physiology and Biophysics* (20th ed.; Philadelphia: W. B. Saunders Co., 1974).

Rushmer, R. F.: *Cardiovascular Dynamics* (3d ed.; Philadelphia: W. B. Saunders Co., 1970).

Shapiro, B. A., Harrison, R. A., and Trout, C. A.: *Clinical Application of Respiratory Care* (Chicago: Year Book Medical Publishers, Inc., 1975).

8 / Physiology of the Cardiovascular System

I. Functions of the Blood
   A. Primary vehicle of transport of substances in the body
      1. Respiratory gases (e.g., oxygen and carbon dioxide)
      2. Circulating antibodies and leukocytes involved in the body's defense mechanisms
      3. Platelets and clotting factors involved in hemostasis
      4. Cellular nutrients to all of the cells
      5. Cellular waste products away from the cells
      6. Electrolytes, proteins, water and hormones, all of which contribute to the numerous complex functions of blood
II. Anatomical Classification of the Vascular Bed
   A. The typical vascular bed begins with the aorta or pulmonary artery.
   B. Branches from either of these main arteries are called large arteries.
   C. The large arteries continue to branch to medium arteries.
   D. The medium arteries further branch to the arterioles.
   E. The end of the arteriolar bed is marked by a thick band of smooth muscle called the precapillary sphincter.
      1. The precapillary sphincter marks the initial portion of the microcirculation.
   F. The arterioles branch to metarterioles or directly to capillaries.
   G. Distal to the precapillary sphincter are the capillaries.
   H. Many capillaries join to form venules.
   I. Numerous venules join to form small veins, which in turn join to form large veins.
   J. Large veins join the major veins of the body—either the vena cava or pulmonary veins.
III. Functional Divisions of Vascular Bed
   A. Distribution, resistance, exchange and capacitance vessels
      1. Distribution vessels begin with the major arteries and include the large and medium arteries.

        a. These vessels distribute the cardiac output to the various organ systems.

        b. These vessels typically are under an elevated pressure, contain a relatively small percentage of total blood volume and are very elastic.

   2. Resistance vessels begin with the arterioles and end with the precapillary sphincter.

        a. These vessels have the largest proportion of smooth muscle constituting the vascular wall of any of the blood vessels.

        b. Through contraction and relaxation of the smooth muscle, the resistance vessels can regulate the distribution of blood to the various capillary beds.

        c. The resistance vessels are the major source of peripheral resistance and function in arterial blood pressure regulation.

   3. The exchange vessels are the capillaries.

        a. Fluid, gas, nutrient and waste exchange occurs in these vessels.

        b. Exchange of these substances occurs between capillary blood and interstitial fluid. Exchange then occurs from the interstitial fluid to the cells that make up the tissue.

        c. The major process underlying exchange in the capillaries is diffusion.

        d. Due to the vast distribution of capillary beds, the process of diffusion is fast enough to maintain cellular metabolism.

   4. Capacitance vessels include the venules through the large veins and encompass the total venous system.

        a. Capacitance vessels serve as channels for blood return to the heart from the various capillary beds.

        b. These vessels are called "capacitance" or "reservoir vessels" because they contain most (70–75%) of the total blood volume.

        c. The capacitance vessels are typically under low pressure, contain a large blood volume and are relatively inelastic compared to their arterial counterparts.

IV. Vascular System: Systemic and Pulmonary Circulations

  A. Systemic Circulation

    1. Systemic circulation begins with the systemic pump,

the left ventricle, and continues to a typical vascular bed, ending with the right atrium.

  a. Functions of systemic circulation:

    (1) To distribute left ventricular cardiac output so that each region of the body receives an adequate volume of blood per unit time.

    (2) To perfuse individual tissues so that cellular metabolism is maintained.

    (3) To return venous blood to the right side of the heart to maintain right ventricular output.

2. Control of systemic circulation is governed by four major mechanisms: autonomic control, hormonal control, local control and mechanical factors.

  a. The arterial portion of the systemic circulation is basically governed by three mechanisms: autonomic nervous system, hormonal control and local control.

    (1) Arteries and arterioles are innervated extensively and virtually exclusively by postganglionic fibers of the sympathetic nervous system.

    (2) The arterial vasculature of different tissues varies in the degree of sympathetic innervation.

      (a) The largest degree of sympathetic innervation is to the arterial vasculature perfusing the skin.

      (b) The degree of sympathetic innervation steadily decreases through the arterial vasculature perfusing spleen, mesenteric vessels and kidneys.

      (c) A smaller degree of sympathetic innervation exists in the muscles.

      (d) The least degree of sympathetic innervation exists in the vessels perfusing the heart and brain. Furthermore, these vessels have a small degree of parasympathetic innervation.

    (3) Sympathetic stimulation of blood vessels results in smooth muscle contraction and vasoconstriction.

      (a) This principally affects the resistance vessels due to their large component of smooth muscle.

      (b) Tonic sympathetic stimulation of arterial

blood vessels results in a given arteriolar caliber.

   (i) Increased sympathetic stimulation above this tonic level results in vasoconstriction and an increase in resistance to flow through these vessels.

  (ii) Decreased sympathetic stimulation below this tonic level results in vasodilatation and a decrease in resistance to flow through these vessels.

 (iii) Because of differing degrees of sympathetic innervation in the different tissues, general sympathetic stimulation results in varying degrees of vasoconstriction and varying resistance to blood flow from tissue to tissue.

(4) Parasympathetic stimulation of the arterial vasculature of the brain and heart results in smooth muscle relaxation and vasodilatation. This phenomenon results in a decrease in resistance to blood flow.

(5) The adrenomedullary hormones, norepinephrine and epinephrine, both stimulate the alpha receptors and produce vasoconstriction.

(6) Acidosis, hypoxemia, hypercarbia and increased temperature all produce local relaxation of smooth muscle in resistance vessels and resultant vasodilatation.

  b. The capillary bed of the systemic circulation is governed almost exclusively by local factors.

(1) In tissues where capillary blood flow is limited by arteriolar constriction, there is local accumulation of acid and carbon dioxide as well as a deficiency of oxygen.

(2) These local factors result in relaxation of the smooth muscle and local arteriolar dilatation, which re-establishes blood flow.

(3) Blood flow removes the local accumulation of waste products and replenishes oxygen and nutrient supply, resulting in arteriolar constriction, which in turn limits blood flow.

(4) Thus the cycle repeats itself, providing blood

flow to tissues intermittently to maintain cellular metabolism.

c. The veins of the systemic circulation are governed by the autonomic nervous system, hormonal factors and mechanical factors.

(1) The veins are exclusively innervated by postganglionic fibers of the sympathetic nervous system.

(2) The veins have a less extensive innervation than do their arterial counterparts. However, unlike that of the arteries, sympathetic innervation of the venous vasculature does not vary from one tissue to the next.

(a) Thus sympathetic stimulation causes venoconstriction of all veins of the body.

(b) Generalized venoconstriction decreases the venous vascular space, resulting in increased venous return to the heart.

(c) On the other hand, decreased sympathetic stimulation results in a decrease in venous tone and venodilatation.

(d) The generalized venodilatation increases the venous vascular space and decreases venous return to the heart.

(3) The adrenomedullary hormones, epinephrine and norepinephrine, both mimic sympathetic stimulation and produce venoconstriction.

(4) Mechanical factors that affect the veins of the systemic venous system are the thoracoabdominal pump, skeletal muscle pump and semilunar valves.

(a) The thoracoabdominal pump affects the veins by aiding venous return. This is accomplished by exposing the intrathoracic veins to the fluctuating subatmospheric pressure produced by spontaneous ventilation. Coupled with the fact that extrathoracic veins are surrounded by atmospheric or supra-atmospheric pressure, venous return is enhanced.

(b) The veins in the limbs contain semilunar valves that prevent retrograde flow of blood. When skeletal muscle contracts, it compresses the veins, increasing venous pressure.

Because these veins have valves, compression of vessels can squeeze blood in only one direction. This mechanism also is responsible for enhancing venous return.

B. Pulmonary Circulation
1. Pulmonary circulation begins with the pulmonary pump, the right ventricle and continues to a typical vascular bed, ending with the left atrium.
   a. Functions of pulmonary circulation
      (1) To distribute right ventricular output to pulmonary capillaries, matching the alveolar ventilation with an adequate volume of blood per unit time.
      (2) To perfuse the cells of the lung parenchyma with nutrients and rid them of waste products.
      (3) To return blood to the left side of the heart to maintain left ventricular output.
2. Control of pulmonary circulation is governed by the same four mechanisms that affect systemic circulation.
   a. In general, the pulmonary vasculature has less smooth muscle and thinner walls than does its counterpart in the systemic circulation.
   b. This makes pulmonary circulation prone to mechanical factors, e.g., intrathoracic and alveolar pressures, and the effects of gravity on distribution of blood flow.
   c. Pulmonary vasculature responds to sympathetic stimulation just as does the systemic circulation, but to a much lesser extent.
   d. Three local factors that have profound effects on pulmonary resistance vessels are decreased alveolar Po_2, hypoxemia and acidemia. All three cause pulmonary vasoconstriction, with increased resistance to blood flow.
   e. Adrenomedullary hormones produce pulmonary vasoconstriction but to a milder degree than in systemic circulation.
   f. Thus most of the control of pulmonary circulation depends on passive response to mechanical factors as well as on local factors. This is in contrast to the dominance that the sympathetic nervous system displays in controlling systemic circulation.

C. In comparing systemic and pulmonary vascular resistance, the following equation can be applied:

1.
$$R = \frac{\Delta P}{\dot{Q}}. \tag{1}$$

where R = vascular resistance expressed in mm Hg/liter/minute

ΔP = change in pressure across the circulation or pressure gradient expressed in mm Hg

$\dot{Q}$ = cardiac output or flow expressed in liters/minute.

2. Systemic vascular resistance equals

a.
$$R = \frac{\overline{LVP} - \overline{RA}}{\dot{Q}} \tag{2}$$

where $\overline{LVP}$ = mean left ventricular pressure

$\overline{RA}$ = mean right atrial pressure

$\dot{Q}$ = cardiac output.

b. Replacing the factors with representative normal values results in

$$R = \frac{(90 - 5) \text{ mm Hg}}{5 \text{ L/minute}} = 17 \text{ mm Hg/L/minute.} \tag{3}$$

3. Pulmonary vascular resistance equals

a.
$$R = \frac{\overline{RVP} - \overline{LA}}{\dot{Q}}. \tag{4}$$

where $\overline{RVP}$ = mean right ventricular pressure

$\overline{LA}$ = mean left atrial pressure

$\dot{Q}$ = cardiac output.

b. Replacing the factors with representative normal values results in

$$R = \frac{(16 - 6) \text{ mm Hg}}{5 \text{ L/minute}} = 2 \text{ mm Hg/L/minute.} \tag{5}$$

4. By these calculations, systemic vascular resistance equals 17 mm Hg/liters/minute and pulmonary vascular resistance equals 2 mm Hg/liters/minute. This relationship results in systemic vascular resistance being about

eight and one-half times pulmonary vascular resistance. Systemic vascular resistance is normally six to ten times pulmonary vascular resistance.

V. Basic Function of the Heart
  A. To impart sufficient energy to the blood to provide circulation through the vascular system.
    1. As has been discussed, vascular resistance of systemic circulation is much greater than that of pulmonary circulation. Therefore the left side of the heart must create greater pressures than the right side to bring about a given flow.
    2. The major principle of circulation (blood flow) is that, for circulation to exist, there must be a pressure gradient. The heart must create that pressure gradient across the respective parts of the vasculature. Therefore, for a given vascular resistance, blood flow is a direct function of the pressure gradient generated by the heart.

VI. Electric Conduction System of the Heart
  A. Sinoatrial (SA) node
    1. The SA node is located in the right atrium just inferior and posterior to the entrance of the superior vena cava.
    2. It is commonly referred to as the pacemaker of the heart—its *primary function*.
    3. The SA node has an intrinsic rate of depolarization of 70–80 per minute.
    4. The rate of depolarization ordinarily is under the control of the sympathetic and parasympathetic nervous systems.
      a. Sympathetic stimulation of the SA node increases the rate of depolarization—positive chronotropism.
      b. Parasympathetic stimulation of the SA node decreases the rate of depolarization—negative chronotropism.
    5. The wave of depolarization initiated from the SA node travels outwardly through the atrial musculature in concentric circles, thus depolarizing the atria and ultimately the atrioventricular node.
    6. For all practical purposes, the left and right atria depolarize simultaneously.
  B. Atrioventricular (AV) node
    1. The AV node is located in the right atrium between the opening of the coronary sinus and interatrial septum.

2. Histologically it is comprised of cells identical to those of the SA node.
3. The *function* of the AV node is threefold:
   a. Backup cardiac pacemaker because of its intrinsic depolarization rate of 40–60 per minute
   b. The only electrical bridge between atria and ventricles
   c. Responsible for delaying impulse from atria to ventricles
4. The AV node becomes continuous with the common bundle branch (bundle of His) and is the only normal pathway for electric conduction between atria and ventricles. The fibroskeleton of the heart electrically separates atrial from ventricular muscle. The AV node and common bundle penetrate the cardiac fibroskeleton.
5. That the tissue of the AV node slows the rate of electrical conduction accounts for the time delay between atrial and ventricular depolarization. This time delay also allows optimal ventricular filling prior to ventricular contraction (systole).
6. The rate of conduction of electrical impulses through the AV node is under the control of the sympathetic and parasympathetic nervous systems.
   a. Sympathetic stimulation decreases conduction time and allows overall increases in cardiac rate.
   b. Parasympathetic stimulation increases conduction time of the AV node. Strong parasympathetic stimulation may actually block all or a portion of the impulses originating from the atria.
C. Common Bundle Branch
   1. It is also known as the AV bundle or bundle of His.
   2. It is located on the right side of the interventricular septum and penetrates the right fibrous trigone.
   3. Its *function* is twofold:
      a. To conduct impulses from the AV node to left and right bundle branches.
      b. To penetrate the fibroskeleton of the heart, electrically bridging atrial conduction system to ventricular conduction system.
   4. The common bundle branch travels inferiorly in the interventricular septum for about 10–12 mm and then divides into one right and two left bundle branches.

   D. Right and left bundle branches

       1. The right bundle branch appears simply as a continuation of the common bundle branch and follows an inferior course toward the apex of the heart.

       2. The left bundle branch penetrates the interventricular septum and divides into an anterior and posterior left bundle branch. Both bundle branches course inferiorly on the left side of the interventricular septum.

       3. The *function* of the three major bundle branches is to conduct electric impulses from the common bundle branch to the Purkinje fibers.

   E. Purkinje fibers

       1. The Purkinje fibers are very fine ramifications of the bundle branches, which terminate on the endocardial layer of the heart.

       2. They are located throughout the entire endocardial layer of both ventricles and conduct the electrical impulses from the bundle branches to the ventricles. Depolarization of the ventricles begins when impulses leaving the Purkinje fibers invade the endocardial layer.

       3. The wave of depolarization travels from the endocardial layer outward toward the epicardium and also from the apex toward the base of the ventricles.

   F. Summary of pathway of normal electrical conduction

       1. Impulses originate in right atrium by spontaneous depolarization of SA node.

       2. Impulses are conducted through atrial muscle, which results in depolarization of right and left atria and AV node.

       3. The impulse is delayed at AV node and then conducted through the cardiac fibroskeleton by AV node and common bundle branch.

       4. The impulse is then conducted from common bundle branch through right and left bundle branches to Purkinje fibers.

       5. The impulses exit from Purkinje fibers and cause depolarization of ventricle from inside out and from apex to base.

       6. Design of the electrical conduction system of the heart allows simultaneous depolarization of right and left atria totally separate from simultaneous depolarization

of right and left ventricles. This fact has important implications for mechanical function of the heart.

VII. Electrocardiogram (ECG or EKG)

A. The ECG is the measurement of current generated by the heart at the surface of the body. It depicts depolarization and repolarization of atria and ventricles.

B. The ECG is used in assessing the electrical activity of the heart, which should be clearly delineated from the mechanical activity of the heart.

C. Each portion of the cardiac cycle is responsible for generating a specific type of electrical impulse. These impulses are repetitious and produce characteristic patterns in an ECG recording.

D. The four major electrical cardiac events are atrial depolarization, atrial repolarization, ventricular depolarization and ventricular repolarization.

1. The polarized state is the normal resting state of cardiac muscle fiber. The extracellular charge is positive with respect to the intracellular charge.

2. Depolarization is the process of reversing the normal state of polarity. Depolarization thus causes the extracellular charge to be negative with respect to the intracellular charge. This is largely because inflow of extracellular sodium ions is faster than outflow of intracellular potassium ions. Reversal of the cellular membrane charge is thus transmitted along cardiac muscle fiber, depolarizing subsequent fibers. If muscle fibers are normal, this electrochemical stimulation results in mechanical activity (shortening of muscle fibers and cardiac contraction).

3. Repolarization is the process of re-establishing the normal state of polarity, i.e., re-establishing a positive extracellular charge with respect to the intracellular charge. The re-establishment of the resting cellular membrane charge is transmitted along cardiac muscle fiber, repolarizing subsequent fibers. If muscle fibers are normal, this electrochemical stimulation results in lengthening of muscle fibers and cardiac relaxation.

(*Note:* It is a mistake to assume that the mechanical activity of the heart is normal simply because the electric activity [ECG] is normal.)

    E. Electric deflections of ECG in normal sequence: P wave, QRS complex and T wave

        1. The P wave is produced by atrial depolarization and usually is 0.06–0.11 second in duration.

        2. The QRS complex is produced by ventricular depolarization and usually is 0.03–0.10 second in duration. Repolarization of the atria occurs simultaneously with ventricular depolarization and is masked by the overwhelming electric event of the QRS complex.

        3. The T wave is produced by ventricular repolarization and usually is 0.14–0.26 second in duration.

    F. Q–T, P–R, R–R and QRS intervals

        1. Q–T interval: Time from the beginning of ventricular depolarization to completion of ventricular repolarization. This interval normally is 0.26 to 0.49 second in duration.

        2. P–R interval: Time from the beginning of atrial depolarization to the beginning of ventricular depolarization. The P–R interval normally is 0.12 to 0.21 second in duration.

        3. R–R interval: Time from the peak of one QRS complex to the next QRS complex. It is used to measure the total cardiac cycle time and normally is 0.6 to 1.0 second in duration.

        4. QRS interval: Normally 0.03–0.10 second in duration. Times outside of this range may indicate abnormalities of conduction system of the ventricles.

VIII. Mechanical Events of the Cardiac Cycle

    A. Electric events of the heart are precursors of the mechanical events of the heart.

        1. If the heart is normal, depolarization of the atria causes atrial contraction (systole).

        2. Depolarization of the ventricles causes ventricular contraction (systole).

        3. Repolarization of the atria causes atrial relaxation (diastole).

        4. Repolarization of the ventricles causes ventricular relaxation (diastole).

    B. Atrial systole

        1. Mechanical left and right atrial systole begins at the peak of the P wave of the ECG.

        2. The decrease in size of the respective atria causes left

atrial pressure to rise about 7 to 8 mm Hg and right atrial pressure 5 to 6 mm Hg. The pressure differential from atria to ventricles causes blood to flow from the atria through the respective AV orifices to the ventricles.

3. Normal mean right and left atrial pressures are 0–8 mm Hg and 2–12 mm Hg, respectively.

4. Atrial systole accounts for 20–40% of the total ventricular volume. This figure dpends on heart rate and atrial contractility. The remaining 60–80% of ventricular volume is a result of passive filling by venous return.

5. The atria are very weak pumps in comparison to the ventricles and should be thought of as thin-walled blood reservoirs for the respective ventricles. The 20–40% of ventricular volume added by atrial systole is simply a priming of the ventricles prior to ventricular systole. Atrial systole is not essential for adequate ventricular filling, as can be demonstrated by atrial fibrillation or complete heart-block.

6. Atrial systole increases the end-diastolic volume of each ventricle to about 145 ml. It also increases the end-diastolic pressure of the right and left ventricles to 2–8 mm Hg and 4–12 mm Hg, respectively. The ventricles are now prepared for their subsequent contraction.

C. Ventricular systole and atrial diastole

1. Mechanical left and right ventricular systole begins at the peak of the R wave of the ECG and coincides with atrial diastole.

2. Ventricular contraction increases intraventricular pressure. When pressure in the respective ventricles exceeds atrial pressure, the tricuspid and mitral valves close, producing the S_1, or first heart sound.

3. Aortic and pulmonic semilunar valves have been closed during ventricular diastole because pressure in the aorta and pulmonary artery has exceeded left and right ventricular pressure.

4. With both AV and semilunar valves closed, the ventricles are functionally closed chambers. Contraction of the ventricle decreases their size and rapidly increases intraventricular pressure.

5. The first portion of ventricular systole is called isovolumetric contraction. It is characterized by both the AV and semilunar valves being closed and by a rapid in-

crease in intraventricular pressure without a concomitant change in intraventricular blood volume.

6. The second portion of ventricular systole is called the period of ejection. Ejection begins when left and right intraventricular pressure exceeds the pressure in the aorta and pulmonary artery, respectively. It should be noted that this point is the diastolic pulmonary artery and aortic pressure. Previous to ventricular systole, blood has been steadily leaving both the pulmonary and systemic (aortic) arterial system, and intra-arterial pressure has been steadily dropping. The lowest intra-arterial pressure attained occurs just prior to actual ventricular ejection and is called diastolic pressure of the respective arteries. Normal diastolic pressure for the aorta and pulmonary artery is 60–90 mm Hg and 5–16 mm Hg, respectively.

7. The period of ejection is characterized by opening of the semilunar valves.

    a. During this time intraventricular pressure steadily increases above intra-arterial pressure, causing blood to leave the ventricles.

    b. Intraventricular pressure attains its maximum value (ventricular systolic pressure), followed by an increase in intra-arterial pressure to its maximum value (arterial systolic pressure).

    c. Normal right and left ventricular systolic pressure is 15–28 mm Hg and 90–140 mm Hg, respectively.

    d. Normal pulmonary artery and aortic systolic pressure is 15–28 mm Hg and 90–140 mm Hg, respectively.

    e. When ejection is complete, intra-arterial pressure and retrograde blood flow cause closing of aortic and pulmonic semilunar valves. This produces the second, or S_2, heart sound.

8. The total period of ejection causes a stroke volume of 70 ml to be added to each arterial system by the respective ventricles.

9. It should be noted that the end-diastolic volume of each ventricle is 145 ml and the stroke volume 70 ml. This results in a residual blood volume of each ventricle equal to 75 ml. The residual volume is called the end-systolic volume. All previous blood volume values are based on the normal resting heart.

10. Closure of aortic and pulmonic semilunar valves marks the beginning of ventricular diastole.

D. Ventricular diastole
   1. Mechanical left and right ventricular diastole begins after completion of the T wave of the ECG.
   2. Ventricular diastole begins with closure of the pulmonic and aortic semilunar valves and ends with onset of atrial systole.
   3. Tricuspid and mitral valves have remained closed all through the preceding ventricular systole and remain closed in early ventricular diastole. This is because intraventricular pressure exceeds intra-arterial pressure.
   4. The ventricles are functionally closed chambers with all cardiac valves remaining closed. Relaxation of the ventricular myocardium precipitates a large decrease in intraventricular pressure without a change in intraventricular blood volume.
   5. When right and left intraventricular pressures drop below the respective intra-atrial pressures, the tricuspid and mitral valves open. This results in a rapid filling of each ventricle by intra-atrial blood, followed by passive distention of the ventricles by blood returning from the lung and periphery.
   6. It should be noted that blood will continue to passively fill the ventricles through the AV valves, which remain open until the onset of ventricular systole. This slow but steady addition to ventricular volume is evidenced by a small increase in intra-atrial and intraventricular pressures.
   7. The ventricular filling occurring during ventricular diastole accounts for 60–80% of the end-diastolic volume.
   8. The entire myocardium remains relaxed until the onset of the P wave and atrial systole initiate another cardiac cycle.

E. Summary of Mechanical Events of the Cardiac Cycle
   1. After the P wave of the ECG, the atria contract, propelling blood through the open AV valves to the ventricles.
   2. During the height of the following QRS complex, the ventricles contract in unison. It is during this same time that atrial relaxation occurs.
   3. Intraventricular pressure soon rises above atrial pressure and causes the AV valves to close. This prevents

retrograde flow of the blood from the ventricles to atria. Closure of the AV valves produces the S_1 heart sound.

4. Intraventricular pressure continues to rise rapidly and soon exceeds intra-arterial pressure. This causes the semilunar valves to open and provides blood flow from the ventricles to the arteries.

5. Relaxation of the ventricles occurs after completion of the T wave of the ECG.

6. As the ventricles relax, intraventricular pressure drops below the respective intra-arterial pressures. This causes the semilunar valves to close, preventing retrograde flow of blood from arteries to respective ventricles. Closure of semilunar valves produces the S_2 heart sound.

7. Intraventricular pressure continues to drop until intraventricular pressure falls below intra-atrial pressure. This causes the respective AV valves to open and provides blood flow from atria to ventricles.

8. Blood returning from pulmonary and systemic circulations continues to flow through the atria and open AV valves passively, filling the relaxed ventricles. This passive filling continues until the onset of the subsequent atrial contraction, which begins the next cardiac cycle.

IX. Cardiac Output

A. The amount of blood pumped out of each ventricle is termed the cardiac output.

B. The cardiac output of the right and left ventricles is equal and identical over a period of time.

C. The cardiac output (CO) is equal to the stroke volume (SV) times the heart rate (HR):

$$CO = SV \times HR \tag{6}$$

1. The cardiac output is conventionally expressed in liters per minute.

a. The normal range of cardiac output in a resting individual is 4–8 liters per minute.

b. *With stress or exercise, the cardiac output can increase five to six times its normal resting value.*

2. The stroke volume is the amount of blood ejected from the ventricle with each ventricular systole.

a. The stroke volume is expressed in milliliters per contraction.

      b. The normal range for the stroke volume of a resting individual is 60 – 130 ml per contraction.
3. The heart rate is the number of times the heart contracts per minute.
      a. The normal range for the heart rate of a resting individual is 60 – 100 contractions per minute.
4. Example:
    An individual with a stroke volume equal to 70 ml per contraction, and a heart rate of 80 contractions per minute would have a cardiac output equal to 5,600 ml per minute or 5.6 liters per minute by the following calculation:

$$\frac{70 \text{ ml}}{\text{contraction}} \times \frac{80 \text{ contractions}}{\text{minute}} = \frac{5600 \text{ ml}}{\text{minute}} \text{ or } \frac{5.6 \text{ L}}{\text{minute}}. \tag{7}$$

5. The cardiac output of different individuals varies greatly according to body size. Therefore, cardiac output is frequently expressed in terms of body size and is then called the cardiac index.
      a. The cardiac index is equal to the cardiac output in liters per minute per body surface area in square meters.
      b. The cardiac index becomes a more meaningful value when comparing cardiac outputs of different individuals.
      c. Since cardiac index is a more consistent value among different individuals, it has a narrower normal range of 2.5 – 4 liters per minute per square meter.
6. It should be evident that increases in cardiac output are brought about by increases in the heart rate and/or stroke volume, and that decreases in cardiac output are brought about by decreases in heart rate and/or stroke volume.
D. Control of heart rate
1. It should be recalled that heart rate is set by the pacemaker of the heart (SA node). The number of times per minute that the SA node depolarizes is largely governed by neural and chemical factors.
2. The neural factors that affect heart rate are mediated through the two divisions of the autonomic nervous system, i.e., parasympathetic and sympathetic nervous systems.

a. Parasympathetic impulses are conducted to the SA node through the X cranial (vagus) nerve.
   (1) Parasympathetic effects on the SA node are inhibitory and decrease the heart rate.
   (2) The result of decreasing the heart rate is called negative chronotropism. Thus the parasympathetic nervous system exhibits negative chronotropic effects.
b. Sympathetic impulses are conducted to the SA node through sympathetic nerve fibers originating from the upper thoracic (T1–T5) segment of the spinal cord.
   (1) Sympathetic effects on the SA node are excitatory and increase the heart rate.
   (2) The result of increasing the heart rate is called positive chronotropism. Thus the sympathetic nervous system exhibits positive chronotropic effects.
c. The sympathetic and parasympathetic nervous systems are generally considered antagonists. However, in bringing about changes in heart rate, the two divisions of the autonomic nervous system complement each other.
   (1) However, each nervous system can perform both positive and negative chronotropism. Under certain clinical conditions, heart rate is altered by selective activities of one division of the autonomic nervous system.
   (2) In general, the parasympathetic nervous system is the dominant division of the neural input into the SA node. This is evidenced by total autonomic blockade, resulting in mild tachycardia.
d. Neural control of heart rate also is mediated through higher brain centers, e.g., cerebral cortex and hypothalamus.
   (1) The cerebral cortex is responsible for changes in heart rate in response to emotional factors, e.g., anxiety, fear, anger and grief.
   (2) The hypothalamus appears responsible for changes in heart rate in response to alterations in both local and environmental temperature.

3. Major chemical factors that affect heart rate: electrolytes, exogenously administered drugs and hormones
   a. The three major electrolytes having effects on the heart rate are potassium, sodium and calcium.
      (1) Excess potassium and sodium have the effect of decreasing the heart rate.
      (2) Excess calcium causes an increase in the heart rate.
      (3) Potassium and sodium imbalance can alter cardiac membrane permeability and thus slow or speed the rate of electric conduction through the myocardium.
      (4) However, only electrolyte *imbalance* brings about such changes in heart rate.
   b. Classes of drugs that have their effect on heart rate by either mimicking or inhibiting the activity of the sympathetic or parasympathetic nervous system:
      (1) Sympathomimetics such as isoproterenol or epinephrine mimic the activity of the sympathetic nervous system and cause positive chronotropism.
      (2) Sympatholytics such as dichloroisoproterenol or propranolol inhibit the activity of the sympathetic nervous system and cause negative chronotropism.
      (3) Parasympathomimetics such as metacholine, pilocarpine or neostigmine mimic the activity of the parasympathetic nervous system and cause negative chronotropism.
      (4) Parasympatholytics such as atropine inhibit the activity of the parasympathetic nervous system and cause positive chronotropism.
   c. The major hormones that affect the heart rate are the adrenomedullary hormones.
      (1) The adrenal medulla secretes epinephrine and norepinephrine into the circulating blood.
      (2) These two naturally occurring catecholamines have direct positive chronotropic effects on the heart.
4. *Heart rate is under many influences,* ranging from conscious control by the cerebral cortex to exogenously

administered pharmacologic agents. The most important regulatory control of heart rate is mediated through the autonomic nervous system.

E. Control of stroke volume
   1. Size of stroke volume: Governed by preload, afterload and state of contractility of ventricles
      a. *Preload:* Degree of ventricular diastolic filling before ejection begins, or the presystolic ventricular loading force
         (1) Frank-Starling's law states that the more the heart is filled during diastole the greater the subsequent force of contraction. This results in increased stroke volume.
         (2) This relationship is primarily related to presystolic myocardial fiber length.
         (3) Presystolic fiber length is directly related to end-diastolic volume, for it is the actual intraventricular blood volume coupled with the compliance characteristics of the ventricle that results in myocardial fiber stretch.
         (4) Since myocardial fiber length is virtually impossible to measure in the intact heart, it would seem that end-diastolic volume is an appropriate parameter for assessing preload.
            (a) The first factor affecting end-diastolic volume is the presence of a total blood volume sufficient for an effective vascular volume to vascular space relationship. There must be an adequate blood volume within the vascular space for the heart to circulate blood effectively. It is the *relationship* between vascular volume to vascular space that is crucial, not the absolute values of either vascular volume or vascular space.
            (b) The state of the venous tone is the second factor affecting end-diastolic volume. The relationship between vascular volume and vascular space is essential to insure adequate venous return and ventricular filling. It should be noted that 60–80% of ventricular filling is accomplished by passive return of blood from the veins. The state of venous tone regulates

venous vascular space, and it is therefore as crucial as blood volume in determining adequacy of venous return.

(c) The third major factor that affects end-diastolic volume is force of atrial systole. As mentioned, 20–40% of ventricular filling is accomplished by atrial systole. This is not of critical importance in the normal heart but becomes paramount in any cardiac dysfunction where ventricular compliance is decreased (i.e., ventricular hypertrophy or myocardial infarction).

(d) The fourth major factor that affects end-diastolic volume is compliance of the ventricle. As mentioned, this factor is not of importance in the normal heart, but decreases in ventricular compliance require a greater filling pressure per unit volume change. Thus increased filling pressure is necessary or the end-diastolic volume will have a reduced value.

(e) End-diastolic volume is an acceptable parameter for assessing preload; however, this too is difficult to measure with any accuracy in the intact heart. The most easily measured parameter that reflects preload is ventricular end-diastolic pressure.

(5) Given a constant ventricular compliance, it may be inferred that ventricular end-diastolic pressure should correlate well with ventricular end-diastolic volume. Accepting the latter as true, myocardial fiber length can be expressed as a function of end-diastolic pressure.

(a) In clinical practice, preload is assessed by measuring ventricular end-diastolic pressure.

(b) Right ventricular preload is assessed by end-diastolic pressure measurements taken from a CVP catheter as central venous pressure (see Section XI on Hemodynamic Monitoring).

(c) Left ventricular preload is assessed by end-diastolic pressure measurements taken from a pulmonary artery catheter as a pulmonary wedge pressure (see Section XI on Hemodynamic Monitoring).

(d) In general, the higher the end-diastolic pressure (preload) the greater the subsequent ventricular contraction and resulting stroke volume.

(6) The Frank-Starling relationship is the basis for (1) matching cardiac output to venous return (2) balancing output of right and left ventricles. For example, if venous return to the right atrium has suddenly increased because increased venous tone has altered the vascular volume/vascular space relationship:

(a) Increased venous return to the right ventricle would increase the right ventricular end-diastolic volume.

(b) Increased end-diastolic volume would result in an increased myocardial fiber length.

(c) Increased myocardial fiber length would in turn result in an increased force of contraction of the right ventricle.

(d) Increased force of contraction of the right ventricle would result in an increased right ventricular stroke volume, all other factors remaining equal.

(e) It should be noted that two phenomena have occurred. (1) Venous blood has been mobilized back to the heart and the increased venous return has been matched by an increase in right ventricular stroke volume. This is one of the major ways that cardiac output is increased. (2) Right ventricular output now exceeds left ventricular output.

(f) Increased right ventricular output will result in increased venous return to left atrium and left ventricle.

(g) In similar fashion, increased venous return to the left ventricle increases left ventricular end-diastolic volume.

(h) The increased end-diastolic volume would result in increasing the left ventricular myocardial fiber length. This in turn would result in an increase in the force of contraction of the left ventricle.

(i) The increased force of contraction of the left ventricle would result in an increased left ventricular stroke volume.

(j) At this point venous blood has been mobilized from the venous reservoirs and has resulted in increased output from both the right and left sides of the heart. Furthermore, left ventricular output is in equilibrium with right ventricular output—all in accordance with Frank-Starling's law of the heart.

(k) The regulatory function of the Frank-Starling mechanism is frequently referred to as "autoregulation" in that it is an intrinsic factor based on the architecture of the myocardial fibers, which automatically regulate cardiac output to equal venous return. Thus it has led physiologists over the years to make the statement that "within the physiologic limits of the heart, it will pump out all the blood it receives without allowing a backup of blood into the venous system."

b. *Afterload:* Resistance to flow from the ventricles

(1) The work the heart must perform in order to pump blood out of the ventricles and into the circulation depends on three major factors: resistance of the semilunar valves, blood viscosity and arterial blood pressure.

(a) As resistance of the semilunar valves (i.e., pulmonic or aortic stenosis) increases, afterload will be increased.

(b) As blood viscosity increases (i.e., hyperproteinemia or polycythemia), afterload will be increased.

(c) As arterial blood pressure increases (pulmonary or systemic hypertension), afterload will be increased.

(d) Decreases in any of these three parameters result in decreasing the afterload.

    (2) Increases in afterload result in increases of ventricular work:

        (a) The greater the resistance against which the ventricle must contract to eject blood, the more slowly it contracts.

        (b) Increased afterload results in a decreased stroke volume, which initially increases end-systolic volume. The normal venous return will then be added to the already increased end-systolic volume and increase end-diastolic volume above normal. This allows a more forceful contraction against an increased afterload as a result of the Frank-Starling mechanism. This enables the ventricle to pump a given stroke volume against an increased afterload. *This compensation is at the expense of an increase in ventricular size.* The larger the heart the greater the work necessary to develop the myocardial tension required to produce a given intraventricular pressure (La Place's law).

        (c) Both the slower rate of contraction and the increased ventricular size result in greater oxygen requirements to perform a given amount of work than that of the normal heart.

    (3) Thus increases in afterload may or may not cause a decrease in stroke volume, but will cause increases in myocardial work.

    (4) Decreases in afterload, commonly called "afterload reduction," may or may not cause an increase in stroke volume, but will cause decreases in myocardial work.

    (5) In general, the poorer the cardiac function the more dependent is the stroke volume on afterload.

        (a) Increases in afterload tend to decrease stroke volume in the patient with poor cardiac function.

        (b) Increases in afterload do not cause decreases in stroke volume in the patient with normal cardiac function.

(c) Decreases in afterload tend to increase stroke volume in the patient with poor cardiac function.

(d) Decreases in afterload generally do not cause increases in stroke volume in the patient with normal cardiac function.

(6) In the absence of valvular disease, afterload is clinically assessed by measuring mean arterial blood pressure.

(a) Right ventricular afterload is assessed by mean pulmonary artery measurements taken via a pulmonary artery catheter.

(b) Left ventricular afterload is assessed by mean systemic arterial pressure measurements taken via an intra-arterial (systemic) catheter.

c. *State of ventricular contractility:* Force with which the ventricles contract.

(1) The force of contraction of the ventricles at any given preload and afterload depends on the state of contractility.

(a) An increase in the state of ventricular contractility for a given preload and afterload is termed positive inotropism.

(b) A decrease in the state of ventricular contractility for a given preload and afterload is termed negative inotropism.

(c) The net effect of positive inotropism is generally a greater volume output per unit time.

(d) The net effect of negative inotropism is generally a smaller volume output per unit time.

(2) Ventricular contractility is altered by the sympathetic and parasympathetic nervous systems, blood gases (PO_2, PCO_2), pH, hormones and exogenously administered drugs.

(3) The sympathetic nervous system extensively innervates the atrial and ventricular myocardium.

(a) Postganglionic nerve fibers of the sympathetic nervous system release norepinephrine to beta receptor sites of the atrial and ventricular myocardium.

(b) This increases contractility of the myocardium — positive inotropism. Thus the sympathetic nervous system displays positive inotropic effects.

    (c) Alterations in sympathetic discharge to the myocardium are believed to constitute the most important regulatory control of ventricular contractility.

(4) The parasympathetic nervous system only minutely innervates the atrial myocardium, and the ventricular myocardium is innervated even more sparsely.

    (a) Postganglionic nerve fibers of the parasympathetic nervous system release acetylcholine to the muscarinic receptor sites of the atrial and ventricular myocardium.

    (b) As previously mentioned, due to the scantiness of parasympathetic innervation, the result is only a mild decrease in myocardial contractility, or a slight negative inotropism. Thus the parasympathetic nervous system displays minor negative inotropic effects.

(5) Effects of blood gases on myocardial contractility:

    (a) Mild decreases in PO_2 result in increased contractility, whereas severe drops in PO_2 result in decreased myocardial contractility.

    (b) Increases in PCO_2 result in decreased contractility, whereas decreases in PCO_2 result in increased myocardial contractility.

    (c) Metabolic or respiratory acidosis results directly in decreased contractility, whereas metabolic and respiratory alkalosis may alter contractility through electric conduction dysfunction and arrhythmia.

(6) The most important hormones affecting myocardial contractility are the adrenomedullary hormones.

    (a) As previously stated, the adrenal medulla secretes epinephrine and norepinephrine into the circulating blood.

    (b) These two naturally occurring catecholamines have direct positive inotropic effects on the myocardium.

      (c) The major differences between the effects of the catecholamines and direct sympathetic stimulation are that the effects of catecholamines take longer to establish but last longer.

      (d) This is true of the effect of catecholamines on both contractility and heart rate.

   (7) The following exogenously administered drugs can alter myocardial contractility.

      (a) The sympatholytics (e.g., propranolol) produce negative inotropic effects through beta receptor blockade.

      (b) The sympathomimetics (e.g., isoproterenol or epinephrine) produce positive inotropic effects through beta receptor stimulation.

      (c) Some antiarrhythmics (e.g., quinidine or procainamide) produce negative inotropic effects.

      (d) Derivatives of digitalis produce positive inotropic effects.

   (8) Myocardial contractility is an elusive parameter to assess clinically. However, controversial attempts have been made to quantitate it.

   (9) It should be remembered that the stroke volume is under a gamut of influences. However, any stroke volume is determined by the interrelation of preload, afterload and the state of ventricular contractility.

F. Techniques of measuring cardiac output

  1. Fick method

    a. The total amount of oxygen available for tissue utilization must be equal to arterial oxygen content (Ca_{O_2}), expressed in volumes percent, times the volume of blood presented to the tissues per unit time ($\dot{Q}$ or cardiac output), expressed in liters per minute:

$$\text{Total } O_2 \text{ available} = (\dot{Q}) \times (Ca_{O_2}). \tag{8}$$

    b. The total amount of oxygen returned to the lung from the tissues must be equal to the mixed venous oxygen content ($C\bar{v}_{O_2}$) times the volume of blood presented to the lung per unit time ($\dot{Q}$ or cardiac output):

$$\text{Total } O_2 \text{ returned} = (\dot{Q}) \times (C\bar{v}_{O_2}). \tag{9}$$

c. Therefore, total tissue extraction of oxygen per unit time ($\dot{V}_{O_2}$) must be equal to the total oxygen available minus the total oxygen returned:

$$\dot{V}_{O_2} = (\dot{Q}) \times (C_{a_{O_2}}) - (\dot{Q}) \times (C\bar{v}_{O_2}). \tag{10}$$

d. Eq. 10 may be simplified by extracting the common factor of ($\dot{Q}$) and rewriting it as follows:

$$\dot{V}_{O_2} = (\dot{Q}) \times (C_{a_{O_2}} - C\bar{v}_{O_2}). \tag{11}$$

e. Eq. 11 is called the Fick equation and, by solving for cardiac output ($\dot{Q}$), it becomes

$$\dot{Q} = \frac{\dot{V}_{O_2}}{C_{a_{O_2}} - C\bar{v}_{O_2}}. \tag{12}$$

f. Thus by measuring total oxygen consumption per minute and arterial and mixed venous oxygen content in volumes percent, the cardiac output can be easily calculated by Eq. 12.

(1) Total oxygen consumption generally is calculated by analysis of exhaled gases.

(2) Arterial oxygen content requires systemic arterial blood sampling.

(3) Mixed venous oxygen content requires pulmonary arterial blood sampling.

g. Example: Given a

$$\dot{V}_{O_2} = \frac{280 \text{ cc of O}_2}{\text{minute}}$$

$$C_{a_{O_2}} = \frac{20 \text{ cc of O}_2}{100 \text{ cc blood}} \text{ or } 20 \text{ vol}\%$$

$$C\bar{v}_{O_2} = \frac{15 \text{ cc of O}_2}{100 \text{ cc blood}} \text{ or } 15 \text{ vol}\%,$$

then the cardiac output must equal 5.6 liters per minute by the following calculation:

$$\dot{Q} = \frac{\dfrac{280 \text{ cc of O}_2}{\text{minute}}}{\dfrac{20 \text{ cc of O}_2}{100 \text{ cc blood}} - \dfrac{15 \text{ cc of O}_2}{100 \text{ cc blood}}}$$

$$\dot{Q} = \frac{5600 \text{ cc of blood}}{\text{minute}} \text{ or } \frac{5.6 \text{ L of blood}}{\text{minute}}.$$

    h. The cardiac output determination obtained by using the Fick equation is considered the most accurate. The Fick method is therefore the standard by which other methods of cardiac output determinations are compared for accuracy.

2. Dye dilution method
    a. A dye (typically indocyanine green) that can be analyzed by a spectrophotometer is used as an indicator.
    b. A known amount (mg) of dye is injected rapidly into the right atrium or pulmonary artery.
    c. The dye is allowed to mix in the pulmonary circulation, and a continuous representative sampling of blood is drawn from the sampling catheter located in a major systemic artery.
    d. Blood samples are analyzed by spectrophotometer for concentration of dye, and the concentrations are plotted on a graph against time.
    e. Knowing the number of milligrams of dye injected and plotting the measured concentrations against time allow calculation of the cardiac output ($\dot{Q}$) by the following equation:

$$\dot{Q} = \frac{d_o}{\overline{d_c} \times t} \qquad (13)$$

where $\dot{Q}$ = cardiac output

    d_o = mg of dye injected

    $\overline{d_c}$ = mean concentration of dye

    t = time from appearance to disappearance of dye at sampling site.

3. Thermal dilution method
    a. This technique uses a four-lumen pulmonary artery catheter (Swan-Ganz catheter) with a port about 30 cm proximal from the end of the catheter.
    b. This proximal port usually lies in the right atrium and is used for injection of a known volume (usually 10 cc) of fluid (D5W) at a known temperature (usually 0 C).

c. At the distal end of the catheter is a device, a thermister, which senses changes in temperature. This device normally resides in a branch of the pulmonary artery.

d. The bolus of cold solution is injected into the right atrium. The right ventricle is used as the mixing chamber, and the blood is continually sampled by the thermister for changes in temperature.

e. The changes in blood temperature can be plotted on a graph against time.

f. The principle underlying cardiac output determination by thermal dilution is identical to that previously described for dye dilution.

g. Knowing the volume of the injected solution and the blood and solution temperatures and plotting the changes in blood temperature against time allow calculation of the cardiac output by the following equation:

$$\dot{Q} = \frac{V \times (T_b - T_s)}{\overline{T_b} \times t} \tag{14}$$

where $\dot{Q}$ = cardiac output

V = volume of solution injected

T_b = temperature of blood

T_s = temperature of solution injected

$\overline{T_b}$ = mean change in temperature of blood

t = time from appearance to disappearance of temperature change at sampling site.

X. Control of Arterial Blood Pressure

A. Under normal circumstances, arterial blood volume exceeds arterial vascular space. This relationship results in an intravascular pressure dictated by the absolute arterial blood volume and the elastic properties of the arterial vasculature.

B. The arterial system is continually receiving blood (inflow) from the left ventricle as cardiac output and continually allowing blood to leave the arterial system (outflow) as arterial runoff.

C. It is the balance or imbalance between cardiac output

(inflow) and arterial runoff (outflow) that results in any given arterial blood volume.

D. The relationship between arterial blood volume and arterial vascular space is the primary determinant of arterial blood pressure.

E. Thus by the equation $P = Q \times R$, it can be demonstrated that cardiac output ($\dot{Q}$) and peripheral resistance are directly related to arterial blood pressure (P). Arterial blood pressure is dependent on alteration of the blood volume to vascular space relationship by cardiac output and/or peripheral resistance, as follows:

   1. Increases in peripheral resistance (i.e., vasoconstriction) result in decreasing the arterial runoff. If cardiac output remains the same, then inflow exceeds outflow from the arterial vasculature. This results in an increase in the arterial blood volume to arterial vascular space relationship and a concomitant increase in arterial blood pressure.

   2. Decreases in peripheral resistance (i.e., vasodilatation) result in decreasing the arterial blood pressure by the exact opposite mechanism.

   3. Increases in cardiac output result in increasing the rate of inflow to the arterial system. If peripheral resistance remains the same, then inflow exceeds outflow from the arterial vasculature. This results in an increase in the arterial blood volume to arterial vascular space relationship and an increase in arterial blood pressure.

   4. Decreases in cardiac output result in decreasing arterial blood pressure by the exact opposite mechanism.

   5. It should be noted that in the four examples above the imbalance between inflow and outflow is only temporary. It is by these mechanisms that arterial blood pressure can be increased or decreased. Once the desired arterial pressure is attained, the balance between inflow and outflow will maintain the pressure at that level.

F. As has been described, cardiac output and peripheral resistance are for a large part under neural control. Therefore it becomes apparent that regulation of arterial blood pressure is mediated through neural alterations in cardiac output and peripheral resistance.

G. Neural regulation of arterial blood pressure is mediated

through autonomic fibers that originate from an area of the medulla oblongata. This area of the medulla is sometimes called the "cardiovascular center."

H. The cardiovascular center may be functionally divided into four subcenters: The vasomotor excitatory (vasoconstrictor) center, vasomotor inhibitory (vasodilator) center, cardiac excitatory center and cardiac inhibitory center.

   1. The vasomotor excitatory center influences the arterioles through the sympathetic nervous system. The degree of vasoconstriction or vasodilatation is directly related to the amount of sympathetic stimulation.

   2. The vasomotor inhibitory center does not influence the arterioles directly but acts by inhibiting the activity of the vasomotor excitatory center.

   3. The cardiac excitatory center influences the heart through the sympathetic nervous system. Sympathetic stimulation originating from this center results in positive inotropic and chronotropic effects.

   4. The cardiac inhibitory center influences the heart through the parasympathetic nervous system. Parasympathetic stimulation originating from this center results in a negative chronotropic effect and a mild negative inotropic effect.

I. The cardiovascular center in the medulla receives sensory input from the entire body. The most important sources of sensory input are the exteroceptors, higher brain centers, local factors, peripheral chemoreceptors and baroreceptors.

   1. Exteroceptors (e.g., proprioceptors, thermal receptors and pain receptors) are sources of sensory input. Stimulation of the proprioceptors, pain receptors and thermal receptors through muscular activation, pain and heat, respectively, results in an increase in heart rate. This potentially will increase arterial blood pressure. Cold and muscular inactivity slow the heart rate and potentially decrease arterial blood pressure.

   2. Higher brain centers (e.g., cerebral cortex and hypothalamus) have medullary input.

      a. Emotional factors alter blood pressure by mediation through the cerebral cortex. Fear or anger usually increases the blood pressure by stimulating the vasomotor and cardiac excitatory centers. This stimulation results in vasoconstriction and an increase in heart rate. However, decreases in blood pressure can be mediated through the cerebrum by stimulation of the vasomotor inhibitory center, as in fainting or blushing.

b. The hypothalamus mediates its control on the vasomotor inhibitory center in response to increases in body temperature. This causes vasodilatation of the vessels of the skin and loss of body heat. A decrease in body temperature will result in vasoconstriction of the vessels of the skin with heat conservation as mediated through the hypothalamus.

c. Direct stimulation of the anterior portion of the hypothalamus produces bradycardia and a decrease in arterial blood pressure, whereas stimulation of the posterior portion of the hypothalamus produces tachycardia and an increase in arterial blood pressure.

3. The vasomotor inhibitory and excitatory centers are sensitive to local and direct effects of pH and Pco_2 of arterial blood perfusing these centers.

a. Local increases in arterial pH and decreases in Pco_2 cause depression of the vasomotor excitatory center by the vasomotor inhibitory center. This results in vasodilatation, decrease in peripheral resistance and decrease in arterial blood pressure.

b. Local decreases in arterial pH and increases in Pco_2 cause direct excitation of the vasomotor excitatory center. This results in vasoconstriction, increase in peripheral resistance and increase in arterial blood pressure.

c. A local drop in Po_2 of arterial blood potentiates the vasoconstrictor effect but alone has no local effect.

4. Peripheral chemoreceptors (aortic and carotid bodies) are responsible for initiating the vasomotor chemoreflex.

a. Hypoxemia, hypercapnia and acidemia all stimulate the peripheral chemoreceptors.

b. The stimulated chemoreceptors in turn send an increased number of afferent impulses to the vasomotor excitatory center, with resultant vasoconstriction. This increases peripheral resistance and arterial blood pressure.

c. When hypoxemia and hypercapnia or hypoxemia and

acidemia exist, the chemoreceptors display a synergistic effect. That is, the stimulation arising from the chemoreceptors secondary to two simultaneous stimuli is greater than the mathematical sum of the two stimuli when they act alone. This results in a more profound vasoconstriction and increase in blood pressure.

5. Baroreceptors are by far the most important short-acting regulator of arterial blood pressure.
   a. Baroreceptors (pressoreceptors) are stretch receptors located in the arch of the aorta and carotid sinus.
   b. They respond to changes in pressure, which stretch them to different degrees. The greater the pressure the greater the number of impulses the baroreceptors will send.
   c. With a drop in arterial blood pressure, the number of impulses sent by the baroreceptors decreases. This decreased number of inhibitory impulses causes the vasomotor excitatory and cardiac excitatory centers to become more active. This results in increased cardiac output and increased peripheral resistance, thus restoring arterial blood pressure to normal.
   d. With an increase in arterial blood pressure, the number of impulses sent out by the baroreceptors increases. This increased number of inhibitory impulses causes the vasomotor excitatory center to become depressed directly and indirectly through increased activity of the vasomotor inhibitory center. In addition, the increased number of inhibitory impulses depresses the cardiac excitatory center and stimulates the cardiac inhibitory center, resulting in a decreased heart rate. Thus peripheral resistance and cardiac output decrease, restoring normal blood pressure.

XI. Hemodynamic Monitoring
   A. Systemic arterial blood pressure is expressed as a systolic pressure divided by a diastolic pressure.
      1. Systolic pressure is the highest pressure attained in the artery and is determined by three major factors:
         a. Stroke volume
            (1) Increased stroke volume generally causes an increased systolic pressure.

       (2) Decreased stroke volume generally causes a decreased systolic pressure.

  b. Rate of blood ejection from left ventricle

       (1) An increased rate of left ventricular ejection generally results in increased systolic pressure.

       (2) A decrease in the rate of ejection generally results in decreased systolic pressure.

  c. Elasticity of the arterial tree

       (1) Increased arterial elasticity generally results in an increased systolic pressure.

       (2) Decreased arterial elasticity generally results in a decreased systolic pressure.

2. Diastolic pressure is the lowest pressure attained in the artery and is determined by three major factors:

  a. Magnitude of preceding systolic pressure

       (1) In general, the higher the preceding systolic pressure the higher the resulting diastolic pressure.

       (2) The lower the preceding systolic pressure the lower the resulting diastolic pressure.

  b. Length of ventricular diastolic interval

       (1) The longer the diastolic interval the greater the time available for blood to leave the arterial system and the lower the resultant diastolic pressure.

       (2) The shorter the diastolic interval the higher the diastolic pressure by the opposite mechanism.

  c. State of peripheral resistance

       (1) The greater the peripheral resistance the lower the rate of arterial runoff and the higher the resultant diastolic pressure.

       (2) The lower the peripheral resistance the higher the rate of arterial runoff and the lower the resultant diastolic pressure.

3. In general, measurement of arterial blood pressure assesses left ventricular function by systolic pressure, and peripheral resistance by diastolic pressure. It should be recalled that one factor responsible for systolic pressure is stroke volume and a factor responsible for diastolic pressure is the state of peripheral resistance.

4. Thus it is assumed that the greater the difference between systolic and diastolic pressure the greater the

resultant flow. The difference between systolic and diastolic pressures is called the pulse pressure.

a. By the equation

$$\dot{Q} = P \times \frac{1}{R} \tag{15}$$

increases in systolic pressure indicate increases in the pressure gradient (P) across the systemic circulation, and decreases in diastolic pressure indicate decreases in peripheral resistance (R).

b. Therefore, widening of pulse pressure is generally thought to indicate increased blood flow (Q).

c. By the opposite mechanism, narrowing of pulse pressure is generally thought to indicate decreased flow.

d. It should be noted that a widening of pulse pressure can occur without increased blood flow. Also, normal blood flow can exist with a narrow pulse pressure. These phenomena occur by alterations in the other factors (i.e., diastolic interval, arterial elasticity) that determine systolic and diastolic pressure. Thus it is imperative to assess all factors responsible for systolic and diastolic pressure before blindly stating that an increased or decreased pulse pressure represents increased or decreased blood flow in a given patient.

5. Systolic pressure is commonly used as an indicator of left ventricular afterload, thus representing the resistance (in terms of pressure) that the left ventricle must pump against.

6. The mean arterial pressure (MAP) represents the average pressure over one complete systolic and diastolic interval.

a. The MAP can be directly measured or estimated by the formula:

$$\text{MAP} = \frac{(2 \times \text{diastolic pressure}) + (\text{systolic pressure})}{3}. \tag{16}$$

b. The MAP is the average pressure in the arterial tree over a given time and thus generally is used as an assessment of the average pressure to which the arterial system is exposed.

c. Thus the pressure gradient across the systemic circulation is generally expressed as MAP − CVP, where CVP equals central venous pressure (see XI, B).

7. Both arterial blood pressure and mean arterial blood pressure can be directly measured by an intra-arterial line (catheter). Arterial blood pressure can be indirectly measured by use of a sphygmomanometer and the MAP calculated from the obtained values.
8. Normal values for arterial blood pressure in the adult are as follows:

    Systolic: 140–90 mm Hg
    Diastolic: 90–60 mm Hg
    Mean: 70–105 mm Hg

B. The CVP usually is expressed as a single number representing the mean right atrial pressure (RAP).
   1. The numerical pressure value of CVP will be the result of the following factors:
      a. The pump capabilities of the right side of the heart in part determine the CVP. If the right ventricle pumps what it receives, blood will not back up in the atrium and the CVP should be normal. If the right side of the heart is not pumping adequately, there will be a backup of blood in the atrium that will be reflected as an elevated CVP.
      b. The venous tone determines CVP in that venous tone is responsible for determining the venous vascular space. It thus has major implications in venous return and filling pressure of the right atrium.
      c. Blood volume, which in part determines CVP, must be adequate to fill the venous vascular space, or venous return to the heart will be impeded.
      d. If the pump capabilities of the right side of the heart are adequate, the CVP will directly reflect the venous vascular volume (blood volume) to venous vascular space relationship. Fluid therapy and diuresis are frequently gauged in terms of the CVP's reflection of this relationship.
   2. The CVP is commonly used as an indicator of right ventricular preload when measured as right ventricular end-diastolic pressure (RVEDP).
      a. RVEDP represents compliance of the right ventricle.
      b. RVEDP also represents the filling pressure necessary for adequate right ventricular function.
   3. The CVP is measured directly through a catheter insert-

ed in a peripheral vein, its tip residing in the right atrium.

4. Normal values for CVP in the adult are 0–8 mm Hg.

C. Pulmonary artery pressure (PAP) is expressed as a systolic pressure divided by a diastolic pressure.

1. Systolic pressure is the highest pressure attained in the pulmonary artery and is determined by the same three factors that determine systolic pressure in the systemic arterial system:
   a. Size of stroke volume
   b. Rate of blood ejection from right ventricle
   c. Elasticity of pulmonary arterial tree

2. Diastolic pressure is the lowest pressure attained in the pulmonary artery and is determined by the same three factors that determine diastolic pressure in the systemic arterial system:
   a. Magnitude of preceding systolic pressure
   b. Length of right ventricular diastolic interval
   c. State of peripheral resistance of pulmonary arterial tree

3. In general, measurement of PAP assesses right ventricular function by systolic pressure, and pulmonary arterial resistance by diastolic pressure. Thus PAP is used in precisely the same fashion as systemic arterial pressure. In this light, it should be noted that all factors contributing to systolic and diastolic PAP should be fully assessed before inferences concerning blood flow are made from these values.

4. Systolic pressure of the pulmonary artery is commonly used as an assessment of right ventricular afterload, thus representing the resistance (in terms of pressure) that the right ventricle must pump against.

5. The mean pulmonary artery pressure ($\overline{\text{PAP}}$) represents the average pressure over one complete systolic and diastolic interval.
   a. The ($\overline{\text{PAP}}$) is the average pressure in the pulmonary artery over a given time and is used as an assessment of the average pressure head (or front) that the pulmonary arterial system is exposed to.
   b. Thus the pressure gradient across the pulmonary circulation is generally represented by the expression $\overline{\text{PAP}}$ – PWP, where PWP equals the mean left atrial or pulmonary wedge pressure (see XI, D).

6. Both the PAP and $\overline{PAP}$ are directly measured by use of a pulmonary artery catheter. The pulmonary artery catheter is inserted through a peripheral vein and traverses the right atrium and ventricle, its tip residing in the pulmonary artery.
7. Normal values for pulmonary arterial blood pressure in the adult are as follows:

Systolic:	15–28 mm Hg
Diastolic:	5–16 mm Hg
Mean:	10–22 mm Hg

D. Pulmonary wedge pressure (PWP) is expressed as a single number representing the mean left atrial pressure $(\overline{LAP})$.
1. The numerical pressure value of PWP will be the result of the following factors.
   a. The pump capabilities of the left side of the heart in part determine PWP. If the left ventricle pumps what it receives, blood will not back up into the atrium and PWP should be normal. If the left ventricle is not pumping adequately, there will be a backup of blood into the atrium that will be reflected as an elevated PWP.
   b. Blood return to the left atrium is due largely to an adequate blood volume to pulmonary venous (venomotor tone) vascular space relationship.
   c. If the left ventricle is pumping adequately, PWP is dependent on the forementioned vascular volume to vascular space relationship.
2. The PWP is commonly used as an indicator of left ventricular preload when measured as the left ventricular end-diastolic pressure (LVEDP).
   a. LVEDP represents compliance of the left ventricle.
   b. LVEDP also represents the filling pressure necessary for adequate left ventricular function.
3. The PWP is measured directly through a pulmonary artery catheter by inflation of a balloon that occludes that branch of the pulmonary artery. Pressure readings are taken from the tip of the catheter, which is distal to the balloon. The pressure reflects back pressure from the left atrium.
4. Normal values for PWP in the adult are 2–12 mm Hg.

BIBLIOGRAPHY

Anthony, C. P., and Kolthoff, N. J.: *Textbook of Anatomy and Physiology* (8th ed.; St. Louis: C. V. Mosby Co., 1971).

Ayres, S. M., Giannelli, S. J., and Mueller, H. S.: *Care of the Critically Ill* (2d ed.; New York: Appleton-Century-Crofts, 1974).

Crowley, L. V.: *Introductory Concepts in Anatomy and Physiology* (Chicago: Year Book Medical Publishers, Inc., 1976).

Gray, H., and Goss, C. M.: *Gray's Anatomy of the Human Body* (29th ed.; Philadelphia: Lea & Febiger, 1973).

Guyton, A. C.: *Textbook of Medical Physiology* (5th ed.; Philadelphia: W. B. Saunders Co., 1976).

Jacob, S. W., and Francone, C. A.: *Structure and Function in Man* (3d ed.; Philadelphia: W. B. Saunders Co., 1974).

Little, R. C.: *Physiology of the Heart and Circulation* (Chicago: Year Book Medical Publishers, Inc., 1977).

McLaughlin, A. J.: *Essentials of Physiology for Advanced Respiratory Therapy* (St. Louis: C. V. Mosby Co., 1977).

Ruch, T. C., and Patton, H. D.: *Physiology and Biophysics* (20th ed.; Philadelphia: W. B. Saunders Co., 1974).

Rushmer, R. F.: *Cardiovascular Dynamics* (3d ed.; Philadelphia: W. B. Saunders Co., 1970).

Schroeder, J. S., and Daily, E. K.: *Techniques in Bedside Hemodynamic Monitoring* (St. Louis: C. V. Mosby Co., 1976).

Shapiro, B. A., Harrison, R. A., and Trout, C. A.: *Clinical Application of Respiratory Care* (Chicago: Year Book Medical Publishers, Inc., 1975).

9 / Oxygen and Carbon Dioxide Transport

I. Carriage of Oxygen in the Blood
  A. Oxygen is carried in two distinct compartments in the blood:
     1. Physically dissolved in plasma.
     2. Chemically attached to hemoglobin molecule.
  B. Volume physically dissolved in plasma
     1. According to the Bunsen solubility coefficient for oxygen, 0.023 ml of oxygen can be dissolved in 1 ml of plasma for every 760 mm Hg P_{O_2}.
     2. Simplifying this factor to the number of milliliters of oxygen per milliliter of plasma per mm Hg P_{O_2}:

$$0.023 \text{ ml} O_2/760 \text{ mm Hg} =$$
$$0.00003 \text{ ml } O_2/\text{mm Hg } P_{O_2}/\text{ml plasma.} \qquad (1)$$

     3. Since the oxygen content normally is expressed in volumes percent, multiplying 0.00003 ml of oxygen per milliliter of plasma by 100 gives the factor:

$$(0.00003 \text{ ml } O_2/\text{ml plasma})(100) =$$
$$0.003 \text{ ml } O_2/100 \text{ ml plasma/mm Hg } P_{O_2}. \qquad (2)$$

     4. Thus multiplying the P_{O_2} of blood by 0.003, the number of milliliters of oxygen physically dissolved in every 100 ml of blood (Vol%) is determined:

$$(P_{O_2})(0.003) = \text{ml of oxygen physically dissolved.} \qquad (3)$$

  C. Hemoglobin (Hb): Structure and carrying capacity
     1. Composition of normal hemoglobin molecule
        a. Four porphyrin rings, called hemes, each with a central iron atom.
        b. Four polypeptide chains: two alpha chains and two beta, called the globin portion of the molecule.
        c. Each of the iron atoms of the heme is bonded via four covalent bonds to the porphyrin ring, one covalent bond to the globin portion and one bond available to combine with oxygen.

135

    d. On the porphyrin ring, amino groups $(R-NH_2)$ allow chemical combination of carbon dioxide with the hemoglobin molecule.

    e. Also, the terminal imidazole $(R-NH)$ groups are available to buffer H^+ (see Chapter 10, Section III).

       (1) Hemoglobin's buffering capacity is second only to that of HCO_3^-/H_2CO_3 buffer system.

       (2) The buffering capacity of the hemoglobin molecule depends upon attachment of oxygen to the iron portion of the molecule.

       (3) Oxygenated hemoglobin acts as a stronger buffer than does unoxygenated hemoglobin.

       (4) Thus the buffering capacity of arterial blood is greater than that of venous blood.

    f. Carbon monoxide attaches chemically at the iron site with an affinity 200 to 250 times that of oxygen.

2. The molecular weight of hemoglobin is about 64,500 gm.

3. Since oxygen attaches to each of the four iron atoms in the hemoglobin molecule, four gram molecular weights of oxygen combine with 64,500 gm of hemoglobin.

4. Simplifying and restating #3, one gram molecular weight of oxygen combines with 16,125 gm of hemoglobin.

5. Since one gram molecular weight of oxygen at STP will occupy 22.4 L:

$$\frac{22,400 \text{ ml of } O_2}{16,125 \text{ gm of Hb}} = 1.34 \text{ ml of } O_2/\text{gm of Hb.} \qquad (4)$$

6. At 100% saturation, 1.34 ml of oxygen can combine with each gram of hemoglobin.

7. The actual volume of oxygen carried attached to hemoglobin is equal to

$$\text{(Hb content)}(1.34)(HbO_2\% \text{ sat.}) =$$
$$\text{vol\% of } O_2 \text{ carried attached to Hb.} \qquad (5)$$

D. Oxygen content

    1. The total oxygen content of blood is equal to the volume of oxygen physically dissolved in plasma plus the amount chemically combined with hemoglobin.

    2. Mathematically the above statement is equal to

$$O_2 \text{ content in vol\%} =$$
$$(Po_2)(0.003) + \text{(Hb content)}(1.34)(HbO_2\% \text{ sat.}) \qquad (6)$$

E. Oxyhemoglobin dissociation curve (Fig 9 – 1)
  1. The overall sigmoidal shape of the curve is a result of the varied affinities of the four oxygen-bonding sites on the hemoglobin molecule.
    a. In general, the affinity of the last site bound is considerably less than the other three sites.
    b. In general, the affinity for the first site is less than the second or third sites.
  2. The steep aspect of the curve is that portion where minimal changes in PO_2 normally will cause significant increases in HbO_2 % saturation and therefore O_2 content.
    a. Increasing the saturation from 50% to 75% normally necessitates only a 13 mm Hg PO_2 increase, whereas increasing the saturation from 75% to 100% normally necessitates well over a 100 mg Hg PO_2 increase.
  3. P_{50} is defined as that PO_2 at which the hemoglobin is 50% saturated with oxygen. Normally the P_{50} is equal to 27 mm Hg (Fig 9 – 2).
    a. An increased P_{50} indicates a shift of the oxyhemoglobin

Fig 9–1. – Volume of oxygen, dissolved, as oxyhemoglobin, and total oxygen are indicated. Overall sigmoidal shape of the curve demonstrates varying bonding affinities for oxygen molecules as oxyhemoglobin saturation is increased. (From Shapiro, B. A., Harrison, R. A., and Walton, J. R.: *Clinical Application of Blood Gases* [2d ed.; Chicago: Year Book Medical Publishers, Inc., 1977]. Used by permission.)

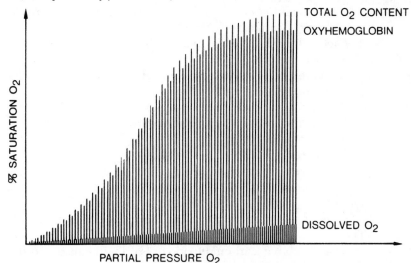

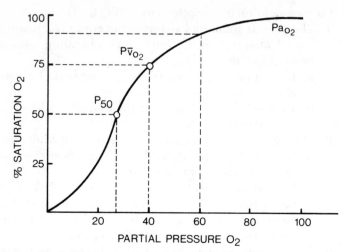

Fig 9–2. — Partial pressure at which hemoglobin is 50% saturated is 27 mm Hg. This is referred to as P_{50}. Normal venous Po_2 of 40 mm Hg and 75% oxyhemoglobin saturation are also indicated. A Po_2 of 60 mm Hg results in 90% saturation of the hemoglobin, whereas the normal arterial Po_2 of 97 mm Hg results in 97% saturation of the hemoglobin. (From Shapiro, B. A., Harrison, R. A., and Walton, J. R.: *Clinical Application of Blood Gases* [2d ed.; Chicago: Year Book Medical Publishers, Inc., 1977]. Used by permission.)

dissociation curve to the right, resulting in a decreased hemoglobin affinity for oxygen.
    b. A decreased P_{50} indicates a shift of the oxyhemoglobin dissociation curve to the left, resulting in an increased hemoglobin affinity for oxygen.
   4. Factors that shift the oxyhemoglobin curve to the right
    a. Increased Pco_2
    b. Increased $[H^+]$ or decreased pH
    c. Increased temperature
    d. Increased 2, 3-DPG (2, 3-diphosphoglycerate)
   5. Factors that shift the oxyhemoglobin curve to the left
    a. Decreased Pco_2
    b. Decreased $[H^+]$ or increased pH
    c. Decreased temperature
    d. Decreased 2, 3-DPG
 F. *The Bohr effect:* The effect of carbon dioxide or $[H^+]$ on uptake and release of oxygen from the hemoglobin molecule. The effect is relatively mild in extent.
   1. As seen above, carbon dioxide or $[H^+]$ will cause a shift in the oxyhemoglobin dissociation curve.

2. At the systemic capillary bed, increased carbon dioxide and [H+] moving into the blood decreases hemoglobin affinity for oxygen and increases the volume of oxygen released at the tissue level.

3. At the pulmonary capillary bed, decreased carbon dioxide and [H+] levels increase hemoglobin affinity for oxygen, thus increasing the volume of oxygen picked up at the pulmonary level.

G. Oxygen consumption
   1. The volume of oxygen consumed by the average adult is 5 vol%, or 250 ml of oxygen per minute.

II. Carriage of Carbon Dioxide in the Blood
   A. Carriage in plasma occurs in three distinct ways (Fig 9–3):
      1. Carbon dioxide is dissolved in plasma as PCO_2, which is in equilibrium with PCO_2 in red blood cells.
      2. Carbon dioxide is carried predominantly as bicarbonate (HCO_3^-) formed in the red blood cells and by the kidney. The HCO_3^- levels in plasma are in equilibrium with the HCO_3^- in red blood cells.
         a. Plasma carbon dioxide will react minimally with water, forming carbonic acid, which will dissociate into H^+ and HCO_3^-:

$$CO_2 + H_2O \leftrightarrows H_2CO_3 \rightleftarrows H^+ + HCO_3^-. \qquad (7)$$

         b. The H^+ formed is buffered in the plasma and therefore causes only a mild decrease in venous pH.

Fig 9–3.—Overall scheme for O_2 and CO_2 transport in blood. See text for explanation.

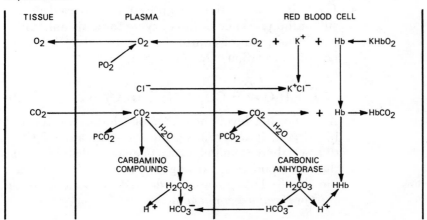

  c. The above reaction's point of equilibrium is shifted to the left in the plasma, therefore favoring formation of reactants.
  d. The mathematical relationship between CO_2 and H_2CO_3 is

$$(P_{CO_2} \text{ mm Hg})(0.0301) = H_2CO_3 \text{ mEq/L or mM/L.} \qquad (8)$$

3. Carbon dioxide is attached to plasma proteins as carbamino compounds.
  a. Carbon dioxide reacts with the terminal amino groups on the plasma proteins ($R-NH_2$):

$$R-N\begin{matrix} H \\ \diagup \\ \diagdown \\ H \end{matrix} + CO_2 \rightleftarrows R-N\begin{matrix} H \\ \diagup \\ \diagdown \\ COO^- \end{matrix} + H^+ \qquad (9)$$

  (R—indicates the remainder of the plasma protein)

  b. Most of the H^+ liberated is buffered and therefore causes only a mild decrease in the pH of venous blood.
  c. The ionization state of the amino groups will affect their ability to bond with carbon dioxide. If the NH_2 groups are oxidized to NH_3^+, their ability to combine with carbon dioxide is significantly decreased.
B. Carriage of carbon dioxide in the red blood cells occurs in three distinct ways (see Fig 9–3).
  1. As dissolved P_{CO_2} in equilibrium with plasma P_{CO_2}
  2. As HCO_3^- formed in the red blood cell
    a. The following reaction is significantly increased as a result of the presence of the enzyme carbonic anhydrase (CA). The point of equilibrium is shifted to the right, favoring formation of the products:

$$CO_2 + H_2O \overset{CA}{\rightleftarrows} H_2CO_3 \rightleftarrows H^+ + HCO_3^-. \qquad (10)$$

    b. As increasing levels of HCO_3^- are formed in the red blood cell, it will diffuse into the plasma. As HCO_3^- diffuses, there is an imbalance of electric charges inside the red blood cell, causing Cl^- to move into the red blood cell. This process is referred to as the *chloride shift* or *Hamburger phenomenon*.

3. Carbon dioxide is attached to the terminal amino $(R-NH_2)$ groups of the hemoglobin molecule. This reaction is the same as Eq. 9 above. Again, the H^+ released from the formation of HCO_3^- must be buffered.

   a. In the red blood cells the primary buffer is the imidazole groups on the hemoglobin molecule.

   b. The ability of the imidazole groups to buffer is affected by oxyhemoglobin saturation. With oxygen bound to the heme, the imidazole groups possess a greater ability to buffer H^+. Without oxygen attached to the heme, the imidazole groups have a decreased ability to buffer H^+.

   c. As oxygen attaches to the heme, more $R-NH_2$ groups will exist in the $R-NH_3^+$ form. The tendency for carbon dioxide to attach to the $R-NH_3^+$ form is less than to the $R-NH_2$ form.

III. The Haldane Effect (Fig 9–4)

   A. Figure 9–4 is a representation of the Haldane effect, which can be defined as the effect of oxygen on carbon dioxide uptake and release.

   B. As PO_2 increases at the pulmonary capillary bed, the ability of hemoglobin to carry carbon dioxide is decreased because more amino groups exist in the oxidized $R-NH_3^+$ state. This allows large volumes of carbon dioxide to be released at the pulmonary capillary bed.

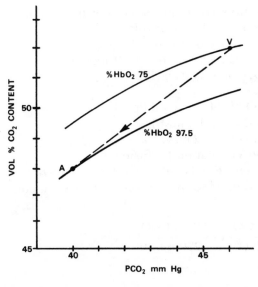

Fig 9–4. — Effect of oxyhemoglobin saturation on volume of CO_2 carried in blood. The carrying capacity of blood for CO_2 is decreased as oxyhemoglobin saturation is increased (Haldane effect). The *arrow* from *V* to *A* depicts change of CO_2 content from venous to arterial blood.

C. As the P_{O_2} decreases at the tissue level, the ability of hemoglobin to carry carbon dioxide is increased because more amino groups exist in the reduced $R-NH_2$ form. This allows large volumes of carbon dioxide to be picked up at the tissue capillary bed (see Fig 9–4).

D. The Haldane effect facilitates carriage of the normal 4 vol% (200 ml/min) of carbon dioxide to be picked up from the tissue and released at the lung.

IV. Quantitative Distribution of Carbon Dioxide
   A. Percentage of carbon dioxide carried in each compartment:
      1. 90% of carbon dioxide in blood exists as HCO_3^-.
      2. 5% of carbon dioxide in blood exists as carbamino compounds.
      3. 5% of carbon dioxide in blood exists as dissolved P_{CO_2}.
   B. Percentage of carbon dioxide exhaled coming from various compartments:
      1. 60% of carbon dioxide exhaled was initially carried as HCO_3^-.
      2. 30% of carbon dioxide exhaled was initially carried as carbamino compounds.
      3. 10% of carbon dioxide exhaled was initially carried as dissolved P_{CO_2}.

V. Total CO_2
   A. Total CO_2 is expressed as the sum of HCO_3^- plus dissolved CO_2.
   B. Total CO_2 may be expressed in millimoles per liter (mM/L), milliequivalents per liter (mEq/L) or vol%.
   C. $(P_{CO_2})(0.0301)$ equals mM/L or mEq/L of H_2CO_3
   D. Vol% of CO_2 equals (mEq/L)(2.23) or (mM/L)(2.23)
   E. mM/L or mEq/L CO_2 equals vol%/2.23
   F. In arterial blood
      1. Total $CO_2 = [HCO_3^-] + [\text{dissolved } P_{CO_2}]$
      2. 25.2 mM/L = 24 mM/L + 1.2 mM/L
      3. 56.2 vol% = 53.52 vol% + 2.68 vol%

VI. Respiratory Quotient and Ventilation/Perfusion Ratio
   A. The respiratory quotient (RQ) is defined as the volume of carbon dioxide produced divided by the volume of oxygen consumed per minute:

$$RQ = \frac{4 \text{ vol\% } CO_2}{5 \text{ vol\% } O_2} \text{ or } \frac{200 \text{ ml } CO_2}{250 \text{ ml } O_2} = 0.8.$$

B. The $\dot{V}/\dot{Q}$ ratio is equal to the minute alveolar ventilation divided by the minute cardiac output:

$$\dot{V}/\dot{Q} = \frac{4 \text{ L alveolar minute volume}}{5 \text{ L minute cardiac output}} = 0.8.$$

BIBLIOGRAPHY

Bendixen, H. H., et al.: *Respiratory Care* (St. Louis: C. V. Mosby Co., 1965).

Cherniack, R. M., Cherniack, L., and Naimark, A.: *Respiration in Health and Disease* (2d ed.; Philadelphia: W. B. Saunders Co., 1972).

Comroe, J. H.: *Physiology of Respiration* (2d ed.; Chicago: Year Book Medical Publishers, Inc., 1974).

Egan, D. F.: *Fundamentals of Respiratory Therapy* (3d ed.; St. Louis: C. V. Mosby Co., 1977).

Guyton, A. C.: *Textbook of Medical Physiology* (5th ed.; Philadelphia: W. B. Saunders Co., 1976).

Murray, J. F.: *The Normal Lung* (Philadelphia: W. B. Saunders Co., 1976).

Nunn, J. F.: *Applied Respiratory Physiology* (London: Butterworth & Co. (Publishers), Ltd., 1969).

Shapiro, B. A., Harrison, R. A., and Trout, C. A.: *Clinical Application of Respiratory Care* (Chicago: Year Book Medical Publishers, Inc., 1975).

Shapiro, B. A., Harrison, R. A., and Walton, J. R.: *Clinical Application of Blood Gases* (2d ed.; Chicago: Year Book Medical Publishers, Inc., 1977).

West, J. B.: *Respiratory Physiology: The Essentials* (Baltimore: William & Wilkins Co., 1974).

Young, J. A., and Crocker, D.: *Principles and Practice of Respiratory Therapy* (2d ed.; Chicago: Year Book Medical Publishers, Inc., 1976).

10 / Blood Gas Interpretation

I. Law of Mass Action

A. The basic chemical and mathematical relationships involved in blood gas interpretation are based on the law of mass action (also referred to as the law of electrolyte dissociation and law of chemical equilibrium).

B. *The law of mass action* states that when a weak electrolyte is placed into solution, only a small percentage of it will dissociate, the vast majority remaining undissociated. Determining the product of the molar concentrations of the dissociated species and dividing that by the molar concentration of the undissociated weak electrolyte results in the dissociation constant for that weak electrolyte. This constant holds true for the particular electrolyte in the solution in which it was dissolved at the temperature at which it was originally determined.

C. The law of mass action as applied to carbonic acid (H_2CO_3) dissolved in plasma at 37 C:

1. H_2CO_3 will dissociate into $H^+ + HCO_3^-$

$$H_2CO_3 \rightleftarrows H^+ + HCO_3^-. \tag{1}$$

2. Taking the molar concentration of H^+ and multiplying it by the molar concentration of HCO_3^- and dividing this by the molar concentration of H_2CO_3, the dissociation constant for H_2CO_3 in plasma is calculated:

$$\frac{[H^+][HCO_3^-]}{[H_2CO_3]} = K. \tag{2}$$

3. K for the above reaction in blood is equal to 7.85×10^{-7}.

II. Henderson-Hasselbalch Equation (Standard Buffer Equation)

A. This equation is based totally on the law of mass action.

B. Any weak electrolyte may be placed into the Henderson-Hasselbalch equation.

C. Taking Eq. 2 from above and
1. Rearranging it and solving for [H^+]
2. Taking the log to the base 10 of each side of the equation

3. Then multiplying the equation by -1, the result is

$$-\text{Log } [H^+] = -\log K + \log \frac{[HCO_3^-]}{[H_2CO_3]} \tag{3}$$

D. In Eq. 3 the $-\log [H^+]$ is equal to the pH. The $-\log K$ is equal to the pK of the buffer.
   1. The pK of a buffer determines the optimal pH for *maximum* dissociation of the buffer.
   2. The $-\log$ of 7.85×10^{-7} is equal to 6.10.
   3. The pK 6.10 is the pH at which the HCO_3^-/H_2CO_3 buffer system functions most efficiently.
   4. As the pH of the solution in which HCO_3^-/H_2CO_3 is buffering deviates from 6.10, its buffering capabilities decrease.
E. Thus Eq. 3 may be rewritten as

$$pH = pK + \log \frac{[HCO_3^-]}{[H_2CO_3]} \tag{4}$$

   or

$$pH = 6.10 + \log \frac{[HCO_3^-]}{[H_2CO_3]}. \tag{5}$$

F. Eq. 4 and Eq. 5 are the classic Henderson-Hasselbalch buffer equations as applied to the HCO_3^-/H_2CO_3 buffer system.
G. In arterial blood the following are true about Eq. 5:
   1. Normally HCO_3^- concentrations are equal to 24 mEq/L or 24 mM/L.
   2. Normally H_2CO_3 concentrations are equal to 1.2 mEq/L or 1.2 mM/L.
   3. The log of $HCO_3^-/H_2CO_3 \left(\dfrac{24}{1.2}\right)$ is equal to 1.3.
   4. Substituting 1.3 into Eq. 5 gives the normal arterial pH of 7.40:

$$pH = 6.10 + 1.3 = 7.40. \tag{6}$$

   5. There normally exists a 20:1 ratio between HCO_3^- and H_2CO_3. When this ratio is altered, the pH of the blood will then be altered. For example:
      a. If the ratio decreases to 10:1, the blood has become more acidotic.

   b. If the ratio increases to 30:1, the blood has become
      more alkalotic.
H. Clinically, HCO_3^- and H_2CO_3 concentrations are extremely
   time consuming and costly to determine.
   1. Since the $(PCO_2) \times (0.0301)$ is equivalent to the H_2CO_3
      levels, this value can be substituted into Eq. 5' for
      H_2CO_3:

$$pH = 6.10 + \log \frac{[HCO_3^-]}{(PCO_2)(0.0301)}. \tag{7}$$

   2. The pH of the blood is easily measured.
   3. $[HCO_3^-]$ is always a calculated value when blood gas
      results are reported.
III. Purpose of Buffer Systems
   A. Buffer systems play a major role in determining the pH of a
      given solution.
   B. Buffer systems minimize changes in the pH of a solution
      when H^+ or OH^- is added to the solution.
      1. In the HCO_3^-/H_2CO_3 system, H^+ added to the solution
         will react with HCO_3^-, creating more H_2CO_3 and mini-
         mizing the change in free $[H^+]$ and pH:

$$H^+ + HCO_3^- \rightarrow H_2CO_3. \tag{8}$$

      2. In the HCO_3^-/H_2CO_3 system, OH^- added to the solution
         will react with free H^+, causing dissociation of H_2CO_3,
         thus minimizing the change in free OH^- and pH:

$$OH^- + H^+ \rightarrow H_2O \tag{9}$$

      causing

$$H_2CO_3 \rightarrow H^+ + HCO_3^-. \tag{10}$$

      3. Statements 1 and 2 above will occur with maximum effi-
         ciency at the pK of the buffer (6.10). The buffering effi-
         ciency will continually decrease, the further the pH of
         the solution deviates from the pK.
   C. The total buffering capacity of the body can be broken
      down approximately as follows:
      1. 60% by the HCO_3^-/H_2CO_3 system
      2. 30% by hemoglobin buffering system
      3. 10% by all other blood buffers (e.g., phosphates, plasma
         proteins, ammonia)

IV. Actual versus Standard HCO_3^-
   A. Actual HCO_3^-: Value calculated from actual, measured PCO_2 and pH of arterial blood.
      1. Value normally given with arterial blood gas results.
      2. Indicative of nonrespiratory acid–base imbalances.
   B. Standard HCO_3^-: Value calculated from measured pH and PCO_2 of venous blood after PCO_2 of blood has been equilibrated to 40 mm Hg.
      1. Value usually reported with electrolyte studies by clinical laboratory.
      2. Indicative of a change in acid–base balance, but not precise as to magnitude of the abnormality or whether the problem is respiratory or nonrespiratory.
 V. Base Excess (BE)
   A. Base excess (BE) is the number of milliequivalents per liter of total body base above or below the normal of 54 mEq/L.
   B. The normal range is from +2 to −2 mEq/L above or below 54 mEq/L.
   C. Base excess is a relatively accurate index of the extent of nonrespiratory acid–base abnormalities.
   D. Base excess calculations are based on
      1. $[HCO_3^-]$
      2. pH
      3. Hemoglobin levels
VI. Normal Ranges for Blood Gases
   A. *Absolute* normals: Arterial blood
1. pH	7.40
2. PCO_2	40 mm Hg
3. PO_2	100 mm Hg
4. HCO_3^-	24 mEq/L
5. Base excess	0
6. Hemoglobin content	14 gm%
7. Oxyhemoglobin saturation	97.5%
8. Oxygen content	19.8 vol%
9. Carboxyhemoglobin saturation	0%
   B. *Normal* ranges: Arterial blood
1. pH	7.35–7.45
2. PCO_2	35–45
3. PO_2	80–100
4. HCO_3^-	22–27 mEq/L
5. Base excess	±2

    6. Hemoglobin content   12–15 gm%
    7. Oxyhemoglobin saturation   ≧95%
    8. Oxygen content   >16 vol%
    9. Carboxyhemoglobin saturation   <2%

C. *Absolute normals:* Venous blood
    1. pH   7.35
    2. P_{CO_2} 46 mm Hg
    3. P_{O_2} 40 mm Hg
    4. HCO_3^- 27 mEq/L
    5. Oxyhemoglobin saturation   75%

D. *Clinical ranges:* Arterial blood
    1. pH   7.30–7.50
    2. P_{CO_2} 30–50 mm Hg
    3. The ranges for arterial blood values given in Section VI-B indicate the "normal" variation in arterial pH and P_{CO_2}. Slight variations outside these normal ranges may not indicate a clinically significant change.
    4. The clinical ranges above indicate an acceptable pH and P_{CO_2} from a *patient management* point of view. Results outside these ranges indicate situations requiring clinical intervention.

VII. Mathematical Interrelationships Between pH, P_{CO_2} and HCO_3^-
    A. If the constants and log relationship are eliminated in the HCO_3^-/H_2CO_3 buffer equation, the equation may be simplified to

$$pH \approx \frac{HCO_3^-}{P_{CO_2}}. \tag{11}$$

This relationship demonstrates the mathematical interrelationship between these variables.
    B. In general, under all clinical circumstances the pH will be a result of the HCO_3^- and P_{CO_2} levels.
    C. In a pure respiratory abnormality where the HCO_3^- remains essentially constant, the P_{CO_2} and pH are indirectly related:

$$HCO_3^- \approx (pH)(P_{CO_2}). \tag{12}$$

    D. In a pure metabolic abnormality where the P_{CO_2} remains essentially constant, the HCO_3^- and pH are directly related:

$$PCO_2 \approx \frac{HCO_3^-}{pH}. \tag{13}$$

VIII. Compensation for Primary Acid–Base Abnormalities
  A. Compensation involves the various mechanisms used by the body to normalize the pH after a primary acid–base abnormality. Compensation does not imply correction of the primary abnormalities.
  B. Compensation for primary respiratory acid–base imbalances is via the kidney (Fig 10–1).
    1. In the cells of the kidney tubule system, carbonic anhydrase is present to increase the hydration of CO_2 to H_2CO_3, which dissociates to $H^+ + HCO_3^-$.
    2. As shown in Figure 10–1, as CO_2 enters the kidney cell, the above reaction rapidly takes place. Following this, HCO_3^- formed moves into the blood and H^+ moves into the glomerular filtrate to be buffered. As each H^+ moves

Fig 10–1.—Overall mechanism of regulation of plasma HCO_3^- levels by the kidney. The volume of HCO_3^- moved into the blood is directly related to plasma PCO_2 levels. The three primary kidney buffers, HPO_4^{-2}, HCO_3^- and NH_3 are illustrated. For further discussion refer to text. (From Shapiro, B. A., Harrison, R. A., and Walton, J. R.: *Clinical Application of Blood Gases* [2d ed.; Chicago: Year Book Medical Publishers, Inc., 1977]. Used by permission.)

BASIC PHYSIOLOGY OF BLOOD GASES

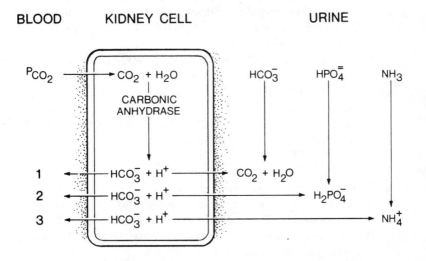

into the glomerular filtrate, a Na^+ will be reabsorbed into the bloodstream.

   3. In the glomerular filtrate, the H^+ will be buffered by
     a. HCO_3^-
     b. HPO_4^{-2} (dibasic phosphate)
     c. NH_3 (ammonia)

   4. By volume, most of the H^+ excreted in urine is buffered by the phosphate groups.

   5. The mechanism depicted in Figure 10–1 demonstrates that the amount of HCO_3^- moving into the blood is basically dependent on PCO_2 levels.
     a. If PCO_2 levels increase, more HCO_3^- is formed and moves into the blood. This normalizes the acidic pH caused by the increased PCO_2 levels.
     b. If PCO_2 levels decrease, less HCO_3^- is formed and moves into the blood. This normalizes the alkalotic pH caused by the decreased PCO_2 levels.

   6. Compensation by the kidney is relatively complete, but the mechanism may take hours to normalize the pH (in some cases up to 24–48 hours).

  C. Compensation for primary metabolic acid–base imbalances by the respiratory system (see Chapter 5).

IX. Effect of Arterial PCO_2 Changes on pH
  A. The most efficient pH for buffering to occur in blood is 6.10.
  B. Since normal arterial pH is 7.40, the blood buffers acid more efficiently than it does base. In acidosis the pH moves closer to the pK of blood (6.10) and therefore H^+ is buffered more efficiently.
  C. For every acute *20 mm Hg PCO_2 increase*, there should be approximately a 0.10 pH unit decrease from 7.40.
    1. PCO_2 60: pH 7.30
    2. PCO_2 80: pH 7.20
  D. For every acute *10 mm Hg PCO_2 decrease*, there should be approximately a 0.10 pH unit increase from 7.40.
    1. PCO_2 30: pH 7.50
    2. PCO_2 20: pH 7.60

X. Pharmacologic Adjustment of pH
  A. In severe metabolic acid–base disturbances, it is sometimes necessary to adjust the pH pharmacologically.
  B. Metabolic alkalosis is occasionally treated by administering ammonium chloride (NH_3Cl).

   C. Metabolic acidosis is treated by administering sodium bicarbonate ($NaHCO_3$).
     1. Bicarbonate administration
       a. The base excess indicates the number of milliequivalents per liter of deficit in body base.
       b. To determine total body deficit of base, an estimate of extracellular fluid volume is made. One third of an individual's normal body weight in kilograms is a reasonable estimate of extracellular volume in liters.
       c. Thus an individual weighing 75 kg, with a base excess of -15 mEq/L would have (75/3)(15) or 375 mEq total body deficit in base.
       d. Since 375 mEq is purely an estimate, normally half that amount is administered rapidly, followed by a reassessment of the acid-base status.

XI. Interpretation of Arterial Blood Gases
   A. Interpretation of arterial blood gases follows three steps:
     1. Interpretation of acid–base status
       a. *Classic textbook* method of blood gas interpretation (Table 10–1)
       b. *Clinical method* of blood gas interpretation (Table 10–2)

TABLE 10–1.—CLASSIC TEXTBOOK METHOD OF
BLOOD GAS INTERPRETATION

STATUS	pH	PCO_2	HCO_3^-	B.E.
RESPIRATORY ACIDOSIS				
Uncompensated	↓ 7.35	↑ 45	Normal	Normal
Partially compensated	↓ 7.35	↑ 45	↑ 27	↑ +2
Compensated	7.35–7.45	↑ 45	↑ 27	↑ +2
RESPIRATORY ALKALOSIS				
Uncompensated	↑ 7.45	↓ 35	Normal	Normal
Partially compensated	↑ 7.45	↓ 35	↓ 22	↓ −2
Compensated	7.40–7.45	↓ 35	↓ 22	↓ −2
METABOLIC ACIDOSIS				
Uncompensated	↓ 7.35	Normal	↓ 22	↓ −2
Partially compensated	↓ 7.35	↓ 35	↓ 22	↓ −2
Compensated	7.35–7.40	↓ 35	↓ 22	↓ −2
METABOLIC ALKALOSIS				
Uncompensated	↑ 7.45	Normal	↑ 27	↑ +2
Partially compensated°	↑ 7.45	↑ 45	↑ 27	↑ +2
Compensated°	7.40–7.45	↑ 45	↑ 27	↑ +2

°In general, partially compensated or compensated metabolic alkalosis is rarely seen clinically because of the body's mechanism to prevent hypoventilation, as outlined in Chapter 5.

TABLE 10–2.–CLINICAL METHOD OF
BLOOD GAS INTERPRETATION

STATUS	pH	PCO_2	HCO_3^-	B.E.
VENTILATORY FAILURE				
(Respiratory Acidosis)				
Acute	↓ 7.30	↑ 50	Normal	Normal
Chronic	7.30–7.50	↑ 50	↑ 27	↑ +2
ALVEOLAR HYPERVENTILATION				
(Respiratory Alkalosis)				
Acute	↑ 7.50	↓ 30	Normal	Normal
Chronic	7.40–7.50	↓ 30	↓ 22	↓ −2
METABOLIC ACIDOSIS				
Uncompensated	↓ 7.30	Normal	↓ 22	↓ −2
Partially compensated	↓ 7.30	↓ 30	↓ 22	↓ −2
Compensated	7.30–7.40	↓ 30	↓ 22	↓ −2
METABOLIC ALKALOSIS				
Uncompensated	↑ 7.50	Normal	↑ 27	↑ +2
Partially compensated°	↑ 7.50	↑ 50	↑ 27	↑ +2
Compensated°	7.40–7.50	↑ 50	↑ 27	↑ +2

°In general, partially compensated or compensated metabolic alkalosis is rarely seen clinically because of the body's mechanism to prevent hypoventilation, as outlined in Chapter 5.

    2. Assessment of hypoxemia
        a. For patients on 21% oxygen and under 60 years of age
            (1) Mild hypoxemia: Arterial PO_2 < 80 mm Hg
            (2) Moderate hypoxemia: Arterial PO_2 < 60 mm Hg
            (3) Severe hypoxemia: Arterial PO_2 < 40 mm Hg
        b. For individuals over age 60, 1 mm Hg should be subtracted from the lower limits of mild and moderate hypoxemia for each year over 60. At any age a PO_2 less than 40 mm Hg indicates severe hypoxemia.
        c. Patients on FI_{O_2} greater than 0.21
            (1) Uncorrected hypoxemia: Arterial PO_2 less than room air acceptable limit.
            (2) Corrected hypoxemia: Arterial PO_2 between minimal acceptable room air limit and 100 mm Hg.
            (3) Excessively corrected hypoxemia: Arterial PO_2 greater than 100 mm Hg.
    3. Assessment of tissue hypoxia
        a. At present there is no direct method of assessing tissue hypoxia; it must be clinically assessed indirectly.
        b. Adequate tissue oxygenation
            (1) Carriage of normal volume of oxygen by arterial blood

      (2) Relatively normal acid base status

      (3) Adequate tissue perfusion

   c. Likelihood of tissue hypoxia

      (1) Severe hypoxemia

      (2) Severe acidosis

      (3) Decreased cardiac output or tissue perfusion

XII. Clinical Causes of Acid-Base Abnormalities

  A. Ventilatory failure (respiratory acidosis)

    1. Primary causes

      a. Cardiopulmonary disease, particularly the end stage of chronic obstructive pulmonary disease (COPD).

      b. CNS depression by drugs, trauma or lesion.

      c. Neurologic or neuromuscular disease resulting in profound weakness of ventilatory muscles.

      d. Fatigue following any acute pulmonary disease.

  B. Alveolar hyperventilation (respiratory alkalosis)

    1. Primary causes

      a. Hypoxemia: Its primary effect on the respiratory system is hyperventilation (acute or chronic pulmonary disease).

      b. Compensation for primary metabolic acidosis.

      c. CNS stimulation by drugs, trauma or lesion.

      d. Emotional disorders (e.g., pain, anxiety or fear).

  C. Metabolic acidosis

    1. Primary causes

      a. Lactic acidosis

        (1) In the absence of oxygen as final electron acceptor in the electron transport chain, aerobic metabolism is decreased.

        (2) An increase in anaerobic metabolism results which increases formation of lactic acid, a nonvolatile organic acid.

        (3) By improving the oxygenation state of the patient, lactic acidosis is reversed.

      b. Ketoacidosis

        (1) Primary causes

          (a) Uncontrolled diabetes mellitus

          (b) Starvation

          (c) High fat content in the diet for extended periods

        (2) In all cases insufficient volumes of glucose enter the cell, resulting in an increase in metabolism of body fats.

(3) The metabolic end products of fat metabolism are ketoacids (acetone and beta hydroxybuteric acid).

(4) The patient in a diabetic acidosis is generally hyperventilating significantly and their breath has a sweet, acetone odor.

(5) In most cases the patient needs glucose, and in the case of diabetes insulin is also needed.

c. Renal failure

(1) Decreased renal function inhibits the body's primary mechanism for maintaining blood HCO_3^- levels and excretion of H^+.

(2) Thus free $[H^+]$ increases and free $[HCO_3^-]$ decreases.

d. Ingestion of base-depleting drugs or acids

D. Metabolic alkalosis:

1. Primary causes

a. Hypokalemia

(1) Extracellular K^+ levels normally are 3.5–5.5 mEq/L, the intracellular K^+ levels are about 140 mEq/L.

(2) Intra- and extracellular Na^+ levels are approximately the opposite. The levels of Na^+ and K^+ in extra- and intracellular fluid normally are maintained by an active transport mechanism.

(3) The major extracellular cation that could respond to an intracellular deficiency in K^+ would be H^+.

(4) Thus if extracellular K^+ levels decrease

(a) Intracellular K^+ moves to the extracellular space.

(b) This movement causes intracellular electric imbalance.

(c) This imbalance is corrected by an influx of H^+.

(d) As a result, there is an extracellular decrease in free H^+ levels, or alkalosis.

(5) Hypokalemia presents clinically with

(a) Metabolic alkalosis

(b) Cardiac arrhythmias

(c) Muscle weakness

b. Hypochloremia

(1) Chloride is the major extracellular anion, followed by HCO_3^- in concentration.

   (2) If extracellular chloride levels decrease, intracellular HCO_3^- moves to the extracellular space to maintain electric balance, causing alkalosis.

   (3) Decreased chloride ion levels inhibit ion exchange at the kidney tubule level, which results in increased K^+ excretion.

   c. Gastric suction or vomiting

   (1) Since gastric contents are very acidic (pH of 1.0 to 2.0), excessive loss of gastric fluid results in alkalosis.

   d. Massive doses of steroids

   (1) Steroids increase reabsorption of Na^+ and accelerate excretion of H^+ and K^+.

   e. Diuretics

   (1) Diuretics cause an increase in the amount of K^+ excreted.

   (2) With excessive or uncontrolled use, hypokalemia may result.

   f. Ingestion of acid-depleting drugs or bases

XIII. Typical Blood Gas Contaminants

   A. Heparin

   1. Sodium heparin is commonly used to prevent coagulation of arterial blood to be used for blood gas analysis.

   2. Ammonium heparin affects pH even in small quantities.

   3. Normal pH of sodium heparin is 6.0 to 7.0.

   4. Concentration used is 1000 units per cc.

   5. P_{CO_2} of sodium heparin is less than 2 mm Hg.

   6. Normally 0.05 cc heparin per 1 cc of blood should be used for anticoagulation.

   7. If the concentration or volume of heparin used is above this level:

   a. pH of blood will decrease.

   b. P_{CO_2} of blood will decrease.

   c. P_{O_2} may be altered depending on the blood's original P_{O_2} in relation to heparin's P_{O_2}.

   d. HbO_2% sat. may be altered depending on the blood's original P_{O_2} and HbO_2% sat.

   e. HbCO% sat. will not be altered.

   f. Hb content will decrease.

   g. HCO_3^- will decrease.

   h. Base excess will decrease.

   i. Oxygen content may be altered.

8. If insufficient heparin levels are used
   a. Machine clotting is very likely.
   b. Results are questionable.
B. Saline and other intravenous solutions alter blood gas values in a manner similar to that of heparin.
C. Air bubbles
   1. pH of blood normally will increase.
   2. P_{CO_2} of blood normally will decrease.
   3. P_{O_2} of blood may be altered depending on blood's original P_{O_2} compared to atmospheric P_{O_2}.
   4. $HbO_2\%$ sat. may be altered depending on blood's original P_{O_2} and $HbO_2\%$ sat.
   5. $HbCO\%$ sat. may increase.
   6. Hb content is unaltered.
   7. HCO_3^- may decrease.
   8. Base excess may decrease.
   9. Oxygen content may be altered.
XIV. Ventilatory versus Respiratory Failure
   A. Ventilatory failure: Purely a blood gas interpretation based on the patient's P_{CO_2} and pH.
   B. Respiratory failure: A clinical diagnosis implying that the respiratory system is incapable of providing normal exchange of gases at the alveolar capillary membrane.
      1. Characteristics
         a. Severe hypoxemia
         b. Acute ventilatory failure
XV. Intrapulmonary Shunting
   A. Shunting: Emptying of unoxygenated blood into left side of the heart. Shunting is generally classified as anatomical shunt, capillary shunt, ventilation/perfusion inequalities and physiologic shunt.
      1. *Anatomical shunt*: normally 2–5%. This is a result of emptying of blood from the following veins into the left side of the heart, causing unoxygenated blood to mix with oxygenated blood:
         a. Bronchial veins
         b. Pleural veins
         c. Thebesian veins
      2. *Capillary shunt:* Perfused but unventilated alveoli.
      3. *Ventilation/perfusion ($\dot{V}/\dot{Q}$) inequalities:* Areas of pulmonary system where perfusion is in excess of ventilation. It should be noted that the extent of shunting pro-

duced by $\dot{V}/\dot{Q}$ abnormalities may be decreased with increased $F_{I_{O_2}}$.

4. *Physiologic shunt:* Sum of anatomical and capillary shunting and $\dot{V}/\dot{Q}$ inequalities.
   a. Physiologic shunt equation
      (1) Definition of terms
          (a) $\dot{V}_{O_2}$: Volume of oxygen consumed per minute
          (b) $\dot{Q}_S$: Shunted cardiac output
          (c) $\dot{Q}_T$: Total cardiac output
          (d) C_{cO_2}: Capillary oxygen content
          (e) Ca_{O_2}: Arterial oxygen content
          (f) $C\bar{v}_{O_2}$: Mixed venous oxygen content
          (g) $P_{A_{O_2}}$: Alveolar oxygen partial pressure
          (h) Pa_{O_2}: Arterial oxygen partial pressure
      (2) The shunt equation is based on the Fick equation, which normally is used to calculate oxygen consumption or cardiac output:

$$\dot{V}_{O_2} = \dot{Q}_T(Ca_{O_2} - C\bar{v}_{O_2}). \qquad (14)$$

      (3) Classic shunt equation:

$$\dot{Q}_S/\dot{Q}_T = \frac{C_{cO_2} - Ca_{O_2}}{C_{cO_2} - C\bar{v}_{O_2}}. \qquad (15)$$

          (a) This equation is difficult to apply clinically in its present form because it is impossible to obtain end capillary blood.
          (b) If enough oxygen is delivered to allow for 100% saturation of hemoglobin in arterial blood, then $C_{cO_2} - Ca_{O_2}$ will be equal to the difference in alveolar and arterial P_{O_2}.
          (c) Thus the numerator on the right side of Eq. 15 would be equal to $(P_{A_{O_2}} - Pa_{O_2})(0.003)$.
          (d) $C_{cO_2} - C\bar{v}_{O_2}$ can be expressed as

$$(Ca_{O_2} - C\bar{v}_{O_2}) + (C_{cO_2} - Ca_{O_2}). \qquad (16)$$

      (1) If, as stated above, $C_{cO_2} - Ca_{O_2}$ is equal to $(P_{A_{O_2}} - Pa_{O_2})(0.003)$ when hemoglobin saturation in arterial blood is equal to 100%, then the denominator in Eq. 15 can be replaced by

$$(Ca_{O_2} - C\bar{v}_{O_2}) + (P_{A_{O_2}} - Pa_{O_2})(0.003).$$

b. The clinical shunt equation thus equals

$$\dot{Q}_S/\dot{Q}_T = \frac{(P_{A_{O_2}} - P_{a_{O_2}})(0.003)}{(C_{a_{O_2}} - C\bar{v}_{O_2}) + (P_{A_{O_2}} - P_{a_{O_2}})(0.003)}. \tag{17}$$

    (1) The clinical shunt equation requires 100% saturation of hemoglobin with oxygen in arterial blood.

    (2) A central venous or pulmonary artery sample is needed to determine $C\bar{v}_{O_2}$.

    (3) If $C\bar{v}_{O_2}$ cannot be determined directly, then a $(C_{a_{O_2}} - C\bar{v}_{O_2})$ difference of 3.5 vol% may be assumed in the patient with a stable cardiovascular system.

B. Clinical situations causing increased shunting
  1. Any pulmonary disorder that causes a decrease in alveolar ventilation, (e.g., pneumonia, atelectasis)
  2. Any cardiovascular disorder that causes increased pulmonary blood flow with normal alveolar ventilation, (e.g. increased cardiac output)

C. Guidelines in assessing shunting in ventilator patients (see Chapter 24, Section V).

D. Alveolar arterial P_{O_2} difference $(A\text{-}aD_{O_2})$
  1. If a patient is receiving 100% oxygen, $A\text{-}aD_{O_2}$ can give an *estimate* of the percent of shunting.
  2. For every 15–20 mm Hg gradient, there exists about a 1% shunt.
  3. Thus with $A\text{-}aD_{O_2}$ of 300 mm Hg on 100% oxygen, there is a 15–20% shunt.

XVI. Deadspace
A. Deadspace: Areas of the pulmonary system where ventilation exceeds perfusion.
B. Definition of terms
  1. V_D: Deadspace volume
  2. V_T: Tidal volume
  3. $F_{A_{CO_2}}$: Fractional concentration of CO_2 in alveolar gas
  4. $F\bar{E}_{CO_2}$: Mean fractional concentration of CO_2 in mixed expired gas
  5. Pa_{CO_2}: Arterial CO_2 partial pressure
  6. $P\bar{E}_{CO_2}$: Mean mixed expired CO_2 partial pressure
C. Deadspace normally is equal to about 20–40% of measured tidal volume. This is a result of the anatomical deadspace of the conducting airways, which usually is equivalent to 1 cc per pound of body weight.

D. Physiologic deadspace is the sum of the anatomical plus the alveolar deadspace plus ventilation/perfusion inequalities.
E. The Bohr equation is the basis for determination of the deadspace to tidal volume ratio:

$$\text{V}_\text{D}/\text{V}_\text{T} = \frac{\text{F}_{\text{A}_{CO_2}} - \text{F}_{\bar{\text{E}}_{CO_2}}}{\text{F}_{\text{A}_{CO_2}}}. \tag{18}$$

F. Enghoff modification of the Bohr equation allows the use of P_{CO_2} in the calculation:

$$\text{V}_\text{D}/\text{V}_\text{T} = \frac{\text{P}_{\text{a}_{CO_2}} - \text{P}_{\bar{\text{E}}_{CO_2}}}{\text{P}_{\text{a}_{CO_2}}}. \tag{19}$$

G. Causes of increased deadspace
 1. Cardiovascular disorders (e.g., shock, myocardial infarction, hemorrhage, pulmonary embolism)
 2. Increases in pulmonary ventilation with normal pulmonary perfusion (e.g., mechanical ventilation)
H. Guidelines for assessing deadspace in the ventilator patient (see Chapter 24, Section V)
XVII. Minute Volume to P_{CO_2} Relationship
 A. Normally, arterial P_{CO_2} levels are indirectly related to minute ventilation:

P_{CO_2} Level	Minute Ventilation
40 mm Hg	5 L
30 mm Hg	10 L
20 mm Hg	20 L

 B. As an individual's minute volume doubles, the P_{CO_2} usually decreases by 10 mm Hg.
 C. When deadspace increases, there is a disparity in the normal minute volume-P_{CO_2} relationship. With doubling of the minute volume, a 10 mm Hg decrease in P_{CO_2} is *not* seen. In severe deadspace-producing diseases (pulmonary emboli), minute volumes may be as much as four times normal without a significant decrease in P_{CO_2}.
 D. In shunt-producing situations, P_{CO_2} responds appropriately with the changes in minute volume under most circumstances.
 E. In both shunt- and deadspace-producing situations, the P_{O_2} may be below normal.

BIBLIOGRAPHY

Bendixen, H. H., et al.: *Respiratory Care* (St. Louis: C. V. Mosby Co., 1965).

Burton, G. G., Gee, G. N., and Hodgkin, J. E.: *Respiratory Care: A Guide to Clinical Practice* (Philadelphia: J. B. Lippincott Co., 1977).

Comroe, J. H.: *Physiology of Respiration* (2d ed.; Chicago: Year Book Medical Publishers, Inc., 1974).

Davenport, H. W.: *The ABC's of Acid-Base Chemistry* (6th ed.; Chicago: University of Chicago Press, 1974).

Egan, D. F.: *Fundamentals of Respiratory Therapy* (3d ed.; St. Louis: C. V. Mosby Co., 1977).

Filey, G. F.: *Acid-Base and Blood Gas Regulation* (Philadelphia: Lea & Febiger, 1972).

Guyton, A. C.: *Textbook of Medical Physiology* (5th ed.; Philadelphia: W. B. Saunders Co., 1976).

Harrison, R. A., et al.: Reassessment of the assumed A-V oxygen content difference in the shunt calculation, Anesth. Analg. 54:198, 1975.

Masterton, W. L., and Slowinski, E. J.: *Chemical Principles* (4th ed.; Philadelphia: W. B. Saunders Co., 1977).

Olszowka, A. J., et al.: *Blood Gases, Hemoglobin, Base Excess and Maldistribution* (Philadelphia: Lea & Febiger, 1973).

Rooth, G.: *Acid-Base and Electrolyte Balance* (Chicago: Year Book Medical Publishers, Inc., 1974).

Shapiro, B. A., Harrison, R. A., and Walton, J. R.: *Clinical Application of Blood Gases* (2d ed.; Chicago: Year Book Medical Publishers, Inc., 1977).

Suter, P. M., Fairley, H. B., and Schlobohm, R. M.: Shunt, lung volume, and perfusion during short periods of ventilation with oxygen, Anesthesiology 43:617, 1975.

11 / Pharmacology

I. General Information
  A. Drug: Any chemical compound that may be administered to or used on an individual to aid in diagnosis, treatment or prevention of disease; to relieve pain; or to control or improve any physiologic disorder or pathologic condition.
  B. Pharmacologic nomenclature
    1. Chemical name: Name illustrative of chemical structural formula of the drug.
    2. Generic name: Officially adopted name of the drug in the United States; name used in United States Pharmacopeia.
    3. Trade or proprietary name: Patented name given a particular drug by the manufacturer who introduced it.
  C. Absorption: The specific physical and chemical characteristics of a drug determine the rate of absorption. Routes of administration are listed in order of speed in attaining blood levels after administration.
    1. Intravenous injection (IV)
    2. Via lung (aerosol)
    3. Intramuscular injection (IM)
    4. Subcutaneous injection (Sub. Q.)
    5. Sublingual and rectal absorption
    6. Oral
    7. Topical
  D. Distribution: Movement of the drug to area of desired pharmacologic activity.
    1. Primary mechanism for distribution: Circulatory system.
    2. Topical administration for effect on skin or mucous membrane decreases likelihood of further, undesired distribution.
  E. Metabolism: Actual inactivation of the drug by the body.
    1. Primary organ for detoxification: Liver.
    2. Many drugs may be inactivated by the body's cells or plasma proteins.

F. Excretion: Mechanism for elimination of the drug from the body.
1. Primary organ for excretion: Kidney.
2. Other drugs may be excreted by gastrointestinal or respiratory tract.
G. Side effect: Any physiologic response other than that for which the drug was administered.

II. Wetting Agents/Diluents
A. Isotonic solution: A solution equivalent to 0.9% W/V solution of NaCl. Isotonic solutions are used in respiratory therapy primarily in small volume nebulizers.
B. Hypertonic solution: A solution with a concentration greater than 0.9% W/V solution of NaCl. Hypertonic solutions are used in respiratory therapy primarily for sputum induction.
C. Hypotonic solution: A solution with a concentration of less than 0.9% W/V solution of NaCl. Hypotonic solutions are most commonly used in respiratory therapy in large volume aerosol generators and seem to have less effect on increasing airway resistance than does normal saline or water.
D. Distilled water: Used in respiratory therapy in all types of humidifiers.

III. Proteolytics
A. Trade name: Dornavac (currently unavailable in U.S.).
B. Generic name: Dornase (pancreatic deoxyribonuclease).
C. Mechanism of action: Lyses DNA in purulent secretions (30–70% of purulent secretions are composed of DNA).
D. Concentration: A vial of powder mixed with 2 cc vial of normal saline forms 100,000 units of Dornase.
E. Dosage
1. Standard dosage: 50,000–100,000 units with saline for a total volume of 4 cc two to four times daily for up to 7 days.
2. Maximum dosage: None specified.
F. Indications: Thick, retained, purulent secretions.
G. Contraindications
1. Hypersensitivity
2. Asthma
H. Side effects/hazards
1. Oral irritation
2. Excessive liquefaction of dried, retained secretions
3. Bronchospasm

I. Comments
  1. Extracted from beef pancreas or as metabolic by-product of beta hemolytic streptococcus metabolism.
  2. Should be refrigerated after opening.
  3. Should be used within 24 hours after mixing.
  4. Ineffective on mucoid secretions.
  5. Supplied: In two vials, one containing white powder and the other, 2 cc of normal saline.
  6. If bronchospasm occurs, should be administered with a bronchodilator.

IV. Mucolytics
  A. Trade name: Mucomyst.
  B. Generic name: Acetylcysteine (N-acetyl-L-cysteine).
  C. Mechanism of action: Lyses disulfide bonds holding mucoproteins together, thus increasing fluidity of mucoid sputum.
  D. Concentration: 20% W/V or 10% W/V solution.
  E. Dosage
    1. Standard dosage: 4 cc of 10% W/V or 20% W/V solution.
    2. Maximum dosage: None specified.
  F. Indications: Thick, retained mucoid or mucopurulent secretions.
  G. Contraindications
    1. Hypersensitivity
  H. Side effects/hazards
    1. Bronchospasm
    2. Excessive liquefaction of dried, retained secretions
    3. Stomatitis
    4. Hypersensitivity
    5. Nausea
    6. Rhinorrhea
  I. Comments
    1. Highly recommended that drug be administered in conjunction with bronchodilator.
    2. Should be refrigerated after opening.
    3. Should be used within 96 hours after opening.
    4. Reacts with rubber, some plastics and iron.
    5. Foul smelling.
    6. Should be administered in glass, plastic or nontarnishable metal container.
    7. Ineffective on predominantly purulent secretions.
    8. Supplied in 30 cc, 10 cc and 4 cc vials.

V. Prophylactic Antiasthmatics
- A. Trade name: Aarane or Intal.
- B. Generic name: Cromolyn sodium.
- C. Mechanism of action
  1. Inhibits release of histamine during allergic, IgE-mediated responses on pulmonary mast cells.
  2. Suppresses response of mast cell to antigen-antibody reaction.
- D. Concentration: 20 mg capsules.
- E. Standard dosage: One 20 mg capsule administered via spin-haler three or four times daily.
- F. Maximum dosage: One 20 mg capsule administered via spin-haler three or four times daily.
- G. Indications: Prophylactic maintenance of severe bronchial asthma.
- H. Contraindications: Hypersensitivity.
- I. Side effects/hazards
  1. Local irritation
  2. Bronchospasm
  3. Maculopapular rash
  4. Urticaria
- J. Comments
  1. Ineffective in acute asthmatic attack.
  2. Maximum effect seen after 4 weeks of continuous use.
  3. Sometimes effective in controlling exercise-induced asthma.

VI. Detergent
- A. Trade name: Alevaire.
- B. Generic name: Active agent superinone (trade name, Tyloxapol); also contains sodium bicarbonate and glycerine.
- C. Mechanism of action
  1. Tyloxapol reduces the surface tension of mucoid secretions, thereby increasing fluidity.
  2. Sodium bicarbonate increases the pH of secretions, causing polysaccharides in sputum to lyse.
  3. Glycerine has hydroscopic effect for stabilization of aerosol.
- D. Concentration
  1. Tyloxapol: 0.125% W/V
  2. Sodium bicarbonate: 2% W/V
  3. Glycerine: 5% W/V
- E. Dosage

1. Standard dosage
   a. Intermittent use: 4 – 10 cc undiluted
   b. May be used continuously
2. Maximum dosage: None specified

F. Indications: Thick, retained secretions primarily of mucoid type.

G. Side effects/hazards
   1. May cause bronchospasm in asthmatic patients.

H. Comments
   1. Should be refrigerated after opening.
   2. Should be discarded 72 hours after opening.
   3. Should be kept from direct light.
   4. Supplied in 60 cc and 500 cc bottles.

VII. Surface-Active Agent
   A. Trade name: Ethyl alcohol, ethanol.
   B. Generic name: Ethyl alcohol, ethanol.
   C. Mechanism of action
      1. Has direct surfactant-like effect on surface tension of frothy, serum-like fluid developed in acute pulmonary edema.
      2. Breaking up of frothy secretions allows them to occupy a much smaller volume, improving distribution of ventilation.
   D. Concentration: 20 – 80% solution.
   E. Dosage
      1. Standard
         a. Intermittent: 4 – 10 cc of 50% solution
         b. Continuous: 500 ml of 50% solution over 24-hour period
   F. Indication: Acute pulmonary edema.
   G. Contraindications: Hypersensitivity.
   H. Side effects/hazards
      1. Airway irritation
      2. Bronchospasm
      3. Local dehydration
   I. Comments: Should not be administered in heated aerosol or ultrasonic nebulizer.

VIII. Sympathomimetics: General Considerations
   A. General classification
      1. Alpha effect: Constriction of vascular smooth muscle.
      2. Beta effect: Peripheral relaxation of vascular smooth muscle (minimal).

       a. *Beta one:* Positive inotropic and chronotropic cardiac effects.

       b. *Beta two:* Relaxation of bronchial smooth muscle.

B. Mechanism of action (Fig 11–1)

   1. Beta effect: Stimulates release of membrane-bound adenylcyclase, which increases formation of cyclic 3′5′-AMP (adenosine monophosphate) from ATP (adenosine triphosphate).

   2. Alpha effect: Inhibits membrane-bound adenylcyclase from converting ATP to cyclic 3′5′-AMP.

C. Indications

   1. Constriction of bronchial smooth muscle

   2. Edema of mucous membrane

D. Contraindications

   1. Hyperthyroidism

   2. Hypertension

   3. Tachycardia

E. Side effects/hazards

   1. Palpitations

   2. Tachycardia

   3. Hypertension

   4. Restlessness

   5. Fear

   6. Anxiety

   7. Tension

   8. Tremor

   9. Weakness

   10. Dizziness

   11. Pallor

Fig 11–1.—Increased cyclic 3′5′-AMP levels result in bronchodilation. Beta stimulation increases cyclic 3′5′-AMP levels by release of adenylcyclase, whereas aminophylline increases cyclic 3′5′-AMP levels by inhibiting its metabolism by phosphodiesterase. Alpha stimulation inhibits adenylcyclase release and therefore decreases cyclic 3′5′-AMP levels.

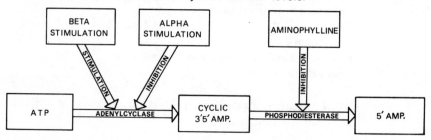

F. Comments
   1. Tolerance is frequently observed (tachyphylaxis).
   2. Synergistic effects may be seen.
   3. Maximally administered every 2 to 3 hours.
   4. Normal duration of effects up to 3 hours.
IX. Specific Sympathomimetics
  A. Isoproterenol HCl
    1. Trade name: Isuprel
    2. Generic name: Isoproterenol HCl
    3. Concentration: 1:100 or 1:200 solution
    4. Effects
      a. Alpha: None
      b. Beta one: Strong
      c. Beta two: Strong
    5. Dosage
      a. Standard
        (1) 0.5 cc of 1:200 solution in 4 cc normal saline
        (2) 0.25 cc of 1:100 solution in 4 cc normal saline
      b. Maximum
        (1) 1 cc of 1:200 solution in 4 cc normal saline
        (2) 0.5 cc of 1:100 solution in 4 cc normal saline
  B. Racemic epinephrine
    1. Trade name: Vaponephrine, Micronephrine
    2. Generic name: Racemic epinephrine
    3. Concentration: 2.25% W/V solution
    4. Effects
      a. Alpha: Medium
      b. Beta one: Weak
      c. Beta two: Medium
    5. Dosage
      a. Standard: 0.5 cc of 2.25% W/V solution in 4 cc normal saline
      b. Maximum: 1 cc of 2.25% W/V solution in 4 cc normal saline
  C. Isoetharine
    1. Trade name: Bronkosol, Dilabron
    2. Generic name: Isoetharine
    3. Concentration: 1% W/V solution
    4. Effects
      a. Alpha: None
      b. Beta one: Weak
      c. Beta two: Medium

    5. Dosage

        a. Standard: 0.5 cc in 4 cc normal saline

        b. Maximum: 1 cc in 4 cc normal saline

D. Epinephrine HCl

    1. Trade name: Adrenalin

    2. Generic name: Epinephrine HCl

    3. Concentration: 1 : 100

    4. Effects

        a. Alpha: Strong

        b. Beta one: Strong

        c. Beta two: Medium

    5. Dosage

        a. Standard: 0.2 cc in 4 cc normal saline

        b. Maximum: 0.5 cc in 4 cc normal saline

E. Phenylephrine

    1. Trade name: Neo-Synephrine

    2. Generic name: Phenylephrine

    3. Concentration: 0.25% W/V

    4. Effects

        a. Alpha: Strong

        b. Beta one: None

        c. Beta two: None

    5. Dosage

        a. Standard: 0.2 cc in 4 cc normal saline

        b. Maximum: 0.5 cc in 4 cc normal saline

    6. Comment

        a. Normally administered only as nasal decongestant by spray or drops.

F. Metaproterenol sulfate

    1. Trade name: Alupent, Metaprel

    2. Generic name: Metaproterenol sulfate

    3. Concentration

        a. 20 mg/tablet (oral dosage)

        b. Metered mist: 0.65 mg/spray

    4. Effects

        a. Alpha: None

        b. Beta one: Very weak

        c. Beta two: Medium

    5. Dosage

        a. Standard

            (1) One tablet four times daily

            (2) Two sprays every 4 to 6 hours

        b. Maximum: None specified

6. Comment
   a. Duration of effects up to 6 hours.

G. Solbutamol
   1. Trade name: Ventolin
   2. Generic name: Solbutamol
   3. Concentration
      a. Metered mist: 0.1 mg/spray (only preparation available in United States).
   4. Effects
      a. Alpha: None
      b. Beta one: None
      c. Beta two: Strong
   5. Dosage
      a. Standard: 2 sprays, every 6 hours
      b. Maximum: None specified
   6. Comment
      a. Duration of effects up to 6 hours.

H. Terbutaline sulfate
   1. Trade name: Bricanyl, Brethine
   2. Generic name: Terbutaline sulfate
   3. Concentration: 0.1% W/V
   4. Effects
      a. Alpha: None
      b. Beta one: Weak
      c. Beta two: Medium
   5. Dosage
      a. 0.25 to 1.0 mg subcutaneously
      b. 0.25 to 0.5 mg in 4 cc normal saline solution via aerosol
   6. Comment
      a. Also available in 5 mg and 2.5 mg tablets.

X. Sympathomimetics Affecting the Cardiovascular System
   A. Norepinephrine
      1. Trade name: Levophed, Noradrenalin
      2. Generic name: Norepinephrine
      3. Effects
         a. Alpha effect: Strong
         b. Beta one effect: Weak
         c. Beta two effect: None
      4. Indications: Hypotension
      5. Administration: Intravenous only
   B. Dopamine HCl
      1. Trade name: Intropin

2. Generic name: Dopamine HCl
3. Effects: Dose dependent
    a. Low dosages
        (1) Increased renal blood flow
        (2) Mild increase in cardiac output
    b. Moderate dosages
        (1) Increased renal blood flow
        (2) Increased cardiac output
    c. High dosages
        (1) Systemic vasoconstriction
4. Indications
    a. Hypotension
    b. Shock
    c. Renal failure
    d. Myocardial infarction
    e. Other hemodynamic problems
5. Administration
    a. Intravenously only in appropriate dilution of non-alkaline solution.

XI. Noncatecholamines Affecting the Sympathetic Nervous System
A. Ephedrine
    1. Trade name: Ephedrine
    2. Generic name: Ephedrine
    3. Mechanism of action: Causes release of epinephrine and norepinephrine stored throughout the body
    4. Effects (lasting up to 6 hours)
        a. Bronchodilatation
        b. Mild cardiac stimulation
        c. Peripheral vasoconstriction
        d. Mild CNS stimulation
    5. Indications
        a. Nonemergency allergic reactions
        b. Chronic asthma
        c. Congestion
    6. Administration: Oral, intramuscular or subcutaneous
B. Theophylline
    1. Trade name: Aminophylline
    2. Generic name: Theophylline
    3. Mechanism of action: Inhibits phosphodiesterase (see Fig 11–1) from converting cyclic 3'5'-AMP to inactive 5'-AMP

4. Effects
   a. Bronchodilatation
   b. Cardiac stimulation
   c. Coronary artery dilatation
   d. Skeletal muscle stimulation
   e. Diuresis
   f. CNS stimulation
5. Indications
   a. Acute and chronic asthma
   b. Abnormal respiratory patterns, (e.g., Cheyne – Stokes)
6. Comments
   a. Administered orally, intramuscularly, intravenously or by suppository.
   b. Causes gastrointestinal discomfort.

XII. General Therapeutic Uses of Sympathomimetics
   A. Control of hemorrhage
   B. Treatment of hypotension
   C. Cardiac stimulation
   D. Treatment of heart block
   E. Treatment of allergic disorders
   F. Treatment of generalized bronchoconstriction
   G. Treatment of mucosal congestion
   H. Treatment of CNS disorders

XIII. Parasympathomimetics
   A. Action: Enhance effects of parasympathetic nervous system.
   B. Classification of effects
      1. *Muscarinic:* Effect on parasympathetic postganglionic fibers, thus stimulating only the parasympathetic nervous system.
      2. *Nicotinic:* Effect on other sites where acetylcholine is the transmitter substance, thus stimulating sites outside the parasympathetic nervous system.
         a. Voluntary muscle
         b. Sympathetic nervous system
         c. CNS
   C. Classification of drug groups
      1. Choline esters (drugs with structure similar to acetylcholine):
         a. Primary effects: Muscarinic with limited nicotinic effects

        b. Primary indications
           (1) Paroxysmal supraventricular tachycardia
           (2) Gastrointestinal disorders
           (3) Urinary bladder disorders
        c. Characteristic drugs
           (1) Methacholine (generic), Mecholyl (trade)
           (2) Bethanechol (generic), Urecholine (trade)
    2. Naturally occurring alkaloids
        a. Primary effect:
           (1) Almost exclusively at muscarinic sites.
        b. Primary indication: Glaucoma
        c. Characteristic drug: Pilocarpine (generic and trade)
    3. Cholinesterase inhibitors
        a. Mechanism of action: Competitive inhibition of cholinesterase.
        b. Primary Effect: Strong stimulation at both nicotinic and muscarinic sites.
        c. Therapeutic uses
           (1) Paralytic ileus
           (2) Atony of urinary bladder
           (3) Glaucoma
           (4) Myasthenia gravis (symptomatic)
           (5) Atropine intoxication
           (6) Reversal of nondepolarizing neuromuscular blocking agents
    4. Characteristic drugs
        a. Neostigmine (generic), Prostigmine (trade)
        b. Pyridostigmine (generic), Mestinon (trade)
        c. Ambenonium (generic), Mytelase (trade)
        d. Edrophonium (generic), Tensilon (trade)
  D. Side effects associated with excessive stimulation of parasympathetic nervous system
    1. Gastrointestinal disorders
    2. Cardiovascular problems
    3. Excessive secretion by exocrine glands, (e.g., mucous, salivary)
XIV. Parasympatholytics
  A. Action: Inhibition of effects of parasympathetic nervous system; only muscarinic sites affected.
  B. Mechanism of action: Competitive inhibition of acetylcholine at muscarinic sites only.

   C. Therapeutic uses
1. CNS disorders
2. Preanesthesia medication
3. Ophthalmologic (pupil dilatation)
4. Upper airway allergies
5. Gastrointestinal disorders
6. Genitourinary tract disorders
7. Common cold
8. Over-the-counter sleeping pills
9. Motion sickness, nausea and vomiting
10. Cardiovascular problems
11. Used with parasympathomimetics for reversal of neuromuscular blocking agents

   D. Side effects
1. Dry mouth
2. Blurred vision
3. Urinary retention
4. Lightheadedness
5. Fatigue

   E. Characteristic drugs
1. Atropa belladonna, atropine (generic)
2. Hyoscine (generic), Scopolamine (trade)

XV. Sympatholytics
   A. Action: Inhibition of the sympathetic nervous system.
   B. Alpha-adrenergic blocking agents
1. Mechanism of action: Direct inhibitory effect at alpha-adrenergic receptor site.
2. Effects
   a. Prevent excitatory responses of smooth muscle and exocrine glands.
   b. Can cause postural hypotension.
   c. Cause an increase in cardiac output and decrease in total peripheral resistance in normal recumbent subjects.
3. Therapeutic uses
   a. Hypertension
   b. Peripheral vascular disease
4. Characteristic drugs
   a. Phentolamine (generic), Regitine (trade)
   b. Azapetine (generic), Ilidar (trade)
   c. Phenoxybenzamine (generic), Dibenzyline (trade)

C. Beta-adrenergic blocking agents
   1. Action: Competitive inhibition at receptor site.
   2. Effects
      a. Cause a negative inotropic and a negative chronotropic effect on heart.
      b. Cause slight bronchoconstriction.
   3. Therapeutic uses
      a. Cardiac arrhythmias
      b. Angina pectoris
      c. Hypertension
   4. Characteristic drug
      a. Propranolol (generic), Inderal (trade)
XVI. Neuromuscular Blocking Agents
   A. Major action: Interruption of transmission of nerve impulse at skeletal neuromuscular junction.
   B. Major categories: nondepolarizing and depolarizing
      1. *Nondepolarizing* agents
         a. Mechanism of action: Competitive inhibition of acetylcholine at skeletal muscle sites.
            (1) The muscle fiber itself is still sensitive to external stimulation.
         b. Effects
            (1) Effects are seen maximally in about 3 to 4 minutes and persist 20 to 40 minutes.
            (2) Hypotension as a result of histamine release seen occasionally with d-tubocurarine.
            (3) Bradycardia occasionally is seen with pancuronium.
            (4) Effects of this group of drugs may be reversed by cholinesterase-inhibiting agents (e.g., neostigmine).
         c. Characteristic drugs
            (1) Tubocurarine (generic), d-Tubocurarine (trade)
            (2) Pancuronium (generic), Pavulon (trade)
      2. *Depolarizing* agents
         a. Mechanism of action
            (1) These agents cause an initial depolarization of the motor end-plates of all voluntary muscle.
            (2) As this wave of depolarization proceeds, a rippling of voluntary muscles occurs, (muscle fasciculation) usually from the head downward. Since these agents are chemically similar to

acetylcholine, they cause continual stimulation of the motor end-plate.

(3) This continual stimulation does not allow time for repolarization; thus the muscle develops a flaccid paralysis.

(4) With time, the depolarizing agent is metabolized by pseudocholinesterase.

b. The muscle fiber itself is still sensitive to external stimulation.

(1) Effects seen in about 30 to 40 seconds and persist 3 to 5 minutes.

(2) Irreversible.

c. Characteristic drugs

(1) Succinylcholine (generic), Anectine (trade)

(2) Decamethonium (generic), Syncurine (trade)

XVII. Steroids

A. Adrenocorticotropic hormone (ACTH) and adrenocorticosteroids

1. Adrenocorticotropic hormone (corticotropin) is produced and released from the adrenohypophysis (anterior pituitary).

2. Mechanism of action

a. Release of ACTH into the blood causes the adrenal cortex to release its steroids into the bloodstream.

b. Release of ACTH is affected directly by corticotropin-releasing factor (CRF), which is secreted by the hypothalamus.

c. Blood level of CRF is indirectly affected by blood steroid levels.

d. Thus there is a cyclic relation between ACTH, CRF and steroid levels (Fig 11 – 2).

e. An increase in steroid levels causes a decrease in CRF levels, which causes a decrease in ACTH levels. This results in a decrease in steroid levels, which causes an increase in CRF levels, etc., thus maintaining a normal equilibrium.

3. Physiologic effects

a. Stimulate glucose formation (i.e., increase blood sugar levels).

b. Diminish glucose utilization.

c. Promote storage of glucose in liver.

d. Regulate rate of synthesis of proteins.

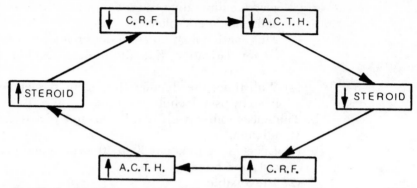

Fig 11–2. —There is a cyclic relationship of corticotropin-releasing factor (CRF), adrenocorticotropic hormone (ACTH) and steroid levels. Normal steroid levels are maintained by this interrelationship. CRF and ACTH levels are directly related; ACTH and steroid levels are also directly related, whereas steroid and CRF levels are indirectly related.

      e. Control distribution of body fat.
      f. Regulate lipid metabolism.
      g. Regulate reabsorption of sodium ions from kidney tubules.
      h. Increase urinary excretion of both K^+ and H^+.
      i. Maintain normal function of skeletal muscles.
      j. Increase hemoglobin and red cell content of blood.
      k. Maintain normal lymphoid tissue.
      l. Prevent or suppress inflammatory responses caused by hypersensitivity.
    4. Therapeutic uses
      a. Allergic asthma
      b. Acute adrenal insufficiency
      c. Chronic adrenal insufficiency
      d. Congenital adrenal hyperplasia
      e. Adrenal insufficiency secondary to anterior pituitary insufficiency
      f. Arthritis
      g. Rheumatic carditis
      h. Osteoarthritis
      i. Acute inflammatory diseases
    5. Side effects
      a. Cushing's disease
        (1) Moon face
        (2) Hirsutism

(3) Muscle wasting

(4) Variable hypernatremia

(5) Hypokalemia

b. Hypertension

c. Aggravation of diabetes mellitus

d. Necrotizing arteritis in rheumatoid patients

e. Aggravation of peptic ulcer

f. Psychotic manifestations

g. Adrenal atrophy

6. Characteristic Drugs

  a. Dexamethasone (Decadron)

    (1) Packaged in 10 cc vial with 4 mg per ml (0.4% W/V).

    (2) Used by aerosol post-extubation to diminish inflammation of larynx and trachea.

    (3) Dosage: 1 mg dexamethasone, 0.5 cc of 2.25% racemic epinephrine and 3 cc normal saline.

  b. Beclomethasone dipropionate (Vanceril)

    (1) Supplied as metered mist of 50 μg/inhalation.

    (2) Used for chronic treatment of bronchial asthma in patients in whom a corticosteroid is indicated.

    (3) Side effects

      (a) Localized (mouth, pharynx, larynx) infection with *Candida albicans* and *Aspergillus niger*.

      (b) Occasional deaths have resulted from ACTH suppression when beclomethasone has been used to replace previous therapies involving corticosteroids with strong systemic activity.

    (4) Dosage:

      (a) Standard: 2 inhalations 3 or 4 times daily

      (b) Maximum: 22 inhalations per day

XVIII. Diuretics

A. Action: Increase rate of urine formation.

B. Site of action of most diuretics: Directly on kidney tubular system — not on glomerular capillaries.

C. Osmotic diuretics

  1. Osmotic diuretics are freely filterable at the glomerulus, are poorly reabsorbed by the renal tubule and are pharmacologically inert.

    2. Mechanism of action
      a. Cause osmotic gradient in urine tubular system, preventing reabsorption of fluid into bloodstream.
      b. Cause osmotic movement of fluid from tissues into plasma.
    3. Most frequently used drugs: Mannitol and urea.

D. Mercurial diuretics
    1. Mechanism of action:
      a. Prevent reabsorption of Na^+ and Cl^- in proximal convoluted tubule, decreasing volume of water reabsorbed.
      b. Promote loss of K^+ and H^+ in distal convoluted tubules.
    2. Effects
      a. May cause metabolic alkalosis with extended use.
      b. Are ineffective in presence of systemic metabolic alkalosis.
      c. Are potentiated in the presence of metabolic acidosis.
    3. Contraindications
      a. Renal insufficiency
      b. Acute nephritis
    4. Characteristic drugs
      a. Mercaptomerin sodium (generic), Thiomerin (trade)
      b. Meralluride (generic), Mercuhydrin (trade)
      c. Mersalyl (generic), Salyrgan (trade)

E. Carbonic anhydrase inhibitors
    1. Mechanism of action: Inhibit effects of carbonic anhydrase in proximal convoluted tubule, increasing amount of HCO_3^- excreted and volume of urine excreted.
    2. Characteristic drugs
      a. Acetazolamide (generic), Diamox (trade)
      b. Dichlorphenamide (generic), Daranide (trade)

F. Thiazides
    1. Mechanism of action: Inhibits reabsorption of 5–10% of Na^+ and Cl^- at distal convoluted tubules.
    2. Cause an excessive loss of K^+.
    3. Not affected by acid–base imbalances.
    4. Can be administered in tablet form.
    5. Characteristic drugs

       a. Chlorothiazide (generic), Diuril (trade)

       b. Hydrochlorothiazide (generic), Hydro-Diuril (trade)

       c. Hydroflumethiazide (generic), Saluron (trade)

       d. Methyclorthiazide (generic), Enduron (trade)

G. Ethacrynic acid (generic), Edecrin (trade); furosemide (generic), Lasix (trade)

    1. Mechanism of action

       a. Inhibit reabsorption of Na^+ and Cl^- primarily at distal convoluted tubules and at proximal convoluted tubules, increasing volume of fluid passed as urine.

       b. Increase volume of K^+ excreted.

    2. Function independently of acid-base balance.

    3. Considered the most potent of all diuretics.

H. Side effects

    1. Loss of potassium

    2. Development of metabolic alkalosis

    3. Aggravation of diabetes mellitus due to impaired glucose tolerance

I. Therapeutic uses

    1. Pulmonary edema

    2. Congestive heart failure

    3. Chronic or acute renal failure

    4. Systemic fluid overload

XIX. Narcotics

A. Primary use: Analgesia

B. Mechanism of action: Unclear, but these drugs affect neurotransmission at specific CNS sites, affect autonomic nervous system transmission and cause some histamine release.

C. General pharmacologic effects

    1. Analgesic

       a. Effective without blocking motor activity or other senses in therapeutic doses.

       b. More effective in relieving continuous dull pain than sharp intermittent pain.

    2. Euphoric: Seen at therapeutic dosages.

    3. Hypnotic: With increasing dosages, more subjective CNS depression.

    4. Metabolic: Transient hyperglycemia.

    5. Urinary tract: Decrease in urinary output.

6. Pupil size: Miosis.
7. Gastrointestinal tract: Constipation because of decreased overall activity.
8. Nausea and vomiting: Direct stimulation of medullary control center.
9. Cardiovascular system
   a. If patient is well oxygenated and in normal acid–base balance, there are no significant effects.
   b. Cardiac arrhythmias may be seen with acid–base abnormalities.
   c. Hypotension may result due to direct effect on venous smooth muscle and release of histamine.
10. Respiratory system
    a. Direct depression of medullary respiratory center response to carbon dioxide changes.
    b. Significant decrease in respiratory rate, tidal volume and minute volume is seen with large dosages.
11. Cough reflex: Decreased as a result of direct depression of medullary cough center.

D. Characteristic drugs
   1. High potency
      a. Morphine (generic and trade)
      b. Oxymorphone (generic), Numorphan (trade)
      c. Heroin
      d. Levorphanol (generic), Levo-Dromoran (trade)
      e. Methadone (generic), Dolophine (trade)
      f. Phenazocine (generic), Prinadol (trade)
   2. Intermediate potency
      a. Meperidine (generic), Demerol (trade)
      b. Alphaprodine (generic), Nisentil (trade)
      c. Pentazocine (generic), Talwin (trade)
      d. Anileridine (generic), Leritine (trade)
      e. Oxycodone (generic), Percodan (trade)
   3. Low potency
      a. Codeine (generic and trade)
      b. Diphenoxylate (generic), Lomotil (trade)
E. Therapeutic uses
   1. Analgesia
   2. Cough control
   3. Emetic
   4. Antidiarrhetic

5. Pulmonary edema
6. Control of patients on ventilators

XX. Narcotic Antagonists
   A. Sole use: To reverse effects of narcotics.
   B. Mechanism of action: Competitive displacement of agonist from receptor site.
   C. Partial antagonists
      1. Cause narcotic-like effects in absence of a narcotic
      2. Cause increased respiratory depression if administered in a non-narcotic overdose (e.g., barbiturates).
      3. Characteristic drugs
         a. Nalorphine (generic), Nalline (trade)
         b. Levallorphan (generic), Lorfan (trade)
   D. Pure antagonists: Have only narcotic antagonist properties. Will not increase respiratory depression in a nonnarcotic overdose.
      1. Characteristic drug
         a. Naloxone (generic), Narcan (trade)
   E. Duration of effect
      1. 45 to 60 minutes *(careful monitoring of overdosed patient must be maintained).*
      2. Narcotic's effect may significantly outlast that of the narcotic antagonist.

XXI. Sedative – Hypnotics
   A. Solid or liquid substances that cause a longer generalized depression of the CNS than do anesthetic gases.
   B. Mechanism of action: Selective depression of ascending reticular activating system, resulting in loss of consciousness.
   C. Physiologic effects
      1. Increased dosages cause behavioral changes.
         a. Sedation: Generalized decreased responsiveness.
         b. Disinhibition: Impaired judgment and loss of self-control.
         c. Relief of anxiety.
         d. Ataxia and nystagmus.
         e. Sleep (hypnosis).
         f. Anesthesia.
      2. EEG pattern changes consistent with generalized CNS depression.
      3. Poor analgesia.

4. Anticonvulsant: (phenobarbital the most effective).
5. Withdrawal state with repeated long-term use and abrupt discontinuance.
6. Habit forming.
7. Voluntary muscle relaxation from spinal cord depression.
8. Depression of respiratory medullary center with larger doses.
9. Profound vasomotor depression and shock with larger doses.
10. No direct effect on myocardium.

D. Side effects
1. Drowsiness
2. Impaired performance and judgment
3. Hangover
4. Drug abuse
5. Withdrawal state
6. Overdose

E. Therapeutic uses
1. Sleep induction
2. Relief of anxiety (sedation)
3. Treatment of neurotic anxiety
4. Relief of depression
5. Voluntary muscle relaxation
6. Anticonvulsant

F. Barbiturates
1. Ultra-short acting: Anesthesia
   a. Hexobarbital (generic), Sombucaps (trade)
   b. Thiopental (generic), Pentothal (trade)
2. Short acting: Primarily for sleep induction
   a. Pentobarbital (generic), Nembutal (trade)
   b. Secobarbital (generic), Seconal (trade)
3. Intermediate acting: Relief of anxiety
   a. Amobarbital (generic), Amytal (trade)
4. Long acting: Anticonvulsant
   a. Phenobarbital (generic and trade)

G. Non-barbiturate sedative: hypnotics
1. Short acting
   a. Methaqualone (generic)
   b. Paraldehyde (generic and trade)
   c. Chloral hydrate (generic)
   d. Flurazepam (generic), Dalmane (trade)

    2. Intermediate acting
      a. Meprobamate (generic), Miltown, Equanil (trade)
      b. Glutethimide (generic), Doriden (trade)
      c. Diazepam (generic), Valium (trade)
    3. Long acting
      a. Chlordiazepoxide (generic), Librium (trade)

XXII. Antipsychotic Tranquilizers

  A. Action: Alterations of psychotic state without inducing sedation or hypnosis.

  B. Increasing dosages cause convulsions.

  C. General effects are subjectively unpleasant.

  D. They are not habit forming.

  E. They show generalized increased electric activity, as evidenced by EEG.

  F. With increasing dosages the patient experiences a state of indifference and apathy, with drowsiness and motor retardation.

  G. Even with very large drug dosages, the patient can be aroused with normal stimulation.

  H. Representative drugs
    1. Chlorpromazine (generic), Thorazine (trade)
    2. Promazine (generic), Sparine (trade)
    3. Triflupromazine (generic), Vesprin (trade)

XXIII. Antimicrobial Drugs

  A. These drugs possess *selective toxicity*—the property of being far more toxic for the parasite than for the host cell.

  B. Mechanism of action and representative drug groups
    1. Inhibition of growth by competitive inhibition of metabolism of microbe's proteins
      a. Sulfonamides (Gantrisin)
      b. P-aminosalicyclic acid (PAS)
    2. Inhibition of cell wall synthesis
      a. Penicillin, ampicillin
      b. Cephalosporins (Keflin, Loridine, Keflex)
      c. Polymyxins
    3. Inhibition of protein synthesis
      a. Chloramphenicol
      b. Tetracycline
      c. Erythromycin
      d. Streptomycin
      e. Kanamycin
      f. Neomycin
      g. Gentamicin

    4. Inhibition of nucleic acid synthesis
      a. Actinomycin
      b. Mitomycin
  C. General principles of antibiotic therapy
    1. Clinical indications of infection should be present.
    2. The specific etiologic diagnosis must be formulated before antibiotic therapy is ordered.
    3. A specimen must be obtained for laboratory culture and sensitivity.
    4. The most indicated antibiotic should be administered.
    5. The antibiotic should be correlated with the results of culture and sensitivity study.
    6. Patient must take full course of antibiotic therapy.
    7. Antibiotics, in general, are not effective against viruses.

XXIV. Miscellaneous Drugs Affecting the Cardiovascular System
  A. Cardiac glycosides (digitalis)
    1. Action
      a. Exhibit a positive inotropic effect on the myocardium.
      b. Normally cause increased cardiac output.
      c. Indirectly cause increased renal blood flow and have a diuretic effect.
      d. Slow impulse conduction through the atrioventricular node and bundle of His.
      e. Exert a direct depressant effect on the SA node, causing decreased heart rate.
    2. Therapeutic use
      a. Primarily used in treatment of congestive heart failure.
    3. Toxic problems are frequent because the therapeutic dose is about one third of the lethal dose.
      a. Toxicity treated with a beta-adrenergic blocking agent propranolol (generic), Inderal (trade)
    4. Representative drugs
      a. Digitoxin (generic), Crystodigin, Purodigin (trade)
      b. Digoxin (generic), Lanoxin (trade)
      c. Lanatoside C (generic), Cedilanid (trade)
      d. Ouabain (generic)
  B. Quinidine
    1. Action
      a. Acts as a depressant to myocardium.

      b. Slows depolarization by increasing time necessary to reach action potential.

      c. Alters cardiac muscle permeability to sodium.

      d. Decreases velocity of electric impulse conduction throughout myocardium.

      e. Has curare-like side effect on skeletal muscle.

    2. Primarily used in treatment of atrial arrhythmias.

    3. Common side effects

      a. Ventricular tachycardia

      b. Premature ventricular contractions

      c. Ventricular fibrillation

      d. Hypotension

  C. Procainamide (generic), Pronestyl (trade)

    1. A local anesthetic derivative with same properties and side effects as Quinidine.

  D. Lidocaine (generic), Xylocaine (trade)

    1. Local anesthetic with myocardial properties similar to those of Quinidine.

      a. Reduces cardiac irritability.

      b. Used primarily to treat or prevent ventricular arrhythmias.

BIBLIOGRAPHY

DeKornfeld, T. J.: *Pharmacology for Respiratory Therapy* (Sarasota: Glenn Educational Medical Services, Inc., 1976).

Egan, D. F.: *Fundamentals of Respiratory Therapy* (3d ed.; St. Louis: C. V. Mosby Co., 1977).

Goodman, L. S., and Gilman, A. (eds.): *The Pharmacological Basis of Therapeutics* (5th ed.; Macmillan Publishing Co., Inc., 1975).

Goth, A.: *Medical Pharmacology* (6th ed.; St. Louis: C. V. Mosby Co., 1974).

Mathewson, H. S.: *Pharmacology for Respiratory Therapists* (St. Louis: C. V. Mosby Co., 1977).

Meyers, F. H., Jawetz, E., and Goldfine, A.: *Review of Medical Pharmacology* (4th ed.; Los Altos, Calif.: Lange Medical Publications, 1974).

Product Information (New York: Breon Laboratories, Inc.).

Rau, J. L.: Autonomic airway pharmacology, Respir. Care 22:263, 1977.

Rau, J. L.: *Respiratory Therapy Pharmacology* (Chicago: Year Book Medical Publishers, Inc., 1978).

Young, J. A., and Crocker, D.: *Principles and Practice of Respiratory Therapy* (2d ed.; Chicago: Year Book Medical Publishers, Inc., 1976).

12 / Neonatal Comparative Anatomy and Disease

I. Embryologic Development of the Lung
   A. Normal gestation: About 38–42 weeks
      1. Premature births: Gestational periods of less than 38 weeks
      2. Postmature births: Gestational periods of more than 42 weeks
   B. Sequential development of the lung
      1. Week 4 of gestation: Lungs start to form as an outpouching of the esophagus.
      2. Week 7 of gestation: Diaphragm starts to form.
      3. Week 10 of gestation: Cartilaginous rings of trachea and lymphatics of the respiratory system start to form.
      4. Week 24 of gestation: Significant development of all cartilaginous support of the conducting airways is developed.
      5. Weeks 24 to 26 of gestation: Lung parenchyma starts to develop. The pulmonary capillary network also develops. In some cases, development is sufficient to support extrauterine life.
      6. Week 28 of gestation: Alveolar ducts and sacs have developed and alveolar type II cells begin to appear. The number of alveoli necessary to support extrauterine life is now present.
      7. At normal birth: The number of alveoli is about 24 million. Alveoli continue to develop after birth until there are about 300 million alveoli at adulthood.
   C. Surfactant development
      1. The first appearance of surfactant is between weeks 22 and 24 of gestation. At this time lecithin and sphingomyelin appear in the pulmonary and amniotic fluid.
      2. As gestation proceeds, the volume of lecithin in the pulmonary fluid increases, whereas sphingomyelin levels remain relatively constant.

3. At about 35 weeks of gestation, lecithin levels increase significantly.

4. Normally, after 35 weeks of gestation, the ratio of lecithin to sphingomyelin (L/S ratio) is above 2:1. An L/S ratio of 2:1 is indicative of pulmonary maturity, i.e., the fetus should be able to support extrauterine life.

5. L/S ratios can be determined intrauterinely by analysis of amniotic fluid (amniocentesis).

6. If L/S amniotic ratios are less than 2:1, incidence of development of the respiratory distress syndrome increases.

7. L/S ratios of less than 1:1 normally are incompatible with extrauterine existence.

II. Fetal Circulation

A. During intrauterine life, gas exchange, nutrient exchange and waste elimination are accomplished in the placenta.

B. The placenta also serves as a rich vascular bed that can accommodate large volumes of blood. The placenta is in part responsible for low systemic vascular resistance in the fetus.

C. The lung is fluid filled to about the FRC level and does not participate in external gas exchange.

D. Lung fluid tends to compress the pulmonary capillary beds. This, coupled with low intrauterine PO_2 causing vasoconstriction, tends to make the pulmonary capillary beds high in vascular resistance.

E. Thus pressures within the heart are completely opposite in utero to those after birth, i.e., pressures within the right side of the heart are greater during fetal life than the pressures within the left side of the heart.

F. In utero, pulmonary blood flow need not be as high as is necessary during extrauterine life.

G. For this reason, blood flow is diverted from the lung by two different routes: foramen ovale and ductus arteriosus.

H. The foramen ovale is a flaplike valve between the right and left atria.

I. The foramen ovale allows blood to flow directly between the right and left atria, bypassing the lung—a right-to-left shunt.

J. Blood flows from right to left atria through the foramen ovale because of the existence of (1) a rudimentary valve called the cristae intervenans, which actually directs and routes blood to the foramen ovale, and (2) a pressure gradient between the right and left sides of the heart.

K. The ductus arteriosus is a fetal communicating vessel between the pulmonary artery and aorta.

L. Blood is pumped from the right ventricle into the pulmonary artery. Since pulmonary artery pressure in utero exceeds systemic (aortic) vascular pressure, much of the blood is directed through (the path of least resistance) the ductus arteriosus, enters the aorta and again bypasses the lung – a right to left shunt.

M. The remainder of the blood passes through the pulmonary capillary bed, through the left side of the heart and out into the aorta.

N. In utero about 10% of cardiac output passes through the lung.

O. The remaining 90% bypasses the lung by either the foramen ovale or ductus arteriosus.

P. Blood in the aorta eventually reaches the umbilical arteries and enters the placenta where it undergoes exchange of gases, nutrients and wastes.

Q. Blood leaves the placenta by the umbilical vein carrying oxygenated blood.

R. The umbilical vein travels to the liver where most of the blood bypasses the liver via the ductus venosus.

S. The ductus venosus drains into the inferior vena cava.

T. The inferior vena cava drains into the right atrium and the blood is again circulated as described, beginning with Section II, I.

III. Circulatory Changes at Normal Birth

A. Following clamping of the cord at birth, the supply of oxygenated blood from the placenta is stopped.

B. In order for the neonate to sustain life, fetal circulation must be altered and blood must perfuse the lung to become oxygenated.

C. There is a significant decrease in pulmonary vascular resistance after birth. This occurs as a result of elimination of fetal lung fluid and the presence of oxygen in the lung.

D. With lung fluid eliminated, the pulmonary capillary bed is no longer compressed by hydrostatic forces.

E. When ventilation begins, oxygen diffuses into the pulmonary capillary blood. As pulmonary capillary blood oxygen tensions begin to rise, the vasoconstriction present in the fetal pulmonary vascular bed is gradually reversed.

F. With pulmonary vascular resistance reduced, larger portions of the cardiac output begin to perfuse the lung.

G. At the same time, there is a significant increase in systemic vascular resistance. This occurs in part from loss of the placenta as a blood reservoir, which also results in a decrease in venous return to the right side of the heart.

H. The increase in peripheral vascular resistance results in an increase in pressure in the left side of the heart.

I. The reduction in venous return and the decrease in pulmonary vascular resistance result in a decrease in pressure in the right side of the heart.

J. Now pressure in the left side of the heart exceeds pressure in the right side. This pressure change causes a functional closure of the foramen ovale.

K. In addition, the rise in oxygen tension in the ductus arteriosus causes it to begin to constrict.

L. Blood flow through the ductus arteriosus is also reversed, due to the change in pressures.

M. The ductus arteriosus usually closes functionally within the first 24 hours of life.

N. The ductus arteriosus anatomically closes within the first 3 weeks of life and becomes the ligamentum arteriosus.

IV. Pulmonary Changes at Birth

A. In order for the neonate to sustain extrauterine life, fetal lung fluid must be eliminated from the lung. This occurs through several mechanisms.

1. The compliant chest wall of the neonate is compressed in the birth canal during the birth process, forcing much of the fluid out of the lung.

2. Fetal lung fluid is low in protein content. When pulmonary blood flow increases at birth, some of the fluid is moved into the blood by osmosis.

3. The lymphatic system also absorbs a portion of lung fluid.

B. The first breath of the neonate is stimulated by several factors.

1. The change in temperature between intrauterine and extrauterine conditions

2. The bright light and sounds in the delivery room

3. The hypoxemia, acidemia and hypercapnia developed during the birth process

C. Intrathoracic pressures of −40 to −90 cwp must be generated to initiate the first breath.

D. During the first several breaths, the inspiratory tidal volume exceeds the expiratory tidal volume. The difference in volumes occurs because the functional residual capacity is being established.

V. Clinical Evaluation of the Neonate

  A. Apgar score: This scoring system evaluates the neonatal cardiopulmonary status after birth.

    1. Apgar scores are normally determined 1 and 5 minutes after birth.

    2. Scores are based on a scale of 0 to 10.

      a. Scores 7–10: Few, if any, supportive measures are needed.

      b. Scores 4–6: Mild to moderate asphyxia; the infant should be suctioned, oxygenated and possibly ventilated.

      c. Scores 0–3: Full cardiopulmonary resuscitation should be initiated.

    3. Scoring is performed in five areas, each area scored from 0 to 2.

      a. Heart rate
        (1) Absent: 0
        (2) Less than 100 per minute: 1
        (3) Greater than 100 per minute: 2

      b. Respiratory rate
        (1) Absent: 0
        (2) Slow, irregular: 1
        (3) Good cry: 2

      c. Muscle tone
        (1) Limp: 0
        (2) Some flexion of the extremities: 1
        (3) Active movement: 2

      d. Reflex irritability to stimulation
        (1) No response: 0
        (2) Grimace: 1
        (3) Cough or sneeze: 2

      e. Color
        (1) Blue or pale: 0
        (2) Pink body, blue extremities: 1

       (3) Completely pink: 2
B. Silverman score: This system evaluates the level of respiratory distress of a neonate.
  1. Scores are based on a scale of 0 to 10.
    a. Scores of 0 to 3: No respiratory distress to mild respiratory distress
    b. Scores of 4 to 6: moderate respiratory distress
    c. Scores of 7 to 10: severe respiratory distress
  2. Scoring is performed in five areas, scored from 0 to 2.
    a. Upper chest movement
      (1) Synchronized movement: 0
      (2) Lag of upper chest on inspiration: 1
      (3) See-saw movement of upper chest: 2
    b. Lower chest movement
      (1) No retractions: 0
      (2) Retractions just visible: 1
      (3) Marked retractions: 2
    c. Xiphoid retractions
      (1) No retractions: 0
      (2) Retractions just visible: 1
      (3) Marked retractions: 2
    d. Dilatation of nares
      (1) None: 0
      (2) Minimal dilatation: 1
      (3) Marked dilatation: 2
    e. Expiratory grunt
      (1) None: 0
      (2) Heard only with stethoscope: 1
      (3) Heard with naked ear: 2
VI. Prenatal Conditions That Increase Neonatal Mortality and Morbidity
  A. Prematurity
  B. Maternal factors
    1. Drug and alcohol abuse
    2. Extreme emotional stress
    3. Obstetric complications
    4. Cigarette smoking
    5. Placental insufficiency
    6. Multiple pregnancy
    7. Third trimester viral infection
    8. First pregnancy late in life
    9. Diabetes

VII. Blood Gases of the Neonate
  A. Blood gases at birth usually show metabolic and respiratory acidosis along with severe hypoxemia.

pH	7.20 – 7.25	HCO_3^-	18 – 19 mEq/L
PCO_2	53 – 58 mm Hg	PO_2	20 – 25 mm Hg

  B. Within the first hour after birth PO_2 in the term infant is about 60 mm Hg and in the premature infant 40 – 60 mm Hg.
  C. Twenty-four hours after birth PCO_2 values range from 35 to 40 mm Hg, but PO_2 values may take weeks to normalize to the 80 – 100 mm Hg range.

VIII. Respiratory Patterns of the Neonate
  A. The respiratory pattern of the neonate usually is rapid and shallow, rates ranging from 30 to 50 per minute depending on gestational age.
  B. The neonate shows little movement of the thoracic cage with ventilation being primarily diaphragmatic in nature. The diaphragm's motion is limited in the neonate due to the large size of the abdominal viscera.
  C. Tidal volumes of the neonate average 6 to 8 ml per kilogram.
  D. Periodic breathing patterns in the premature infant
    1. Periods of apnea lasting 5 – 10 seconds, followed by a period of tachypnea lasting 10 – 15 seconds, are frequently seen.
    2. The neonate's overall ventilatory rate remains at 30 – 50 per minute, but during the actual ventilatory periods the rate accelerates to 50 – 60 per minute.
    3. Periodic breathing patterns occur more often during wakeful states.
    4. The pattern does not develop until after the first 24 hours of life; the more premature the infant the more common the pattern.
    5. This pattern usually is not considered serious if periods of apnea do not exceed 10 seconds.
  E. True apneic spells in very small premature neonates.
    1. Apneic spells are defined as true periods of apnea if longer than 15 – 20 seconds.
    2. A high mortality is associated with apneic spells of this length.
    3. The etiology is unclear but the spells seem to be a result of CNS problems.

IX. Comparative Neonatal Respiratory Anatomy
  A. Neonatal head: Very large, about one fourth of total body

length, in contrast to the adult head, which is about one eighth of body height.

B. Neonatal tongue
   1. Very large in relation to size of oral cavity.
   2. Size is primary factor forcing neonates to be nose breathers. Normally only during crying will an infant actively ventilate through the mouth.
   3. Because of tongue size, nasal continuous positive airway pressure (CPAP) without use of endotracheal intubation can be accomplished.
   4. Positive end expiratory pressure (PEEP) levels up to about 8 – 10 cm H_2O can be used. PEEP levels above this usually cause an oral leak and are difficult to maintain nasally.

C. Neonatal neck: Very short and normally is creased.

D. Neonatal larynx
   1. The length is about 2 cm compared to 5–6 cm in the adult.
   2. The neonatal larynx is funnel-shaped, whereas the diameter of the adult larynx is more or less constant.
   3. The narrowest portion of the neonate's upper airway is the cricoid cartilage; in the adult, the rima glottidis is the narrowest point. The normal diameter of the neonatal glottis is about 7–9 mm anteroposterior, the anteroposterior diameter of the cricoid cartilage about 4–6 mm.
      a. Endotracheal tube size must be based on the diameter of cricoid cartilage.
      b. The larynx is much higher in relation to the oral pharynx and the opening of the larynx more in a straight line than in the adult.
      c. Thus an infant frequently extends the neck when in respiratory distress, whereas the adult will thrust the head forward.

E. Neonatal epiglottis
   1. Stiffer, relatively longer and U or V shaped compared to a flatter and much more flexible epiglottis in the adult.
   2. Located at level of 1st cervical vertebra; in the adult at 4th cervical vertebra.

F. Neonatal trachea
   1. About 4 cm long compared to 10–15 cm in the adult.
   2. Anteroposterior diameter about 3.5 mm, lateral diameter about 5 mm.
   3. Normally located to right of midline.

4. Bifurcation of neonatal trachea at 3d or 4th thoracic vertebra; in the adult at 5th thoracic vertebra.
5. The angle of right and left mainstem bronchi widens with age. At birth the angles from the midline are 10 degrees for the right and 30 degrees for the left; in adulthood the angles are about 30 and 50 degrees, respectively.
6. Cartilage of the trachea may not be fully formed and often is more flexible than in the adult.
   a. As a result, hyperextension of the head may cause compression of the trachea and result in airway obstruction.
   b. Thus during artificial ventilation without an endotracheal tube, the neonate's head should be maintained in a neutral position.

G. Neonatal mainstem bronchi
   1. Short and relatively wide compared to those of the adult.

H. Neonatal thoracic cage
   1. This has nearly equal anteroposterior and transverse diameters, and its general appearance is bullet shaped.
   2. Range of movement is limited, and the ribs are basically fixed in a horizontal position.
   3. The diaphragm is much higher than in the adult because of the size of the abdominal viscera. Diaphragm shows minimal movement during ventilation.
   4. The heart is located in the center of the chest and slightly higher than in the adult. When external cardiac massage is performed, compression should be applied over the middle of the body of the sternum.

X. Body Surface Area
   A. The neonate's body surface area in relation to his size is about nine times that of the adult.
   B. Maintenance of body heat is thus a significant problem in the neonate and even more so in the premature infant.
   C. The skin of the neonate plays a much greater role in water and heat balance than does that of the adult. This is a result of the large body surface area, which allows significant evaporation of water. In the neonate, 80% of body weight is water, in the adult only 55–60%.

XI. Congenital Cardiopulmonary Anomalies in the Neonate
   A. Choanal atresia: Blockage of the opening into the nasopharynx by a membranous tissue, usually with bony implants.

    1. If bilateral, the condition is a respiratory emergency because it inhibits nasal ventilation.

    2. If a nasal suction catheter cannot be passed, choanal atresia should be suspected in a neonate with severe respiratory distress.

    3. Surgical correction is necessary.

B. Esophageal atresia: Malformation of esophagus, with tracheoesophageal fistulas a common complication.

    1. Types

        a. Atresia of upper esophagus, with lower esophagus connected to stomach and trachea.

        b. An intact trachea, but unattached stomach and esophagus.

        c. H-type fistula: A normal trachea and esophagus connected by a small tubelike fistula.

    2. Clinical signs

        a. Accumulation of oral secretions

        b. Continuous or sporadic respiratory distress

        c. Abdominal distention as a result of air entry

    3. Surgical correction is necessary.

C. Diaphragmatic hernia: Result of incomplete development of diaphragm, allowing abdominal organs to enter the thoracic cavity.

    1. Respiratory and cardiovascular stress is pronounced.

    2. Most hernias occur on the left side, frequently causing a shift of the mediastinum and atelectasis.

    3. Surgical correction is necessary.

D. Congenital laryngeal stridor or partial airway obstruction: Result of incomplete development of larynx

    1. May cause mild respiratory distress.

    2. Usually improves with maturing of laryngeal and tracheal cartilage.

E. Tetralogy of Fallot: Congenital cardiovascular anomaly

    1. Ventricular septal defect, allowing blood to enter aorta from both right and left ventricles.

    2. Stenosis of pulmonic valve, which increases with age, causing right ventricular hypertrophy.

    3. Significant right to left shunt, severe hypoxemia, polycythemia and cyanosis.

    4. Surgical correction is necessary.

F. Truncus arteriosus: Cardiovascular congenital anomaly

    1. Ventricular septal defect associated with a common blood vessel leaving both ventricles.

    2. Branching of pulmonary arteries from the common vessel (truncus), which continues as the aorta.

    3. Variable pulmonary blood flow, dependent on level of the stenosis distal to branching of the pulmonary arteries.

    4. Variable pulmonary symptoms, depending on amount of pulmonary circulation.

    5. Both right and left ventricular hypertrophy is common.

    6. Surgical correction is necessary.

G. Complete transposition of the great vessels: Congenital cardiovascular anomaly

    1. Reversed position of aorta and pulmonary arteries (i.e., the aorta comes off the right ventricle and the pulmonary artery comes off the left ventricle).

    2. Frequently a patent ductus arteriosus and atrial septal wall defect.

    3. Surgical correction is necessary.

XII. Infant Respiratory Distress Syndrome (IRDS) (Idiopathic Respiratory Distress Syndrome or Hyaline Membrane Disease)

A. Factors suggestive of IRDS

    1. Premature birth at less than 35 weeks

    2. Low birth weight

        a. Neonates of less than 1000 gm very frequently develop IRDS.

        b. At birth weights of 1000–1500 gm, IRDS is common.

        c. At birth weights of 1500–2000 gm, some infants develop IRDS.

        d. In general, the lower the birth weight the higher the incidence of IRDS.

B. Early signs and symptoms

    1. Expiratory grunting

    2. Sternal and intercostal retractions

    3. Nasal flaring

    4. Cyanosis

    5. Rapid respiratory rates

    6. Edematous extremities

    7. X-Ray: Ground glass appearance with an air bronchogram

C. Physiologic changes

    1. Decreased surfactant production

    2. Increased capillary endothelial cell permeability

    3. Atelectasis

    4. Decreased pulmonary compliance

    5. Increased intrapulmonary shunting

    6. Severe hypoxemia

    7. Decreased functional residual capacity

D. Etiology: Primarily decreased surfactant production as a result of decreased L/S ratio associated with premature birth.

E. Course

    1. Normally a self-limiting process, the first 48-hour period being critical.

    2. Process is totally reversible.

F. Management

    1. Supportive in nature.

    2. Oxygenation with least F_{IO_2} necessary to attain an acceptable P_{O_2}.

        a. Maintenance of P_{O_2} between 50 mm Hg and 70 mm Hg.

        b. Application of PEEP via CPAP in early phases or in moderate cases.

        c. Possible ventilatory support in severe cases or if the infant tires and blood gases show acute or impending ventilatory failure.

    3. Reduction of stress on neonate and decrease of overall level of activity to reduce oxygen consumption to a minimum.

    4. Maintenance of adequate cardiovascular function.

XIII. Bronchopulmonary Dysplasia (BPD)

A. BPD is a disease process associated with ventilator therapy, a high F_{IO_2}, high peak inspiratory pressures and prolonged inspiratory times that causes chronic pulmonary changes.

B. Frequently BPD develops during the course of therapy for IRDS.

C. Pathophysiologic pulmonary changes

    1. Damage to alveolar and bronchiolar epithelium

    2. Bronchiolar metaplasia

    3. Peribronchial and interstitial fibrosis

D. Chronic pulmonary changes show a slow clearing during infancy, and most individuals are clinically and radiologically normal by age 6 months to 2 years.

XIV. Meconium Aspiration

A. Meconium: Normal contents of the intestinal tract of the fetus. Normally it is not passed from fetus' gastrointestinal tract until extrauterine existence.

    1. Composition
      a. Dark brownish-green semisolid material, tarry in texture.
      b. Bile, intestinal secretions and other pancreatic secretions.
    2. Presence in amniotic fluid
      a. In full-term and postmature neonates, meconium may be free in the amniotic fluid, making its aspiration likely.
      b. Whenever meconium is found in the amniotic fluid, its aspiration should be suspected.
      c. It has been *hypothesized* that meconium is passed in utero following an anoxic episode of the fetus.

  B. Aspiration
    1. At birth, all attempts to suction the oral and nasal pharynx should be made before ventilating an infant suspected of meconium aspiration.
    2. Results of irritation to respiratory tract from meconium
      a. Obstruction (check valve type) associated with pneumothorax
      b. Chemical pneumonitis
      c. Bacterial infection
    3. Management: Symptomatic
      a. Aggressive chest physiotherapy and suctioning
      b. Oxygen therapy
      c. In severe cases, possible CPAP and CPPV

XV. Croup
  A. Croup: Inflammation of larynx and trachea, inflammation being confined to subglottic area; also referred to as laryngotracheobronchitis.
  B. Cause: Almost exclusively *viral infection*
    1. Most common causative viruses
      a. Parainfluenza virus
      b. Influenza virus
      c. Adenovirus
  C. Diagnosis: Lateral x-ray of neck in which the epiglottis is seen as normal, whereas the area of the larynx and trachea shows haziness, indicating inflammation.
  D. Clinical manifestations
    1. Normal occurrence between ages of 6 months and 3 years.
    2. Primarily a dry, barking cough.
    3. Inspiratory stridor and noisy, labored breathing.

    4. Onset of symptoms progress over a period of 1 to 2 days before cough reaches maximum severity.

  E. Laboratory analysis: Normal white blood cell count compatible with a viral infection.

  F. Management
    1. Cool aerosol mist
    2. Racemic epinephrine
    3. Systemic hydration
    4. Oxygen therapy
    5. Cough suppressant

XVI. Epiglottitis
  A. Acute inflammation of supraglottic area, having the potential of causing complete upper airway obstruction.
  B. Etiology: *Bacterial, Haemophilus influenzae* being the most frequent agent in children.
  C. Diagnosis
    1. Lateral x-ray of neck, in which the epiglottis appears as a large, round, dense tissue mass covering the opening of the trachea. Subglottic area appears normal.
    2. Visualization of epiglottis should be performed with extreme caution due to increased incidence of spasm of epiglottis and complete obstruction.
  D. Clinical manifestations
    1. Epiglottitis normally occurs in older children (between ages 2 and 8 years).
    2. Primary feature: Rapid onset. Symptoms may progress to the point of partial airway obstruction in about 8 hours.
    3. Patient complains of a sore throat and has noisy, labored breathing, inspiratory stridor, hoarseness and fever.
    4. Speech and cough are muffled due to damping effect by the swollen epiglottis.
  E. Laboratory analysis: Elevated white blood cell count compatible with bacterial infection.
  F. Management
    1. Artificial airway, tracheotomy preferred
    2. Appropriate antibiotic therapy
    3. Symptomatic treatment of fever

BIBLIOGRAPHY

Abramson, H.: *Resuscitation of the Newborn Infant* (St. Louis: C. V. Mosby Co., 1973).

Avery, G. B.: *Neonatology, Pathophysiology and Management of the Newborn* (Philadelphia: J. B. Lippincott Co., 1975).

Avery, M. E.: *The Lung and Its Disorders in the Newborn Infant* (Philadelphia: W. B. Saunders Co., 1974).

Eigen, H.: Croup or epiglottitis: Differential diagnosis and treatment, Respir. Care 20:1158, 1975.

Goodwin, J. W., et al.: *Perinatal Medicine—The Basic Science Underlying Clinical Practice* (Baltimore: Williams & Wilkins Co., 1976).

Keuskamp, D. H. G.: *Neonatal and Pediatric Ventilation* (Boston: Little, Brown and Co., 1974).

Korones, S. B.: *High-Risk Newborn Infants* (St. Louis: C. V. Mosby Co., 1976).

Nowakowski, L.: *Pediatrics: Specific Anatomic Variables, Newborn Respiratory Tract* (Washington, D.C.: Robert J. Brady Co.).

Scarpelli, E. E.: *Pulmonary Physiology of the Fetus, Newborn and Child* (Philadelphia: Lea & Febiger, 1975).

Slonim, N. B., et al.: *Pediatric Respiratory Therapy: An Introductory Text* (Sarasota: Glenn Educational Medical Services, Inc., 1974).

Storer, J. S.: Respiratory problems unique to the newborn, Respir. Care 20: 1146, 1975.

Strang, L. B.: *Neonatal Respiration: Physiologic and Clinical Studies* (Philadelphia: J. B. Lippincott Co., 1974).

William, J. W.: *Handbook of Neonatal Respiratory Care* (Riverside, Calif: Bourns Inc., 1977).

13 / Pulmonary Function Studies

I. Lung Volumes and Capacities
   A. The gas in the respiratory system is divided into four basic lung volumes and four lung capacities. All capacities are composed of two or more lung volumes.
      1. Lung volumes
         a. Residual volume (RV): Amount of gas left in the lung after a maximal exhalation.
         b. Expiratory Reserve Volume (ERV): Amount of gas that can be exhaled after a normal exhalation.
         c. Tidal volume (VT): Amount of gas inspired during a normal inspiration.
         d. Inspiratory Reserve Volume (IRV): Amount of gas that can be inspired above a normal inspiration.
      2. Lung capacities
         a. Total lung capacity (TLC): Volume of gas contained in the lung at maximum inspiration (RV + ERV + VT + IRV).
         b. Inspiratory capacity (IC): Maximum volume of gas that can be inhaled after a normal exhalation (VT + IRV).
         c. Vital capacity (VC): Maximum volume of gas that can be exhaled after a maximal inspiration (ERV + VT + IRV).
         d. Functional Residual Capacity (FRC): Volume of gas that remains in the lung after a normal exhalation (RV + ERV).
   B. Normal lung volumes and capacities for a 165-lb, 6 ft tall, 25-year-old man
      1. TLC = 6000 cc
      2. VC = 4800 cc, about 80% of TLC
      3. IC = 3600 cc, about 60% of TLC
      4. FRC = 2400 cc, about 40% of TLC
      5. RV = 1200 cc, about 20% of TLC
      6. ERV = 1200 cc, about 20% of TLC
      7. VT = 500 cc, about 3 cc per pound of ideal body weight (8–10% of TLC)
      8. IRV = 3100 cc, about 50–55% of TLC

C. All predicted lung volumes and capacities are based on statistical data from a group of individuals of the stated height, age and sex. The acceptable percent deviation from normal in all cases is ± 20%. Thus unless there is greater than 20% variance, the results will be reported as essentially normal.
  1. Volumes determined must be corrected from room temperature to body temperature (Charles' law).

D. Normal vital capacities may be taken from various charts or from the following formulas:
  1. For males:

$$VC = 27.63 - (0.112 \times age) \times (height\ in\ cm). \qquad (1)$$

  2. For females:

$$VC = 21.78 - (0.101 \times age) \times (height\ in\ cm). \qquad (2)$$

E. All lung volumes and capacities depicted in Figure 13–1 can be measured by spirometry except
  1. RV
  2. FRC
  3. TLC

Fig 13–1.—Normal lung volumes and capacities and their relation to each other. Note that with normal spirometry the *RV* (residual volume) cannot be directly determined. Refer to text for further explanation. (From Shapiro, B. A.: *Clinical Application of Blood Gases* [Chicago: Year Book Medical Publishers, Inc., 1977]. Used by permission.)

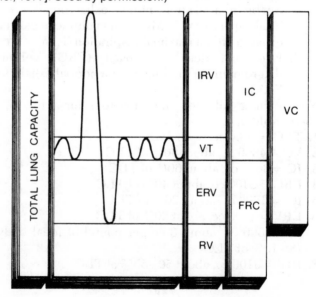

F. Methods of measuring RV, FRC and TLC
  1. Determination of these volumes and capacities is accomplished by using indirect methods of measuring FRC. FRC is measured because it is the most stable of all lung volumes and capacities. Once the FRC is determined, it is used to calculate TLC and RV.
  2. Three basic methods of measuring FRC: nitrogen washout study — open circuit technique; helium dilution study — closed circuit technique; and body plethysmograph — total thoracic gas volume determination.
  a. Nitrogen washout study
    (1) The test is always initiated and concluded at the patient's FRC level.
    (2) The patient is connected to a breathing circuit where he inspires 100% oxygen and the total volume of exhaled gas is collected.
    (3) Normally, the test is carried out for 7 minutes or until the percent nitrogen expired is less than 1%.
    (4) Since nitrogen makes up about 80% of FRC when the subject is breathing room air, the volume of nitrogen in the total exhaled gas will equal about 80% of the FRC.
    (5) Thus the total gas exhaled is measured for volume and percent nitrogen present.
    Example:

Total volume collected (liters)	50 L
Measured nitrogen concentration	5%
Volume of nitrogen in FRC	2.5 L

    (6) The FRC is determined as follows:

$$\frac{2.5\ L}{0.80\ FRC} = \frac{x}{1\ FRC}$$
$$x = 3.2\ L.$$

    (7) The RV is determined by subtracting ERV from FRC.
    (8) The TLC is determined by adding VC to RV.
    (9) Problems associated with nitrogen washout study:
      (a) Atelectasis may result from washout of nitrogen from poorly ventilated, partially obstructed areas.
      (b) Elimination of hypoxic drive in carbon dioxide retainers results in apnea.

(c) Error in determinations if severe airway obstruction present. The error will be on the low side of actual FRC because of poor distribution of ventilation.

b. Helium dilution study

    (1) Since helium is metabolically inert, a given volume of helium may be distributed throughout a lung bellows system without absorption of a significant volume.

    (2) The test is initiated and concluded at patient's FRC level.

    (3) The patient is connected to a rebreathing system and a certain volume (%) of helium is placed into a bellows. The patient breathes through the system until a constant helium percentage is read in the lung bellows system.

    (4) Normally the test takes up to 7 minutes to complete.

    (5) A soda lime absorber is placed in the system to remove carbon dioxide. Oxygen is titrated into the system to meet the patient's oxygen demands.

    (6) At beginning of the test, concentration of helium in the bellows and volume of gas in the bellows are measured.

    (7) At completion of the test, volume of gas in the bellows and concentration of helium in the lung bellows system are measured.

    (8) Calculation of FRC

        (a) The amount of helium in the system is constant.

        (b) Thus

Vol of He at beginning = vol of He at end of test

$$(\text{Vol lung}_B)(\text{conc. lung}_B) + (\text{vol bellows}_B)(\text{conc. bellows}_B) =$$
$$(\text{Vol lung}_E)(\text{conc. lung}_E) + (\text{vol bellows}_E)(\text{conc. bellows}_E). \qquad (3)$$

        (c) If the volume of gas in the bellows at the beginning (B) of the test is 2 L and helium concentration is 10%, and at the end (E) of the test the volume in the bellows is 2.2 L and helium concentration is 3.5%, then the patient's FRC can be calculated using Eq. 3, the unknown being equal to the FRC.

$$(x)(0.0\%) + (2.0 \text{ L})(0.10) = (x)(0.035) + (2.2 \text{ L})(0.035)$$
$$0.0 + 0.2 \text{ L} = 0.035x + 0.077 \text{ L}$$
$$\frac{0.123 \text{ L}}{0.035} = \frac{0.035x}{0.035}$$
$$x = 3.5 \text{ L.}$$

(9) Problem associated with the study: Gas distal to severely obstructed airways may not be measured because of poor distribution of ventilation

c. Body plethysmograph

(1) The patient's total thoracic gas volume is determined. All of the contained gas in the thoracic cavity, even if it is distal to completely obstructed airways, is measured.

(2) The overall calculations are based on Boyle's law.

(3) The total volume of the plethysmograph is known, and the volume displacement of the patient may be determined by body surface area charts. The volume of gas in the box surrounding the patient is determined by subtracting the volume the patient occupies from the volume of the box.

(4) The patient is sealed in the box and ventilates through a mouthpiece with a pressure transducer attachment and a shutter valve allowing obstruction at the mouthpiece.

(5) During the testing, the patient breathes gas from within the box.

(6) At FRC level, the shutter is closed and the patient inspires against an obstruction. As this occurs, proximal airway pressure and pressure in the plethysmograph are measured simultaneously.

(7) Boyle's law is used to determine the final volume in the plethysmograph itself:

$$P_1 V_1 = P_2 V_2 \tag{4}$$

where

P_1 = Original pressure in the plethysmograph is usually equal to atmospheric, or 760 mm Hg

V_1 = Original volume in the plethysmograph minus the volume occupied by patient, e.g., 1000 L

P_2 = Increased pressure in the plethysmograph as

a result of expansion of the thorax, e.g., 760.2 mm Hg

V_2 = Final volume in the plethysmograph

$$(760 \text{ mm Hg})(1000 \text{ L}) = (760.2 \text{ mm Hg})(x)$$

$$\frac{(760 \text{ mm Hg})(1000 \text{ L})}{760.2 \text{ mm Hg}} = x \text{ L}$$

$$x = 999.737 \text{ L.}$$

(8) The difference (V) between V_1 and V_2 is equal to the decreased volume in the plethysmograph after chest expansion. Since this is a sealed system, the change in volume in the plethysmograph is equal to the change in the volume in the patient's thorax. For the example above:

$$V_1 - V_2 = V \tag{5}$$
$$1000 \text{ L} - 999.737 \text{ L} = 0.263 \text{ L.}$$

(9) As the patient breathes in against an obstruction, the volume in the thorax increases and the pressure in the thorax is decreased. Thus, again applying Boyle's law:

$$Pa_1Va_1 = Pa_2Va_2 \tag{6}$$

where

Pa_1 = Proximal airway pressure at resting FRC levels, which would be equivalent to atmospheric (760 mm Hg)

Va_1 = Volume of FRC

Pa_2 = Pressure in airway after inspiring against an obstruction. In this example: 700 mm Hg

Va_2 = Final volume in thorax is equal to original volume Va_1 plus results from Eq. 5 (V). Thus Boyle's law may be written as

$$(Pa_1)(Va_1) = (Pa_2)(Va_1 + V)$$
$$(760 \text{ mm Hg})(x) = 700 \text{ mm Hg} \ (x + 0.263 \text{ L})$$
$$760 \text{ mm Hg} \ x = 700 \text{ mm Hg} \ x + 184.1 \text{ mm Hg–L}$$
$$\frac{60x}{60} = \frac{184.1 \text{ mm Hg–L}}{60 \text{ mm Hg}}$$
$$x = 3.07 \text{ L.} \tag{7}$$

(10) The thoracic gas volume is equal to 3.07 L.

(11) The major source of error in this determination is the additional volume that may be calculated as a result of gas contained in the abdominal cavity or pleural space.

G. Closing volume

1. The closing volume is defined as the terminal portion of a slow exhaled VC that indicates the point at which the most gravity-dependent airways start to collapse.

2. Normally during a maximal exhalation, there is a collapsing of peripheral bronchioles. In disease states, the volume of gas present in the lung when peripheral bronchioles begin to collapse increases.

3. A single-breath nitrogen washout study is used to determine the closing volume.

4. If an individual starts at RV level and inspires maximally, the first part of the inspired gas will move from the conducting airways into the apices. At this time, the apices fill only partially. Gas will then start to fill the bases. Toward the end of inspiration, both bases and apices fill. The lung fills in this manner due to transpulmonary pressure differences between apices and bases. An individual in the standing position has a higher transpulmonary pressure in the apices than in the bases. The lower transpulmonary pressure in the bases is essentially a result of lung position and gravity. Thus the alveoli in the apices are considered slow alveoli: they fill first but empty last; the alveoli in the bases are considered fast alveoli: they fill last but empty first. (For further explanation, see Chap. 6.)

5. In the single-breath nitrogen washout study, the patient breathes 100% oxygen from RV level to TLC, then slowly exhales to RV level.

   a. The initial part of the inspiration will go to the apices. This gas will contain a high nitrogen concentration because the volume will be primarily from the conducting airways, which contains 80% nitrogen.

   b. The next volume of gas will move to the bases. This volume will contain nitrogen, but to a lesser extent than the gas that originally moved to the apices.

   c. Finally, the bases and apices will fill to capacity with 100% oxygen.

   d. At maximal inspiration the nitrogen concentration in the apices is much greater than in the bases.

      e. As the patient slowly exhales, gas leaves the area of the lung where compliance is least, i.e., the bases. The bases will empty until the peripheral bronchioles start to collapse. The volume of gas left in the airways at onset of collapsing is referred to as the closing volume.

      f. As the patient continues to exhale, gas starts to leave the apices where the nitrogen concentration is much higher.

  6. Graphically plotting the nitrogen concentration against the volume exhaled, a graph similar to that in Figure 13–2 results. This graph depicts the four phases of the single-breath nitrogen washout curve.

    a. Phase 1: The nitrogen concentration is zero, indicating that only gas from the conducting airways is being exhaled.

    b. Phase 2: The steep increase in nitrogen concentration indicates that the gas being exhaled is mixed bronchial and alveolar air.

    c. Phase 3: A very slow increase is evident, indicating that mostly alveolar air is being exhaled.

    d. Phase 4: At closing volume, gas is being exhaled primarily from the apices.

  7. Normally the closing volume is expressed as a percentage of the VC.

    a. In young, healthy adults, closing volume is equal to about 10% of VC.

    b. This percentage increases normally with age. An indi-

Fig 13–2.—Single-breath nitrogen washout curve shows the four phases associated with the study. Phase 4 is the volume referred to as the closing volume. Δ %N$_2$ is the percent change in nitrogen concentration between the first 750 cc and 1,250 cc of exhaled gas.

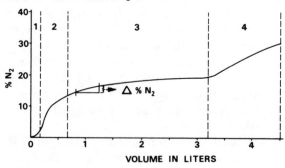

vidual age 60 years or older may have a normal closing volume of 40%.

    c. Increases in closing volume appear to be one of the earliest indications of small airway obstruction.

8. Closing capacity is a term used to express the percentage of the TLC that the closing volume plus the RV represents. Normally in young, healthy adults this is equal to about 30%.

9. Delta %nitrogen ($\Delta\%N_2$) is an expression used to indicate the change in nitrogen concentration between the first 750 ml and 1250 ml exhaled.

    a. In normal, healthy adults it is equal to 1.5% or less.

    b. As the $\Delta\%N_2$ increases, it indicates uneven distribution of ventilation.

II. Flow Rate Studies

  A. Forced vital capacity (FVC)

    1. The following flow rate determinations may be calculated from a FVC curve.

      a. The percentage of the vital capacity that is expired in 1 second ($\%FEV_1$) (Fig 13–3).

        (1) The forced expired volume in 1 second (FEV_1) is divided by the FVC:

$$\%FEV_1 = \frac{FEV_1}{FVC} \times 100. \qquad (8)$$

Fig 13–3.—Determination of $\%FEV_1$ and $\%FEV_3$. See text for explanation.

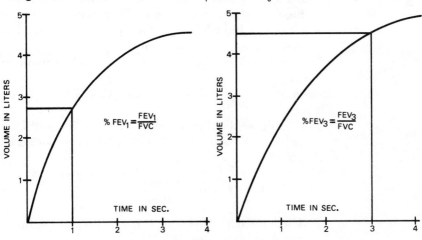

(2) Normally the $\%FEV_1$ is equal to at least 75% of the FVC.

(3) Decreased values basically indicate obstruction of larger airways.

b. The percentage of VC that is expired in 3 seconds ($\%FEV_3$) (see Fig 13-3).

(1) The FEV in 3 seconds (FEV_3) is divided by FVC:

$$\%FEV_3 = \frac{FEV_3}{FVC} \times 100. \tag{9}$$

(2) Normally this is equal to at least 97% of FVC.

(3) Decreased values basically indicate obstruction of smaller airways.

c. Forced expiratory flow (FEF) determined between the first 200 ml and 1200 ml of exhaled volume ($FEF_{200\text{-}1200}$) (Fig 13-4).

(1) The slope of the line between the first 200 cc and 1200 cc of exhaled volume is determined and reported as a flow:

$$\text{Slope in L/sec} = \frac{1\ L}{\text{time}}. \tag{10}$$

(2) The flow in liters per second is then converted to liters per minute:

$$(\text{liters/second})(60\ \text{seconds/minute}) = \text{liters/minute}. \tag{11}$$

(3) Since the graph is determined at room temperature, the flow must be corrected to body temperature.

(4) Normally the $FEF_{200\text{-}1200}$ for a young, healthy adult male is about 350-400 L/min.

(5) Decreased values basically indicate obstruction of larger airways.

d. Maximum midexpiratory flow rate ($MMEFR_{25\text{-}75\%}$) (see Fig 13-4).

(1) The slope of a line between the first 25% and 75% of exhaled volume is determined and reported as a flow:

$$\text{Slope in L/sec} = \frac{\text{volume}}{\text{time}}. \tag{12}$$

(2) The flow in liters/second is then converted to liters per minute (see Eq. 11).

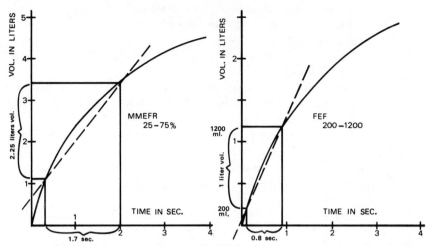

Fig 13–4.—Determination of MMEFR$_{25-75\%}$ and FEF$_{200-1200}$. See text for explanation.

(3) Since the graph is determined at room temperature, the flow must be converted to body temperature.

(4) Normally the MMEFR$_{25-75\%}$ for a young, healthy adult male is 250–300 L/min.

(5) Decreased values basically indicate obstruction of smaller airways.

B. Maximum voluntary ventilation (MVV) or maximum breathing capacity (MBC)

1. This study is used to determine the maximum volume of gas that a patient can ventilate in a minute.

2. The patient is directed to breathe as rapidly and as deeply as possible for 10–15 seconds.

3. The total volume inspired or expired during the stated period is determined.

4. This volume is converted to the volume per minute. For example, if the patient breathed 30 L in 10 seconds, then:

$$\frac{30 \text{ L}}{10 \text{ seconds}} = \frac{x}{60 \text{ seconds}}$$
$$x = 180 \text{ L.} \tag{13}$$

5. Normal MVV for young healthy adult males is 150–200 L/min.

6. Decreased values basically indicate increased airway re-

sistance or obstruction, decreased lung or thoracic compliance or weakness of ventilatory muscles.

C. Peak expiratory flow rate
   1. Peak expiratory flow normally occurs during the early part of exhalation.
   2. Peak flows normally are equal to 400–600 L/min for young, healthy males and 300–500 L/min for young, healthy females.
   3. Decreased peak flows indicate larger airway obstruction.

D. *It is extremely important to remember that all volumes determined must be converted to body temperature and that flow studies are totally patient effort dependent.*

III. Flow Volume Loops
   A. A flow volume loop is the simultaneous measurement of inspiratory and expiratory flows and volumes.
   B. The test is performed by having the patient maximally in-

Fig 13–5.—Normal flow-volume loop with superimposed tidal volume (VT) loop. All normal spirometry values plus peak inspiratory and expiratory flows along with flow at 25%, 50% and 75% of inspiration and expiration may be determined.

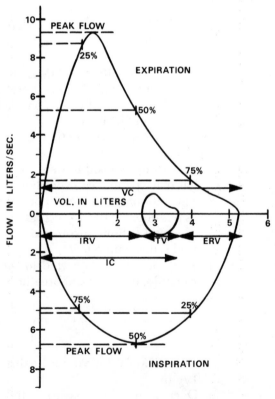

spire, followed by a single forced exhaled vital capacity (VC) and forced inspired VC (VC loop).

C. The following data can be determined from a flow volume loop if a VT loop is superimposed on a VC loop (Fig 13–5).

    1. VC

    2. VT

    3. IRV

    4. ERV

    5. IC

    6. Peak inspiratory and expiratory flows

    7. Inspiratory flows at 25%, 50% and 75% of VC

    8. Expiratory flows at 25%, 50% and 75% of VC

D. The major advantage of flow volume loops is that they give a quick visual impression of the general disease category (Fig 13–6).

IV. Diffusion Studies

A. Diffusion studies are used to determine how rapidly gases can move across the alveolar-capillary membrane.

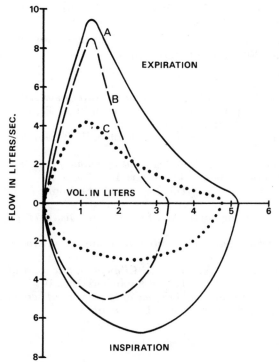

Fig 13–6. — A represents a normal flow-volume loop, B a flow-volume loop in restrictive lung disease and C a flow-volume loop in an obstructive lung disease. Flow-volume loops afford a rapid visual evaluation of the overall disease state.

B. Oxygen and carbon monoxide (CO) are used because of their strong affinity for hemoglobin and poor solubility coefficients.

C. Single-breath method: The patient maximally inhales a mixture of gases containing 0.1–0.3% CO, helium and air, followed by breath-holding for 10 seconds.

D. The pulmonary diffusing capacity for CO (DLCO) is equal to

$$\frac{\text{ml CO transferred/minute}}{\text{mean alveolar CO mm Hg} - \text{mean capillary CO mm Hg}}. \quad (14)$$

E. Normal resting DLCO for the average young adult male is 25 ml/min/mm Hg CO.

F. The DLO_2 may be computed by multiplying the DLCO by 1.23:

$$DLO_2 = DLCO)(1.23). \quad (15)$$

V. Normal Values
   A. Normal values for all studies discussed are based on the averages of many healthy individuals of a particular sex, age and height.
   B. Tables are available that give normal values for all tests for both sexes in all age and height categories.
   C. Determined values are considered normal unless they are greater or less than 20% of predicted values.

BIBLIOGRAPHY

Ayers, L. N., Whipp, B. J., and Ziment, I.: *A Guide to the Interpretation of Pulmonary Function Tests* (New York: Roerig, Division of Pfizer Pharmaceuticals, New York Projects in Health, Inc., 1974).

Cherniack, R. N.: *Pulmonary Function Testing* (Philadelphia: W. B. Saunders Co., 1977).

Comroe, J. H., et al.: *The Lung: Clinical Physiology and Pulmonary Function Tests* (2d ed.; Chicago: Year Book Medical Publishers, Inc., 1962).

Egan, D. F.: *Fundamentals of Respiratory Therapy* (3d ed.; St. Louis: C. V. Mosby Co., 1977).

Hyatt, R. E., et al.: The flow volume curve, Am. Rev. Respir. Dis. 107:191, 1973.

Ruppel, G.: *Manual of Pulmonary Function Testing* (St. Louis: C. V. Mosby Co., 1975).

Shapiro, B. A., Harrison, R. A., and Walton, J. R.: *Clinical Application of Blood Gases* (2d ed.; Chicago: Year Book Medical Publishers, Inc., 1977).

Young, J. A., and Crocker, D.: *Principles and Practice of Respiratory Therapy* (2d ed.; Chicago: Year Book Medical Publishers, Inc., 1976).

14 / Obstructive Pulmonary Diseases

I. General Comments
   A. The acronym COPD is applied to patients with long-term chronic obstructive pulmonary disease, who show persistent airway obstruction normally manifested by decreased expiratory flow rates.
   B. Prevalence
      1. From 1960 to 1970, the increase in deaths from emphysema was about 150%.
      2. In 1970, 30,000 deaths were attributed to emphysema.
      3. In 1970, 324,000 new cases of chronic bronchitis were reported.
      4. There seems to be a much greater incidence of COPD in men than in women.
      5. On autopsy some degree of emphysema appears in a large percentage of the population.
      6. Emphysema is the second leading cause of disability, arteriosclerotic heart disease being first.
   C. General causes of COPD
      1. Smoking
         a. Inhibits ciliary function.
         b. Causes bronchospasm.
         c. Affects macrophage activity.
         d. Affects alveolar septal wall and capillary endothelium.
      2. Air pollutants, both particulate and gaseous.
      3. Occupational exposure to dusts and fumes.
      4. Infection, which may cause decreased pulmonary clearance resulting in increased incidence of recurrent infection.
      5. Heredity
         a. Alpha$_1$ antitrypsin deficiency, which results in emphysematous changes measurable in the third and fourth decades.
         b. Cystic fibrosis.
         c. Asthma

      6. Allergies (e.g., chronic asthma), which can lead to permanent pulmonary changes.

      7. Aging, which causes natural degenerative changes in the respiratory tract resembling emphysematous changes.

D. Physical appearance of patient

      1. *Barrel-chested* as a result of increased air trapping (anteroposterior diameter increased).

      2. Clubbing of digits is frequently exhibited.

      3. Polycythemia, a result of the chronic hypoxemia seen with most chronic pulmonary disease.

      4. Cyanosis, a result of hypoxemia coupled with polycythemia.

      5. Decreased and adventitious breath sounds

      6. Often a hyperresonant chest.

      7. Ventilatory pattern

         a. Increased use of accessory muscles.

         b. Paradoxical movement of the abdomen frequently observed.

         c. Prolonged expiratory time.

      8. Malnutrition.

      9. Loss of appetite, depression, anxiety.

    10. General muscle atrophy.

E. General pulmonary function changes

      1. Frequently an increase in pulmonary compliance.

      2. Increased airway resistance as a result of mucosal edema and bronchiolar wall weakening.

      3. Prolonged expiratory times when #1 and #2 are combined.

      4. Increased FRC.

      5. Increased RV.

      6. Increased RV/TLC ratio.

      7. Increased or normal TLC.

      8. Decreased or normal VC.

      9. Decreased or normal IC and IRV.

    10. Increased ERV.

    11. Decreased flow studies; $\%FEV_1$, $\%FEV_3$, $MMEFR_{25\text{-}75\%}$, $FEF_{200\text{-}1200}$ and MBC may all be reduced.

F. General x-ray findings

      1. Increased anteroposterior diameter.

      2. Flattened diaphragm.

      3. Hyperinflation.

      4. Pulmonary vascular engorgement.

    5. In severe cases or end stage disease, right ventricular hypertrophy also may be seen.

G. Dyspnea

    1. In all patients dyspnea on exertion is one of the first noticeable symptoms.

    2. As the disease process progresses, dyspnea becomes apparent even at rest.

    3. Dyspnea normally increases as work of breathing progressively increases.

    4. The percentage of the oxygen consumed to ventilate is increased, severely limiting the patient's level of physical exertion.

H. Arterial blood gases of COPD and CO_2 retention

    1. Patients may experience a regular, predictable pattern of blood gas changes as the disease progresses.

    2. Because of the pathophysiology of COPD, ventilation/perfusion inequalities develop.

    3. Mismatching of ventilation and blood flow results in hypoxemia. It should be noted that hypoxemia normally is the first measured blood gas abnormality (see Chapter 6, Section VII).

    4. Hypoxemia becomes increasingly worse as the disease process progresses, resulting in stimulation of peripheral chemoreceptors.

    5. Stimulation of peripheral chemoreceptors results in hyperventilation — the body's attempt to correct hypoxemia.

    6. Hyperventilation persists and the kidneys compensate for the acid – base imbalance. Blood gas analysis reveals compensated respiratory alkalosis (chronic alveolar hyperventilation) with hypoxemia.

    7. Hyperventilation continues until oxygen consumption by the patient's respiratory musculature exceeds the benefits received by hyperventilation.

    8. The percentage of total oxygen consumption being used for ventilation becomes greatly increased because the efficiency of the respiratory system is greatly reduced by disease and increased accessory muscle use.

    9. The body can no longer maintain the level of alveolar ventilation necessary to maintain adequate oxygen tensions without severely compromising oxygen delivery to other organs.

    10. An inbred instinct in the survival of any organism is

conservation of energy. Thus the body's instinctive response is to hypoventilate in an attempt to conserve energy.

11. This results in further progression of the hypoxemia.

12. The total oxygen reservoir may be decreased even further. This is counterbalanced to a degree by a reduction in oxygen consumption by the respiratory muscles and a decrease in the patient's overall level of activity.

13. Alveolar ventilation continues to decrease. This is evidenced by increasing CO_2 levels and further development of hypoxemia.

14. With time, the patient begins to retain CO_2. Blood gases at this time would reveal compensated respiratory acidosis (chronic ventilatory failure) with moderate to severe hypoxemia.

15. It is at the point where CO_2 starts to be retained that the patient's primary stimulus to breathe becomes oxygen. This abnormal primary stimulus to ventilation is known as the hypoxic drive.

16. If oxygen were administered in sufficient amounts, the hypoxic stimulus to breathe would be reduced, potentially to the point of apnea.

17. The disease continues to progress with increasing levels of CO_2 retention and more severe hypoxemia.

18. The disease process becomes end stage and terminal. The patient's level of physical activity is severely limited and he is reduced to a pulmonary cripple (see Chapter 5, Sections IX and X).

I. Cor Pulmonale
   1. Congestive heart failure secondary to respiratory disease.
   2. A frequent sequel to chronic bronchitis and cystic fibrosis.
   3. Pathogenesis
      a. Developing pulmonary disease results in increasing hypoxemia, which causes constriction of the pulmonary capillary system.
      b. Constriction causes pulmonary hypertension. The decreased capillary bed seen with advancing pulmonary disease also contributes to development of pulmonary hypertension.
      c. Pulmonary hypertension causes the right side of the

heart to work harder. With time, right ventricular hypertrophy develops.

    d. Right ventricular hypertrophy will result in right-sided heart failure with time and will cause increased venous pressure.

    e. Thus peripheral edema occurs due to increased resistance to venous return and a backup of blood.

    f. Failure of the right side of the heart is more frequently seen in association with pulmonary disease than is left-sided heart failure.

II. Management of COPD
    A. The process is treatable to a certain extent but is not reversible

    B. Management revolves mainly around symptomatic treatment of the presenting problem.

        1. Relief of airway obstruction

          a. Mucosal edema: Sympathomimetics (alpha drugs), steroids and aerosol.

          b. Bronchospasm: Sympathomimetics (beta drugs).

          c. Secretions: Mobilization by aerosol therapy and chest physiotherapy.

        2. Prevention and treatment of bronchopulmonary infection by use of antibiotics and proper patient education.

        3. Improvement of patient's exercise tolerance by general graded body toning and stamina-developing exercises.

        4. Treatment of severe hypoxemia with oxygen therapy.

        5. Maintenance of cardiovascular status by treatment of congestive heart failure.

        6. Avoidance of exposure to all types of airway irritants.

        7. Proper education and psychologic and sociologic support.

III. Emphysema
    A. Characterized by enlargement of air spaces distal to terminal bronchioles, with loss of elastic fibers and destruction of alveolar septal wall.

    B. Etiology

        1. Smoking (high correlation with emphysema).

        2. High correlation with environmental conditions (e.g., air pollution).

        3. Occupational hazards, dust, fumes and similar factors.

        4. Heredity

          a. Alpha$_1$ antitrypsin deficiency, a lack of the enzyme that metabolizes trypsin, a digestive enzyme.

      b. If the trypsin is not metabolized, it will cause destruction of normal pulmonary tissue.

C. Types of emphysema
  1. Centrilobular
    a. Destructive changes primarily in the respiratory bronchioles.
    b. Much higher incidence in men.
    c. Primary lesions appear in upper lobes.
    d. A very high correlation with centrilobular emphysema and smoking; frequently a sequel to chronic bronchitis.
    e. Rare occurrence in nonsmokers.
  2. Panlobular
    a. Changes at alveolar level where destruction of septa predominates.
    b. Effects seemingly generalized in distribution.
    c. Seen with alpha$_1$ antitrypsin deficiency and the natural aging process.

D. Clinical manifestations
  1. Shortness of breath that develops increases very gradually
  2. Nonproductive cough
  3. Frequent respiratory infections
  4. Cyanosis
  5. Barrel-chested appearance
  6. Hyperresonant chest
  7. Polycythemia
  8. Use of accessory muscles

E. Pulmonary function studies: As outlined in Section I.

F. Management: As outlined in Section II.

IV. Bronchitis
  A. Acute bronchitis
    1. Acute inflammation of tracheobronchial tree with production of excessive mucus.
    2. Clinical manifestations
      a. Mucosal edema
      b. Increased sputum production
      c. Hacking paroxysms of cough
      d. Raw, burning substernal pain
    3. Causes
      a. Infectious: viral, bacterial or fungal
      b. Allergic
      c. Chemical, smoke, irritant gases and similar factors

    4. Treatment: Usually by administration of antibiotics, expectorants, aerosol therapy and occasionally antitussives.

    5. Normally a self-limiting process without serious complications or residual effects.

B. Chronic bronchitis

    1. Chronic cough with excessive sputum production of unknown specific etiology for 3 months per year for 2 or more successive years.

    2. Cause basically is frequent acute episodes of bronchitis, which may result from

        a. Smoking (by far the leading cause)

        b. Air pollution

        c. Chronic infections

    3. Clinical manifestations

        a. Onset: Normally insidious with patient rarely aware of its development.

        b. Steps in development

            (1) Smokers cough, followed by a

            (2) Morning cough, leading to

            (3) Continual cough, especially during cold weather and exacerbations.

        c. Sputum

            (1) Normally a slow increase until there is continual abnormal production.

            (2) Sputum usually thick, gray and mucoid until chronic infections develop, then turning mucopurulent.

    4. Pathophysiology

        a. Mucosal glands

            (1) Size increases in relation to wall thickness; normally gland size is about one third of height of bronchial walls.

            (2) In chronic bronchitis, gland size is about two thirds of height of bronchial walls.

            (3) Increase in number of mucus-secreting glands.

        b. Inflammation and edema of airways

    5. X-ray

        a. Early in the disease, x-ray changes are not significant, especially if the disease is associated only with larger airways.

        b. If the disease has moved to the periphery, hyperinflation with a flattened diaphragm may be noticed.

      c. X-ray usually is of little use in establishing diagnosis.

      d. A positive patient history usually is the best diagnostic tool.

  6. Pulmonary function studies

      a. In early stages, all pulmonary function studies may be normal, except for slight decreases in expiratory flow rates.

      b. As the disease process progresses, pulmonary function results are consistent with those presented in Section I.

  7. Treatment

      a. Most important: Removal of patient from irritants.

      b. Aerosol and bronchodilator therapy.

      c. Antibiotics if indicated.

      d. Treatment regime fairly consistent with that outlined in Section II.

V. Bronchiectasis

  A. Permanent abnormal dilatation and distortion of bronchi and/or bronchioles.

  B. Classification

    1. Cylindric (tubular)

      a. Bronchial walls are dilated, with regular outlines.

      b. Least severe type, as bronchiectatic areas drain fairly well.

    2. Fusiform (cystic)

      a. Bronchial walls have large, irregularly shaped distortions with bulbous ends.

      b. Evidence of bronchitis or bronchiolitis often is present.

    3. Saccular

      a. Complete destruction of bronchial walls.

      b. Replacement of normal bronchial tissue by fibrous tissue.

      c. Most severe type and has worst prognosis.

  C. Etiology

    1. Despite controversy, probable contributing factors are as follows:

      a. Recurrent infection, gram-negative infections being prominent.

      b. Complete airway obstruction.

      c. Atelectasis.

      d. Congenital abnormalities.

D. Diagnosis
   1. The bronchogram is the only absolute diagnostic tool.
   2. Bronchoscopy may afford direct visualization of bronchiectatic lesions.
E. Clinical manifestations
   1. Chronic loose cough, often exacerbated by change of position.
   2. Clubbing of fingers.
   3. Recurrent infections.
   4. Increased sputum production of a characteristic three-layer nature upon standing
      a. Top layer: Thin, frothy.
      b. Middle layer: Turbid, mucopurulent.
      c. Bottom layer: Opaque, mucopurulent to purulent with mucous plugs (Dittrich's plugs), sometimes foul smelling.
   5. Hemoptysis (common).
   6. Severe ventilation/perfusion abnormalities.
F. Pulmonary function studies
   1. Cylindric type may show no changes or decreases in expiratory flow rates.
   2. The saccular or cystic type shows decreased flow rates, especially if associated with bronchitis, emphysema or cystic fibrosis.
G. Management
   1. Aggressive bronchial hygiene with aerosol and chest physiotherapy.
   2. Appropriate antibiotic therapy.
   3. Possible lung resection if lesions are localized.
VI. Bronchiolitis
   A. Inflammation of the bronchioles primarily associated with children, age 6 months to 3 years but also may occur in adults, especially those with chronic bronchitis or emphysema.
   B. Etiology: In children primarily the respiratory syncytial virus.
   C. Clinical manifestations in children
      1. Fever.
      2. Cough.
      3. Audible expiratory wheezing.
      4. Increased anteroposterior chest diameter with hyperresonance.

     5. Commonly, subcostal, intercostal and suprasternal retractions.

     6. Sometimes inspiratory and expiratory wheezes as well as rhonchi.

  D. X-ray: Hyperinflation state.

  E. Treatment: Symptomatic; artificial airways and mechanical ventilation sometimes required.

VII. Asthma

  A. Asthma, according to the American Thoracic Society, is "characterized by an increased responsiveness of the trachea and bronchi to various stimuli and is manifested by widespread narrowing of the airways that changes in severity either spontaneously or as the result of treatment."

  B. Categories of asthma

     1. *Allergic* or *extrinsic:* Implies that asthma is a result of an antigen-antibody reaction on mast cells of the respiratory tract. This reaction causes release of histamine and slow-reacting substance of anaphylaxis. These substances then elicit responses associated with an asthmatic attack.

     2. *Idiopathic* or *intrinsic:* Implies that asthma is a result of imbalance of the autonomic nervous system, i.e., response of beta- and alpha-adrenergic sites, as well as cholinergic sites of the autonomic nervous system are not properly coordinated.

     3. *Nonspecific:* Implies that the origin of asthmatic reactions is unknown. The asthmatic attack may follow viral infection, emotional changes or exercise.

  C. Etiology

     1. In general, the complete causes are unknown, but heredity plays a significant role. Allergies and environmental factors also are frequently implicated.

     2. If the disease develops between ages 5 through 15, it usually has an allergic basis.

     3. If onset is after age 30, the disease normally is considered nonspecific.

     4. Incidence

       a. About 5–15% of the population under age 15 are asthmatic.

       b. About 1% of the adult population is asthmatic.

       c. Normally at onset of adolescence, the disease begins to disappear.

D. Diagnosis
   1. Depends on skin testing for antibodies and on patient's and family history.
   2. In allergic asthma, antibody IgE serum levels are about six times that of normal.
   3. In idiopathic asthma, patients show an abnormal response to drug therapy: decreased beta sympathetic response and increased alpha sympathetic response.
   4. In nonspecific asthma, frequent presenting symptoms are nasal polyps and aspirin intolerance.
   5. Eosinophilia of sputum and blood are common.
E. Pathophysiology
   1. Thickening of subepithelial membranes.
   2. Hypertrophy of mucous glands.
   3. Eosinophilic infiltrates common in both sputum and serum.
   4. Decrease in number of pulmonary mast cells.
   5. Mucosal edema and bronchoconstriction.
   6. Increased production of thick viscid secretions.
F. Clinical manifestations
   1. Presenting symptom: Severe respiratory distress.
   2. Rapid, shallow respiratory pattern.
   3. Wheezing that is often audible without a stethoscope.
   4. Weak cough.
   5. Tachycardia and hypertension.
   6. Sometimes diaphoresis.
   7. Cyanosis may be present.
   8. Barrel-chested appearance with hyperresonance.
G. X-ray
   1. During an attack a classic hyperinflation pattern is seen.
   2. Between attacks the chest x-ray may be normal.
H. Pulmonary function studies
   1. During an attack expiratory flow rates and vital capacity are decreased. Bronchodilator therapy during pulmonary function testing often results in a significant improvement in test results.
   2. Between attacks pulmonary function studies may be normal or show decreased expiratory flow rates.
I. Status asthmaticus
   1. Sustained asthmatic attack that does not respond to conventional therapy.
   2. Severe hypoxemia is normally present.

       3. Possible results
         a. Lactic acidosis
         b. Respiratory failure
         c. Mechanical ventilation
         d. Death
  J. Management
       1. Primarily drug oriented
         a. Sympathomimetics
         b. Cromolyn sodium
         c. Steroids
         d. Xanthines
       2. Systemic fluid administration.
       3. Use of IPPB and aerosol therapy is controversial; its use depends on patient tolerance.
       4. Oxygen therapy if hypoxemia is present.
       5. If status asthmaticus results in ventilatory failure, mechanical ventilation is indicated.
VIII. Cystic Fibrosis (Mucoviscidosis)
  A. A generalized genetic abnormality of the exocrine glands resulting primarily in malfunction of pancreas, sweat glands, salivary glands and respiratory mucosal glands.
  B. Etiology and incidence
       1. A non-sex-linked autosomal recessive trait primarily affecting Caucasian race.
       2. About one of every 2,000 Caucasians is born with the disease.
       3. Of cystic males, 95% are sterile.
  C. Prognosis
       1. Extremely poor: Patients usually die before age 25.
       2. A mortality of 90% associated with respiratory complications.
  D. Clinical manifestations
       1. Chronic pulmonary disease
       2. Pancreatic insufficiency
       3. Increased electrolyte concentration in sweat
  E. Clinical symptoms
       1. Gastrointestinal
         a. Pancreatic enzyme deficiency resulting from obstruction of the pancreatic duct in 80–85% of patients.
         b. Very large appetite with little or no weight gain.
         c. Incomplete digestion of food.

      d. Large, bulky, loose stools, pale and foul smelling.
      e. Protruding abdomen.
      f. Intestinal obstruction in 5–10% of patients.
  2. Pulmonary
      a. Initially a dry, hacking cough
      b. With time development of a loose and more productive cough
      c. Eventually paroxysmal coughing
      d. Fatigability
      e. Shortness of breath
      f. Fever
      g. Barrel-chested appearance
      h. Clubbing of fingers
      i. Cyanosis

F. Diagnosis
  1. Positive diagnosis normally is dependent on a "sweat test" or ionophoresis, which measures the chloride content of the sweat. Normally 18 mEq/L of chloride is contained in the sweat. If more than 60 mEq/L of chloride is found, diagnosis is positive.
  2. Increased amount of fat in stool.
  3. Decreased amount of trypsin in stool.
  4. Decreased blood chloride and sodium levels.

G. X-ray
  1. If pulmonary problems are not significant, the chest x-ray may be normal.
  2. As the disease progresses, pulmonary manifestations show a hyperinflation pattern on x-ray.
  3. If end stage cardiac decompensation is present, vascular engorgement and myocardial hypertrophy will be seen.

H. Management
  1. Gastrointestinal problems
      a. Pancreatic enzyme substitutes
      b. Diet: Low fat, high protein and high caloric intake.
      c. Supplemental salt
  2. Respiratory problems
      a. Aggressive bronchial hygiene with aerosol and chest physiotherapy on a daily basis.
      b. Mucolytics to improve clearance of secretions.
      c. IPPB therapy generally not indicated due to presence of bullous lung disease.

    d. Appropriate antibiotic administration, when indicated by infection.

    e. Oxygen therapy if necessary in acute exacerbation and at end stage of disease.

BIBLIOGRAPHY

Abraham, A. S.: The management of patient with chronic bronchitis and cor pulmonale, Heart Lung 6:104, 1977.

Bates, D. V., Macklem, P. T., and Christie, R. V.: *Respiratory Function in Disease* (Philadelphia: W. B. Saunders Co., 1971).

Cherniack, R. M., Cherniack, L., and Naimark, A.: *Respiration in Health and Disease* (2d ed.; Philadelphia: W. B. Saunders Co., 1972).

Committee of the Oregon Thoracic Society, Chronic Obstructive Pulmonary Disease: C.O.P.D. Manual (New York: American Lung Association, 1977).

Gates, A. J.: Bronchiolitis or asthma: Differential diagnosis and treatment, Respir. Care 20:1153, 1975.

Joint Committee of the Allergy Foundation of America and the American Thoracic Society: Asthma; A Practical Guide for Physicians (New York: National Tuberculosis and Respiratory Disease Association, 1973).

Said, S. I.: The Lung in Relationship to Hormones (New York: American Thoracic Society, Basics of Respiratory Diseases, vol. 1 no. 3, 1973).

Tecklin, J. S., and Holsclaw, D. S.: Cystic fibrosis and the role of the physical therapist in its management, Phys. Ther. 53:386, 1973.

Thurlbeck, W. M.: Chronic Bronchitis and Emphysema (New York: American Thoracic Society, Basics of Respiratory Diseases, vol. 3 no. 1, 1974).

Ward, J.: Cromolyn sodium: A new approach to treatment of asthma, Heart Lung 4:415, 1975.

West, J. B.: *Pulmonary Pathophysiology: The Essentials* (Baltimore: Williams & Wilkins Co., 1977).

15 / Restrictive Lung Disease

I. General Comments
   A. A restrictive lung disease is any disease state in which the ability to inhale is affected. Generally the characteristic feature is an inability to expand the lung fully.
   B. Restrictive diseases of pulmonary origin are normally associated with an increase in pulmonary fibrous tissue. The result is an overall increase in pulmonary elastance and a decrease in pulmonary compliance.
   C. Characteristic pulmonary function findings
      1. Decreased or normal VT (tidal volume).
      2. Decreased or normal RV (residual volume).
      3. Decreased or normal ERV (expiratory reserve volume).
      4. Decreased or normal IRV (inspiratory reserve volume).
      5. Decreased TLC (total lung capacity).
      6. Decreased VC (vital capacity).
      7. Decreased IC (inspiratory capacity).
      8. Decreased or normal FRC (functional residual capacity).
      9. In pure restrictive lung diseases flow rate studies usually are normal; flow rate studies may be decreased when obstructive component is present.
     10. Pulmonary and/or thoracic and total compliance is usually severely decreased.
     11. Progressive increase in work of breathing as severity of disease increases.
         a. Initially the alveolar minute volume is normal or increased but, as the disease progresses, the alveolar minute volume progressively decreases.
         b. Arterial blood gases may follow the same pattern as that seen in obstructive lung disease. The presenting symptom may be chronic respiratory alkalosis with hypoxemia but, as the disease progresses, chronic respiratory acidosis with hypoxemia may develop.
   D. Restrictive lung diseases may be categorized as pulmonary, thoracoskeletal, neurologic-neuromuscular or abdominal.

II. Pulmonary Restrictive Lung Diseases
  A. Pulmonary fibrosis: Excessive connective tissue formation.
    1. Cause: Any permanent injury to the lung
    2. Distribution: Localized or diffuse
      a. Causes of localized fibrosis
        (1) Tuberculosis
        (2) Unresolved pneumonias
        (3) Fungal infections
      b. Causes of diffuse fibrosis
        (1) Chronic exposure to various inhalants. Specific pneumoconiosis are listed in Table 15–1.
        (2) Diseases of unknown etiology that often show diffuse fibrosis
          (a) Hamman-Rich syndrome
          (b) Eosinophilic granuloma
          (c) Sarcoidosis
          (d) Familial fibrocystic dysphagia
          (e) Chronic interstitial pneumonia
          (f) Collagen diseases
    3. Clinical presentation
      a. Primary symptom: Progressive dyspnea on exertion and ultimately at rest.
      b. Nonproductive cough.
      c. As disease continues, progressive respiratory impairment and often cor pulmonale.
      d. Physical examination findings
        (1) Clubbing
        (2) Cyanosis

TABLE 15–1.—SPECIFIC PNEUMOCONIOSIS

DISEASE	CAUSATIVE AGENT
Silicosis	Silica dust
Farmer's lung	Moldy hay
Stannosis	Tin dust
Silo-fillers' disease	Nitrogen dioxide
Coal workers' pneumoconiosis	Coal dust
Asbestosis	Asbestos
Berylliosis	Beryllium
Siderosis	Iron dust
Talcosis	Talc
Barritosis	Barium
Aluminosis	Aluminum

(3) Restricted chest wall and diaphragmatic movement

(4) Diffuse, dry, crackling rales

   e. X-ray

(1) Small lung with large heart and elevated diaphragm.

(2) Fine reticular or nodular pattern involving entire lung but predominantly the lower lobes.

   f. Arterial blood gases and pulmonary function studies as outlined in section I.

  4. Treatment

   a. Removal of patient from environment causing the fibrotic changes.

   b. Therapy for underlying disease entity.

   c. Symptomatic management of pulmonary problems, emphasizing

(1) Bronchial hygiene

(2) Overall nutrition

(3) Graded exercise programs

B. Pleural effusion: Accumulation of fluid in pleural space.

  1. Normally the fluid lining of the pleura is produced by the capillary network of the visceral pleural surface, and any excess is removed by the lymphatic system.

  2. Any disturbance in production of this fluid or in its removal can lead to development of pleural effusion.

  3. Primary causes: Inflammation and circulatory disorders

   a. Malignancy

   b. Congestive heart failure

   c. Infection

   d. Pulmonary infarction

   e. Trauma

  4. The effusion compresses the lung on the affected side.

  5. The effusion is gravity dependent and may shift with positional change.

  6. Treatment

   a. Primary: Removal of fluid from pleural space

(1) Thoracentesis or insertion of chest tubes

(2) Fluid allowed to reabsorb into pulmonary lymphatic system.

   b. Treatment of underlying disease state

C. Pneumothorax: Accumulation of air within pleural space.

1. If air enters the pleural space, the pressure within the space changes from subatmospheric to atmospheric or supra-atmospheric pressure.
   a. This increased pressure will compress lung tissue and result in atelectasis.
   b. Ventilation of the lung on the affected side is decreased as a result of elimination of the subatmospheric intrapleural pressure.
2. Types: Open and under tension
   a. In an open pneumothorax, there is no buildup of pressure because the gas is allowed to move freely in and out of the pleural space.
   b. A tension pneumothorax results from presence of a one-way valve, which allows gas only to enter the pleural space—not to leave it. This results in significant increases in pressure within the pleural space.
      (1) Clinical signs
          (a) Increased difficulty in ventilating. If patient is on a ventilator, airway pressure will increase with each breath.
          (b) Patient's vital signs will begin to deteriorate as mean intrathoracic pressure increases.
          (c) Breath sounds will be absent on affected side.
          (d) Affected side will be hyperresonant to percussion.
          (e) Trachea and mediastinum may be shifted toward unaffected side as extent of tension pneumothorax increases.
          (f) Possible pleuritic pain
          (g) Dry hacking cough
          (h) These clinical signs are more predominant if patient is on a mechanical ventilator than if he is ventilating spontaneously. This is due to the greater pressure gradients developed, forcing more gas into the pleural space.
          (i) In all cases a chest tube must be inserted to decompress the thorax.
D. Pulmonary edema: Active movement of fluid across alveolar capillary membrane into alveoli.
   1. Normally a fine balance exists among capillary osmotic (oncotic) pressure, capillary hydrostatic pressure, intersti-

tial hydrostatic pressure and interstitial osmotic (oncotic) pressure.

2. Usually a very small net pressure forces fluid into the interstitial space. This interstitial fluid is drained by the lymphatics.

3. If capillary hydrostatic pressure increases significantly, the net pressure forcing fluid into the interstitial space increases and eventually fluid will move directly into the alveoli.

4. Primary cause: Acute left ventricular failure
   a. The hydrostatic pressure of the pulmonary vascular bed is increased because of the inability of the left side of the heart to accept the blood presented to it.
   b. This increased pressure offsets the normal pressure dynamics at the alveolar capillary membrane.

5. Other causes
   a. Altered alveolar capillary membrane permeability, which may result from inhalation of noxious gases and/or shock.
   b. Decrease in capillary osmotic pressure, which results from decrease in plasma protein levels.

6. Treatment
   a. Primary: Pharmacologic
      (1) Furosemide (Lasix)
      (2) Morphine
      (3) Digitalis
   b. Pulmonary management
      (1) Oxygen at a high $F_{I_{O_2}}$
      (2) IPPB with ethyl alcohol
      (3) PEEP and mechanical ventilation in severe cases

E. Pneumonia: Pneumonitis caused by a microorganism.
   1. Pneumonias are a leading cause of death in the United States and account for 10% of admissions to general medical floors.
   2. Bacterial pneumonia
      a. Common clinical signs and symptoms
         (1) Onset normally is abrupt.
         (2) Very high fevers, with chills, sometimes lasting longer than 20 minutes.
         (3) Large volumes of thick, purulent sputum.
         (4) Frequently tachypnea and tachycardia, sometimes a pleuritic type pain.

          (5) X-ray: Consolidation.

          (6) White blood cell count: Frequently greater than 10,000/cu mm.

          (7) Hypoxemia secondary to shunting.

   3. Nonbacterial (viral or fungal) pneumonia

      a. Clinical signs and symptoms (occasionally mild and frequently undiagnosed).

          (1) Onset normally is very gradual.

          (2) Fevers normally are low grade, chills uncommon.

          (3) Sputum production is minimal, usually thin and mucoid.

          (4) Tachypnea and tachycardia are rare; pleuritic pain uncommon.

          (5) X-ray: Consolidation uncommon.

          (6) White blood cell count: Commonly less than 10,000/cu mm

  4. Treatment

      a. Appropriate antibiotic therapy

      b. Oxygen therapy

      c. Fluid therapy

      d. IPPB, aerosol and chest physiotherapy, if indicated

F. Adult Respiratory Distress Syndrome (ARDS)

  1. Terms representing the same clinical syndrome

      a. Oxygen toxicity

      b. Oxygen pneumonitis

      c. Wet lung

      d. Congestive atelectasis

      e. Stiff lung syndrome

      f. Respiratory lung syndrome

      g. Postpump lung

      h. Posttraumatic pulmonary insufficiency

      i. Shock lung

  2. Clinical features of the syndrome's pathophysiologic processes

      a. Refractory hypoxemia (hypoxemia that does not respond to an increasing $F_{I_{O_2}}$)

      b. Decrease in pulmonary compliance

      c. Decrease in FRC

      d. Chest x-ray: Diffuse alveolar infiltrates throughout entire lung field

      e. Complete reversal of disease process except for any residual fibrotic changes

3. Postmortem pulmonary findings
   a. Beefy lung, which does not collapse on removal from thoracic cavity
   b. Hyaline membrane formation on pulmonary parenchyma
   c. Interstitial edema and fibrosis
   d. Pneumocyte hyperplasia
4. Cause
   a. Probably a reaction of the respiratory tract to high levels of stress for prolonged periods. This stress may be associated with any of the organ systems.
   b. Clinical problems associated with development of ARDS
      (1) Oxygen toxicity
      (2) Chest trauma
      (3) Aspiration
      (4) Chemical irritation of respiratory tract
      (5) Blood transfusion
      (6) Emboli formation
      (7) Sepsis
      (8) Shock
      (9) Radiation injury
      (10) Near drowning
      (11) Pancreatitis
5. Pathophysiology of ARDS resulting from oxygen toxicity
   a. FI_{O_2} maintained above 0.50–0.60 for prolonged periods may cause pulmonary changes.
      (1) Interference with pulmonary enzyme systems, which disrupts pulmonary metabolism.
      (2) Type II alveolar cell dysfunction, which results in altered surfactant production.
      (3) Inhibition of mucociliary activity.
      (4) Increased permeability of capillary endothelium.
      (5) Nitrogen washout and atelectasis (absorption atelectasis).
   b. Primary symptoms noted by patient
      (1) Substernal distress
      (2) Cough
      (3) Nausea and vomiting
      (4) Paresthesia
   c. Functional changes
      (1) Decrease in compliance secondary to

(a) Altered surfactant levels

(b) Dilution of surfactant by transudate

(c) Atelectasis

(2) Decrease in FRC secondary to

(a) Altered surfactant levels

(b) Nitrogen washout atelectasis

(3) Increased work of breathing

(4) Refractory hypoxemia

d. Pathophysiology of ARDS resulting from clinical problems presented in #4 follows the general pattern seen with oxygen toxicity. The actual mechanism by which these changes develop is unclear.

6. Management

a. Maintenance of adequate oxygenation state

(1) Primary concern: Reduce F_{IO_2} below 0.5–0.6 so that compounding effects of oxygen toxicity can be avoided.

(2) Arterial P_{O_2} may be maintained in the 50–60 mm Hg range if hemoglobin level and tissue perfusion state are adequate.

(3) Role of PEEP

(a) Increase FRC

(b) Improve oxygenation state

(c) Decrease work of breathing

b. Steroid therapy: In early stages of management, steroids, especially methylprednisolone sodium succinate (Solu-Medrol), appear to help stabilize endothelial cells and type II pneumocytes if they are administered in large doses for short periods.

III. Thoracoskeletal Restrictive Lung Diseases

A. Deformities of thoracic cage that result in limited movement of the chest demonstrate pulmonary function patterns consistent with restrictive lung disease.

B. If the deformity is severe enough, a significant increase in work of breathing results.

C. Increased work of breathing eventually leads to hypoxemia, hypercapnia and possible heart failure.

D. Most commonly encountered thoracic abnormalities leading to restrictive lung disease

1. Scoliosis: Gradual curvature of vertebral column in lateral plane of body.

a. One of the most common thoracic deformities.

   b. May occur at various levels of the vertebral column.

   c. May develop with age as a result of poor posture.

2. Kyphosis: Posterior curvature of thoracic vertebral column, resulting in a bony hump.

   a. Frequently develops in older individuals with degenerative osteoarthritis.

   b. May develop in individuals with chronic obstructive pulmonary disease.

3. Kyphoscoliosis: Combination of thoracic scoliosis and kyphosis.

   a. In severe cases of kyphoscoliosis, one lung becomes severely compressed, the other overdistended.

   b. Cardiopulmonary disability may be very pronounced in severe kyphoscoliosis.

IV. Neurologic-Neuromuscular Restrictive Lung Diseases

   A. Weakness or paralysis of the muscles of ventilation results in a pulmonary function pattern consistent with restrictive lung disease.

   B. Myasthenia gravis: A disease of the myoneural junction in which transmission of impulses across the motor end plate is inhibited.

      1. Etiology: Unknown. Functionally it appears that acetylcholine is improperly released, synthesized or prematurely hydrolyzed before crossing the neuromuscular junction.

      2. The disease is most common in women in their 20s to 40s, but it affects individuals of both sexes and of all ages.

      3. The disease is manifested by generalized muscle weakness and most commonly demonstrates a descending paralysis.

      4. The primary symptoms normally are ocular, with paralysis descending to eventually affect the muscles of ventilation.

      5. Characteristically the least amount of muscle weakness is felt in the morning, the weakness progressing throughout the day.

      6. The disease normally is managed with the use of parasympathomimetics, atropine and occasionally steroids.

   C. Guillain-Barré syndrome: Polyneuritis primarily affecting the peripheral motor and sensory neurons.

      1. Etiology: Unclear. The disease may be viral or traumatic in nature. An increase in the number of cases has been

reported following vaccination against poliomyelitis and swine flu.

2. The syndrome affects all ages but is more prevalent in adults.
3. The signs and symptoms show an ascending pattern of sensory abnormalities that may progress to actual paralysis.
4. The disease is normally self-limiting and is reversible with time. The amount of residual effects are dependent on the extent of demyelination occurring during the active disease state.
5. Diagnosis is made by the presentation of the disease, a high protein content in the cerebral spinal fluid and the reversible nature of the disease.
6. Treatment is purely symptomatic, the patient frequently requiring ventilatory support.

D. Other neuromuscular or neurologic diseases that may show a restrictive lung disease pattern
   1. Spinal cord diseases
     a. Paraplegia or quadriplegia
     b. Poliomyelitis
   2. Tetanus
   3. Muscular dystrophy
   4. Tick bite paralysis
   5. Congenital myotonia

V. Abdominal Restrictive Lung Diseases
A. Increased size of abdominal contents results in limited movement and elevation of the diaphragm.
B. The limited diaphragmatic movement will demonstrate pulmonary function findings consistent with those of restrictive lung disease.
C. Conditions that may show a restrictive pattern
   1. Abdominal tumors
   2. Obesity
   3. Third trimester pregnancy
   4. Diaphragmatic hernias
   5. Ascites

BIBLIOGRAPHY

Amandus, H. E., et al.: The pneumoconioses: Methods of measuring progression, Chest 63:736, 1973.

Bates, D. V., Macklem, P. T., and Christie, R. V.: *Respiratory Function in Disease* (2d ed.; Philadelphia: W. B. Saunders, 1971).

Bendixen, H. H., et al.: *Respiratory Care* (St. Louis: C. V. Mosby Co., 1965).

Cushing, R.: Pulmonary infections, Heart Lung 5:611, 1976.

Fink, J. N., et al.: Clinical survey of pigeon breeders, Chest 62:277, 1972.

Gracey, D. R.: Adult respiratory distress syndrome, Heart Lung 4:280, 1975.

Kealy, S. L.: Respiratory care in Guillain-Barré Syndrome, Am. J. Nurs. 22:58, 1977.

Lakshminarayan, S., Stanford, R. E., and Petty, T. L.: Prognosis after recovery from adult respiratory distress syndrome, Am. Rev. Respir. Dis. 113:7, 1976.

Safar, P. (ed.): *Respiratory Therapy* (Philadelphia: F. A. Davis Co., 1965).

Selecky, P. A., and Ziment, I.: Prolonged respirator support for the treatment of intractable myasthenia gravis, Chest 65:207, 1974.

Shapiro, B. A., Harrison, R. A., and Trout, C. A.: *Clinical Application of Respiratory Care* (Chicago: Year Book Medical Publishers, Inc., 1975).

Shapiro, B. A., et al.: Case study: Myasthenia gravis, Respir. Care 19:460, 1974.

Shulman, J. A.: Errors and hazards in the diagnosis and treatment of bacterial pneumonias, Ann. Intern. Med. 62:41, 1965.

Solliday, N. H., Shapiro, B. A., and Gracey, D. R.: Adult respiratory distress syndrome, Chest 69:207, 1976.

Ziskind, M. M.: *The Acute Bacterial Pneumonia in the Adult* (New York: American Lung Association, 1974).

16 / Analyzers

I. Oxygen Analyzers
  A. Analyzers that use Pauling's principle of paramagnetic susceptibility of oxygen (Beckman D–2).
    1. The basic principle of operation is the ability of oxygen to be attracted by a magnetic field and cause displacement of nitrogen from the field.
    2. A *dry* gas is drawn into a chamber containing a magnetic field.
      a. The gas is dried by passing through anhydrous silica (blue) gel crystals.
      b. The gas must be dried because water vapor causes interference in the magnetic field and exerts a partial pressure.
    3. As oxygen enters the chamber, it causes an increased magnetic force, resulting in rotation of a nitrogen-filled dumbbell, suspended by a quartz fiber in the magnetic field.
    4. Attached to the dumbbell is a mirror, which reflects a beam of light that indicates degree of rotation of the dumbbell.
    5. Degree of rotation is directly related to partial pressure of oxygen in the system and is indicated on a scale in mm Hg Po_2 and FI_{O_2}.
    6. Since the analyzer measures partial pressure of oxygen, the mm Hg scale is accurate at all altitudes.
    7. The FI_{O_2} scale is accurate only at sea level, unless recalibrated with changes in altitude.
    8. The analyzer accurately measures oxygen partial pressure in all respiratory gas mixtures.
  B. Analyzers that use the thermal conductivity of oxygen (Mira, OEM)
    1. The principle of operation is based on ability of oxygen to cool an electric wire more so than air.
    2. The cooler the electric wire the less resistant the wire is to flow of electrons and the greater the current.

3. The analyzer uses an electric circuit referred to as the *Wheatstone bridge.*
4. The Wheatstone bridge has two reference chambers, which contain room air. A constant cooling effect maintains current at a specific constant level.
5. Two sampling chambers are filled with the gas to be analyzed.
6. During analysis of the gas, difference in current between reference and sampling chambers is compared.
7. The FI_{O_2} of gas being sampled determines this current differential.
8. This analyzer actually measures FI_{O_2}.
   a. Cooling ability of the sample gas is always compared to the constant thermoconductive effect of room air with about 21% oxygen and 79% nitrogen.
   b. Thus no matter what the altitude, there is always a comparison to a fixed oxygen-nitrogen ratio.
9. Gas entering the sample chamber must contain water vapor.
   a. Water vapor is added by using hydrated (pink) silica gel crystals.
   b. The gas is saturated to prevent buildup of a static charge in the system.
10. Only oxygen-nitrogen gas mixtures can be analyzed because the cooling effect of sampled gas is always compared to a reference oxygen-nitrogen mixture.
11. These analyzers cannot be used with a flammable gas mixture because of the electric circuitry.

C. Analyzers operated on polarographic principle (Clark electrode)
   1. Basic overall chemical reaction occurring in electrode system is

$$O_2 + 2H_2O + 4 \text{ electrons} \rightarrow 4OH^-. \tag{1}$$

   2. The analyzer is composed of two electrodes immersed in a potassium chloride electrolyte solution.
      a. At the silver anode, oxidation of chloride ion to silver chloride takes place. This reaction releases electrons, developing a current.
      b. At the platinum cathode, oxygen is reduced to form OH^- ions, thus consuming electrons produced from the anode.

3. In solution, the greater the partial pressure of oxygen the greater the current used.
4. A negative 0.6 polarizing voltage is applied to the anode.
   a. This voltage is needed to maintain direction of current from anode to cathode through the electrolyte solution.
   b. At negative 0.6 volts oxygen is the only respiratory gas that will be readily reduced.
5. The tip of the Clark electrode is covered with a polypropylene membrane that allows slow diffusion of oxygen from blood or gas being analyzed.
6. This analyzer type directly measures partial pressure of the gas. For this reason the analyzer must be carefully calibrated at varying altitudes and to changing atmospheric pressures.
7. The analyzer may be used in all respiratory gas mixtures.
8. Measurement of flow of electrons is referred to as an amperometric principle.

D. Analyzers using a galvanic cell
   1. The galvanic cell is similar to a battery cell that utilizes oxygen to create a current between its electrodes.
   2. Current is continually produced if the cell is exposed to oxygen. Thus the life of the cell is dependent on duration and frequency of use.
   3. The analyzer is composed of two electrodes immersed in a potassium hydroxide electrolyte.
      a. A lead anode, in the presence of oxygen, produces a current as a result of an oxidation reaction with potassium hydroxide.
      b. A gold cathode, in the presence of oxygen, produces the following reaction:

$$O_2 + 2H_2O + 4 \text{ electrons} \rightarrow 4OH^-. \tag{2}$$

   (*Note:* Overall reactions for galvanic cell and polarographic analyzers are the same.)
   4. The current is measured from anode to the cathode, which allows completion of electric circuit.
   5. The greater the partial pressure of oxygen, the greater the measured current.
   6. As with the polarographic analyzer, the galvanic cell measures partial pressure of oxygen.

II. pH Electrode (Sanz)

A. The electrode is composed of two half-cells connected via a potassium chloride electrolyte bridge.
  1. A reference half-cell composed of mercury-mercurous chloride (calomel).
  2. A measuring half-cell composed of silver-silver chloride.
B. The measuring half-cell has two chambers separated by pH-sensitive glass, which allows measurement of voltage differences across the glass.
  1. The enclosed buffer chamber with a buffer of a constant pH surrounds the pH-sensitive glass capillary tube.
  2. The sample chamber capillary tube allows blood to be in contact with the pH-sensitive glass.
C. The reference half-cell is immersed in potassium chloride solution.
  1. Allows completion of basic electrical circuit while providing constant reference voltage.
D. As a result of electric activity on the pH-sensitive glass, a potential difference can be measured.
E. The potential difference is measured on a voltmeter calibrated in pH units.
F. This type of system comparing voltage measurements is termed potentiometric.

III. P_{CO_2} Electrode (Severinghaus)
A. The P_{CO_2} electrode is a modified pH electrode.
B. P_{CO_2} is measured indirectly by determining change in pH of the solution.
C. The electrode is composed of two half-cells, each composed of silver-silver chloride.
D. Functioning of electrode
  1. Carbon dioxide diffuses across a silicon membrane into a $NaHCO_3$ electrolyte.
  2. After entering the solution, carbon dioxide reacts with water to form hydrogen and bicarbonate ions:

$$CO_2 + H_2O \rightarrow H_2CO_3 \rightarrow H^+ + HCO_3^-. \tag{3}$$

  3. The H^+ formed sets up a potential difference across the pH-sensitive glass in the measuring half-cell.
E. All other aspects of the electrode are consistent with the pH electrode.
F. The potential difference is measured on a voltmeter and reflected as mm Hg carbon dioxide.

Note the P_{O_2} electrode (Clark) for blood gas analyzers is covered in section I, C.

BIBLIOGRAPHY

Egan, D. F.: *Fundamentals of Respiratory Therapy* (3d ed.; St. Louis: C. V. Mosby Co., 1977).

McPherson, S. P.: *Respiratory Therapy Equipment* (St. Louis: C. V. Mosby Co., 1977).

Shapiro, B. A., Harrison, R. A., and Walton, J. R.: *Clinical Application of Blood Gases* (2d ed.; Chicago: Year Book Medical Publishers, Inc., 1977).

Young, J. A., and Crocker, D.: *Principles and Practice of Respiratory Therapy* (2d ed.; Chicago: Year Book Medical Publishers, Inc., 1976).

17 / Gas Therapy

I. Medical, Laboratory and Therapeutic Gases and Mixtures
   A. Ethylene (C_2H_4)
   B. Nitrous oxide (N_2O)
   C. Cyclopropane (CH_2)$_3$
   D. Oxygen (O_2)
   E. Nitrogen (N_2)
   F. Carbon dioxide (CO_2)
   G. Helium (He)
   H. Oxygen/nitrogen (21% O_2/79% N_2)
   I. Oxygen/carbon dioxide (90–98% O_2/2–10% CO_2)
   J. Helium/oxygen (40–80% He/20–60% O_2)
II. Flammable Gases
   A. Ethylene
   B. Cyclopropane
III. Nonflammable Gases
   A. Nitrogen
   B. Carbon dioxide
   C. Helium
IV. Gases That Support Combustion
   A. Oxygen
   B. Helium/oxygen
   C. Oxygen/carbon dioxide
   D. Oxygen/nitrogen
   E. Nitrous oxide
V. Gas Cylinders
   A. Cylinder types and composition
      1. Type 3AA: Seamless, high quality heat-treated steel, spun chrome molybdenum
      2. Type 3A: Seamless, low carbon, heat-treated steel (no longer produced)
   B. Cylinder markings: Markings are located at the neck of the cylinder in two groupings.
      1. Group One
         a. Line One: ICC or DOT, 3A or 3AA, 2015*
            (1) ICC or DOT: The organization governing the transport of cylinder

        (2) 3A or 3AA: Cylinder type
        (3) 2015: Maximum working pressure in psi (pounds per square inch)
        (4) *Cylinder can be filled to 10% in excess of maximum working pressure (2200 psi)
    b. Line Two: E, 08687210
        (1) E: Cylinder size
        (2) 08687210: Cylinder serial number
    c. Line Three: NCG
        (1) NCG: Initial of owner
    d. Line Four: B
        (1) B: Inspector's mark
  2. Group Two
    a. Line One: Spun, Cr – Mo
        (1) Spun: Type of end sealing
        (2) Cr – Mo: Chrome molybdenum (type of manufacturing material)
    b. Line Two: USS, 6/50, 6/60, 6/70
        (1) USS: Manufacturer's symbol
        (2) 6/50: Date when cylinder was first hydrostatically tested
        (3) 6/60 and 6/70: Dates when cylinder was retested
    c. Line Three: EE – 10
        (1) EE – 10: Elastic expansion of cylinder in cubic centimeters of volume
C. Cylinder size
  1. Large cylinders using hex nut connections
    a. H or K: 9 in. diameter, 55 in. height
    b. G: 8½ in. diameter, 55 in. height
    c. M: 7⅛ in. diameter, 46 in. height
    d. F: 5½ in. diameter, 55 in. height
  2. Small cylinders using yoke connections
    a. E: 4¼ in. diameter, 30 in. height
    b. D: 4¼ in. diameter, 20 in. height
    c. B: 3½ in. diameter, 16 in. height
    d. A: 3 in. diameter, 10 in. height
D. Cylinder capacities for oxygen
  1. D: 12.7 cu ft
  2. E: 22 cu ft
  3. G: 187 cu ft
  4. H or K: 244 cu ft
E. Maximum filling pressure of 3AA oxygen cylinders: 2015 psi plus 10%.

F. Calculation of duration of flow from cylinders
   1. One cubic foot of gas = 28.3 L
   2. The volume of gas in liters in a full cylinder = cubic foot volume × 28.3 L/cu ft
   3. Dividing the above determined value by the maximum filling pressure of 2200 psi results in the calculation of a factor indicating the number of liters/pound/sq in.:

$$\text{Factor for duration of flow} = \frac{(\text{cu ft vol})(28.3 \text{ L/cu ft})}{2200 \text{ psi}}. \tag{1}$$

   4. For a D size cylinder:

$$\frac{(12.7 \text{ cu ft})(28.3 \text{ L/cu ft})}{2200 \text{ psi}} = 0.16 \text{ L/psi.}$$

   5. Liters per psi factors for oxygen cylinders
      a. D: 0.16 L/psi
      b. E: 0.28 L/psi
      c. G: 2.41 L/psi
      d. H or K: 3.14 L/psi
   6. Calculation of duration of flow in minutes
      a. Gauge pressure multiplied by duration of flow factor (L/psi) equals the number of liters in the cylinder.
      b. Dividing the result of 6a by the flow in liters/minute results in the time in minutes that the cylinder will last:

$$\text{Time in minutes cylinder will last} = \frac{(\text{Gauge pressure})(\text{duration of flow factor})}{(\text{Flow in L/min})}. \tag{2}$$

      c. Example for D cylinder:

$$24 \text{ minutes} = \frac{(1500 \text{ psi})(0.16 \text{ L/psi})}{(10 \text{ L/min})}.$$

      d. It is clinically advisable to subtract 500 psi from the gauge pressure to provide a safety margin before calculating duration of flow.
G. Color code for E cylinders (color coding is mandatory for E size cylinders only)
   1. Oxygen: Green (Universal code: white)
   2. Helium: Brown

3. Ethylene: Red
4. Cyclopropane: Orange
5. Nitrous oxide: Light blue
6. Carbon dioxide: Gray

H. Hydrostatic testing of cylinders
1. Cylinder expansion is determined by measuring water displacement of an empty cylinder compared to that cylinder when filled to 5/3 of its maximum pressure.
2. All cylinders must be retested every 5 to 10 years depending on elastic expansion of the original testing.

I. Cylinder stem pop-off valves
1. Large cylinders use a frangible disc designed to rupture at a pressure of within 5% of cylinder-bursting pressure.
2. Small cylinders use a fusable plug designed to melt at a temperature of 150–170 F.

VI. Regulation of Gas Flow
A. High pressure gas regulator
1. Regulators limit flow in a system by reducing maximum working pressure.
2. Regulators reduce cylinder pressures to a usable working pressure of 50 psi or less.
3. Single-stage regulator
   a. Cylinder pressure is reduced to a working pressure of up to 50 psi in one step or stage.
   b. One high pressure pop-off valve is incorporated in the regulator and set at about 200 psi.
4. Multistage regulator
   a. Cylinder pressure is reduced to a working pressure of up to 50 psi in a series of steps or stages.
   b. A high pressure pop-off valve is incorporated into each stage of the regulator, with the final stage pop-off set at about 200 psi.
5. Preset regulator
   a. Pressure is reduced in one or more stages to a fixed working pressure of 50 psi.
   b. Normally a low pressure gas-regulating device (i.e., Thorpe tube) is incorporated to reduce flows to working levels.
   c. Preset regulators are used without a Thorpe tube when connected to a system utilizing a 50 psi pressure source (i.e., ventilators).

6. Adjustable regulator
   a. Pressure is reduced in one or more stages to a final working pressure adjustable to between 0 and 50 psi.
   b. Normally a Bourdon pressure gauge calibrated in liters/minute measures flow leaving the final stage of the adjustable regulator.
B. Low pressure gas regulators (flowmeters)
   1. Bourdon gauge
      a. A pressure-sensitive gauge uses an expandable copper coil to indicate a pressure reading.
      b. Bourdon gauges can be calibrated to indicate flow and are used as flow-measuring devices.
      c. If back pressure is applied distal to the gauge, it will indicate a flow higher than actual flow.
   2. Thorpe tube flowmeters: The flow of gas is measured by the vertical displacement of a float in an increasing diameter tube. Flow is regulated by a needle valve placed proximal or distal to the float.
      a. Compensated Thorpe tubes are designed to function accurately at a working pressure of 50 psi at 70 F.
         (1) The needle valve is always located distal to the float.
         (2) If back pressure is applied distal to the needle valve, the float will indicate the actual flow delivered.
      b. Uncompensated Thorpe tubes are designed to function at variable working pressures.
         (1) The needle valve is always located proximal to the float.
         (2) If back pressure is applied distal to the float, the float will always indicate a flow lower than the actual flow delivered.
VII. Safety Systems Incorporated in Gas Flow Systems and Cylinders
   A. Pin Index Safety System (PISS)
      1. This is used only on E size cylinders or smaller.
      2. It is used on connections where the maximum working pressure is greater than 200 psig (pounds per square inch gauge).
      3. It incorporates a yoke type of connection where two pins on the regulator connection (yoke) are matched to holes on the cylinder stem.

       4. Ten possible combinations are available, nine currently in use.

       5. Pin positions 2–5 are used for oxygen.

  B. American Standard Compressed Gas Cylinder Valve Outlet and Inlet Connections Safety System

       1. This is used only on cylinders *larger than* E size.

       2. It is used on connections where the maximum working pressure is greater than 200 psig.

       3. It incorporates a hexagonal nut and specific nipple on the regulator fitted to an externally threaded cylinder connection.

       4. For oxygen the connection is CGA–540, 0.903–14 NGO, RH–Ext. A Compressed Gas Association connection no. 540 is used with a 0.903 inch threaded outlet diameter and 14 threads per inch of the National Gas Outlet type. The threads are external and right-handed.

  C. Diameter-Index Safety System (DISS)

       1. Used on all connections distal to the regulator where maximum working pressures are less than 200 psig.

       2. Used for connections of flowmeters to regulators or other connections where frequent equipment changes are made.

       3. It incorporates a hexagonal nut and a nipple designed with two shoulders fitted into a body and externally threaded with two concentric borings.

       4. DISS connection for oxygen is no. 1240 with a 0.5625 inch diameter and 18 threads per inch.

VIII. Agencies Regulating Medical Gases

  A. Food and Drug Administration (FDA): Determines purity standards and labeling for all medical gases listed in the United States Pharmacopeia (USP).

  B. Compressed Gas Association (CGA): Sets standards and makes recommendations to manufacturers and municipal authorities on manufacture of gases and on safety standards for cylinders.

  C. National Fire Prevention Agency (NFPA): Sets standards and makes recommendations to manufacturers and municipal authorities on storage and handling of cylinders.

  D. Department of Transportation (DOT): Regulates interstate transport of cylinders, safety systems on cylinders and hydrostatic testing methods.

IX. Fractional Distillation of Air
   A. The gas is filtered to remove all dust and impurities.
   B. The gas is dried to remove all water vapor.
   C. The gas is compressed to 200 atm. pressure.
   D. The heat of compression is removed by heat exchangers until the temperature returns to ambient.
   E. The gas is then rapidly decompressed with the pressure dropped by 5 atm., allowing tremendous cooling by expansion. This brings the temperature below the boiling point and liquefies all gases in the air.
   F. The temperature of the liquid is then increased and the various gases evaporated and collected at their respective boiling points.

BIBLIOGRAPHY

Burton, G. G., Gee, G. N., and Hodgkin, J. E.: *Respiratory Care: A Guide to Clinical Practice* (Philadelphia: J. B. Lippincott Co., 1977).

Compressed Gas Association: *Handbook of Compressed Gases* (New York: Van Nostrand Reinhold Company, 1966).

Egan, D. F.: *Fundamentals of Respiratory Therapy* (3d ed.; St. Louis: C. V. Mosby Co., 1977).

McPherson, S. P.: *Respiratory Therapy Equipment* (St. Louis: C. V. Mosby Co., 1977).

Young, J. A., and Crocker, D.: *Principles and Practice of Respiratory Therapy* (2d ed.; Chicago: Year Book Medical Publishers, Inc., 1976).

18 / Oxygen Therapy

I. General Characteristics of Oxygen
   A. Colorless
   B. Odorless
   C. Tasteless
   D. Molecular weight: 32 gm
   E. Density at STP: 1.43 gm/L
   F. Boiling point at 1 atm: -297.4 F (-183 C)
   G. Melting point at 1 atm: -361.1 F (-216.6 C)
   H. Critical temperature: -181.1 F (-118.4 C)
   I. Critical pressure: 736.9 psia (pounds per square inch absolute)
   J. Triple point: -361.89 F (-218.7 C) at 0.2321 psia
   K. Forms oxides with all elements except inert gases
   L. Constitutes about 20.95% of atmosphere
   M. Used at cellular level as the final electron acceptor in electron transport chain located in mitochondria of cell
II. Categories of Hypoxia
   A. Anemic hypoxia: Decreased carrying capacity of blood for oxygen
      1. Anemia
      2. Carbon monoxide poisoning
      3. Rarely accompanied by hypoxemia
   B. Stagnant hypoxia: Decreased cardiac output resulting in increased systemic transit time.
      1. Shock
      2. Cardiovascular instability
      3. Regional vasoconstriction
   C. Histotoxic hypoxia: Inability of tissue to utilize available oxygen.
      1. Cyanide poisoning
      2. Rarely accompanied by hypoxemia
   D. Hypoxemic hypoxia: Decrease in diffusion of oxygen across alveolar capillary membrane.
      1. Low inspired $F_{I_{O_2}}$
      2. Ventilation/perfusion inequalities

      3. Increased true shunt

      4. Cardiac anomalies

III. Effects of Hypoxemia

    A. Primary effect: Increase in heart rate and force of contraction.

    B. Increase in tidal volume and respiratory rate.

    C. Constriction of pulmonary vascular bed.

    D. Generalized vasoconstriction of vascular beds supplying skin, muscles and abdominal viscera.

    E. Vasodilatation may be seen in vascular beds supplying heart and brain.

IV. Indications for Oxygen Therapy

    A. Hypoxemia

      1. Oxygen therapy increases alveolar PO_2, thus increasing the pressure gradient for oxygen diffusion into bloodstream.

      2. Increasing the pressure gradient may cause an increase in Pa_{O_2}.

    B. Excessive work of breathing

      1. Hypoxemia stimulates peripheral chemoreceptors, causing an increase in rate and depth of ventilation and increasing work of breathing.

      2. Oxygen therapy, by increasing alveolar PO_2, may increase arterial PO_2. This will reduce stimulation of peripheral chemoreceptors and reduce work of breathing.

    C. Excessive myocardial work

      1. The primary compensatory response to hypoxemia is an increase in force and rate of contraction of the heart.

      2. Oxygen therapy may correct hypoxemia and decrease the stimulus to increase cardiac output.

V. Hazards of Oxygen Therapy

    A. Retrolental fibroplasia (RLF)

      1. RLF is a fibrotic process occurring behind the lens of the eye, causing blindness. Fibrotic changes prevent penetration of light to the retina.

      2. RLF is primarily confined to the premature neonate receiving oxygen and maintained with arterial PO_2 above 80–100 mm Hg for extended periods (exact Pa_{O_2} levels necessary for development of RLF have not been established).

      3. Elevated PO_2 levels cause severe vasoconstriction of blood vessels leading to retina, resulting in fibrotic changes.

    B. Oxygen toxicity

      1. A series of reversible pathophysiologic changes occurs

over the lung fields, with predominance in lower lobes. Oxygen toxicity is primarily a result of exposure to high concentrations of oxygen for prolonged periods.

2. In general, a FI_{O_2} of 0.50 or greater for prolonged periods shows an increased incidence of oxygen toxicity. Oxygen toxicity may develop at a lower FI_{O_2}.

3. Pulmonary changes
   a. *Exudative phase:* Seen early in development of oxygen toxicity when increased permeability of capillary endothelial cells results in alveolar congestion, intra-alveolar hemorrhage and a fibrinous exudation (development of a hyaline membrane).
   b. *Proliferative phase:* Characterized by hyperplasia and dysfunction of type II alveolar pneumocytes, thickening of the alveolar capillary membrane and early changes associated with fibrosis.

4. Signs and symptoms
   a. Normally the first symptoms involve substernal burning discomfort, cough, paresthesia, nausea and vomiting.
   b. As a result of type II alveolar cell dysfunction, pulmonary surfactant production is interfered with and/or its effectiveness is reduced.
   c. X-ray results are similar to those associated with a diffuse patchy atelectasis or pneumonitis.
   d. Pulmonary compliance is decreased, work of breathing is increased, FRC levels are decreased and refractive hypoxemia is present (see Chapter 15, Section II).

C. Oxygen-induced hypoventilation
   1. This is observed in patients with chronic CO_2 retention or CNS depression.
   2. The increased Pa_{O_2} decreases or eliminates the hypoxic drive, inducing greater levels of hypoventilation.
   3. Intermittent use of oxygen therapy may cause arterial P_{O_2} to fall below pretreatment levels.

D. Absorption atelectasis
   1. Nitrogen is metabolically inactive and exists in about 80% by volume of alveolar gas. Nitrogen assists in maintaining alveolar stability.
   2. High FI_{O_2} replaces nitrogen with oxygen.
   3. In poorly ventilated alveoli, oxygen would be continually absorbed by the bloodstream but may not be replaced by

normal ventilation. As a result, alveolar size would continually decrease.

4. As alveoli reach their critical volume, collapse would occur, resulting in atelectasis.

5. This commonly occurs in patients with small tidal volumes and/or poor distribution of ventilation due to airway obstruction.

VI. Oxygen Delivery Systems

A. In general, delivery systems are divided into two categories: high flow and low flow.

B. High flow systems

1. The patient's entire inspired atmosphere is consistently and predictably delivered by the system.

2. To maintain a consistent $F_{I_{O_2}}$, the apparatus should deliver a total flow at least *three times* the patient's measured minute volume.

a. Normal I:E ratios are 1:2. This ratio indicates that total inspiratory time per minute is 20 seconds, i.e., the patient's entire minute volume will be inspired in a 20-second period. Three times the patient's minute volume indicates the flow necessary over a 1-minute period to meet the patient's 20-second inspiratory time demands.

b. Normal peak inspiratory flows are about 3 times the patient's measured minute volume.

c. This flow usually will provide adequate volume in the face of a changing ventilatory pattern.

3. The flow from the system always must be at least three times the patient's measured minute volume to insure a consistent $F_{I_{O_2}}$.

4. Typical high flow systems

a. Ventimasks: Deliver a specific $F_{I_{O_2}}$ normally up to 40% (Table 18–1).

b. Mechanical aerosol systems: Set up singly or in tandem to deliver high humidity along with a specific $F_{I_{O_2}}$ (see Table 18–1).

c. Cascade-type humidifier system

(1) Volume and concentration of gas determined by titration of compressed air and oxygen or use of oxygen blender.

(2) Virtually any $F_{I_{O_2}}$ available.

(3) Virtually any flow available.

TABLE 18–1.—ENTRAINMENT RATIOS AND OUTPUTS
OF SPECIFIC VENTURI SYSTEMS

SYSTEM	$F_{I_{O_2}}$	ENTRAINMENT RATIO	FLOW AT WHICH OPERATED	TOTAL FLOW (L/MIN)
Ventimasks	0.24	1–25	3	78
	0.28	1–10	3	33
	0.31	1–7	3	24
	0.35	1–5	6	36
	0.40	1–3	6	24
Mechanical	0.60	1–1	10	20
aerosol	0.70	1–0.6	10	16

        (4) Extremely versatile, may be applied to a patient via an aerosol mask or standard artificial airway attachment.

    d. Determination of $F_{I_{O_2}}$ with any combined flow system:

$$(1)$$
$$F_{I_{O_2}} = \frac{(F_{I_{O_2}} \text{ system A})(\text{flow of A}) + (F_{I_{O_2}} \text{ system B})(\text{flow of B}) + \text{etc.}}{\text{total flow of combined systems}}$$

C. Low flow systems

    1. The total minute volume is not delivered by the apparatus.

    2. The $F_{I_{O_2}}$ delivered to the patient depends on

        a. Flow of gas from equipment

        b. Patient anatomical reservoir (oral and nasal cavity)

        c. Reservoir of equipment

        d. Patient respiratory rate, tidal volume and I : E ratio

    3. The $F_{I_{O_2}}$ delivered with any low flow system is extremely variable and unpredictable.

    4. If the patient's minute volume were to increase on a particular piece of equipment, his $F_{I_{O_2}}$ *would decrease.* The patient would entrain a larger percentage of room air in his minute volume.

    5. If the patient's minute volume were to decrease on a particular piece of equipment, his $F_{I_{O_2}}$ *would increase.* The patient would entrain a smaller percentage of room air in his minute volume.

    6. *The circumstances in which the $F_{I_{O_2}}$ is determined are very specific, showing the lack of accurate predictability of the $F_{I_{O_2}}$ in an actual clinical setting.* Below is an example calculation of a patient's $F_{I_{O_2}}$ when breathing with a cannula at 6 L/min.

a. Ventilatory parameters
   (1) Respiratory rate: 20/min
   (2) Tidal volume: 500 cc
   (3) I:E ratio: 1:2
   (4) Inspiratory time: 1 second
   (5) Volume of patient's anatomical reservoir, (volume of oral and nasal cavity): 50 cc
b. Volume delivered by cannula per second
   (1) Flow is 6 L/min, which equals 6000 cc/min
   (2) 100 cc/sec is thus delivered to patient.
c. Volume of 100% oxygen inspired per breath
   (1) 100 cc is delivered by cannula in the 1-second inspiratory time.
   (2) 50 cc volume of oxygen is accumulated in anatomical reservoir prior to inspiration (accumulates during expiratory pause).
   (3) If 150 cc is inspired from (1) and (2) above, then 350 cc of room air would need to be entrained. Since about 20% of room air is oxygen, 70 cc of oxygen is entrained.
   (4) The total amount of oxygen per tidal volume is equal to 220 cc:

$$100 \text{ cc} + 50 \text{ cc} + 70 \text{ cc} = 220 \text{ cc}. \tag{2}$$

d. The percentage that the 220 cc of inspired oxygen constitutes of the patient's total tidal volume (V_T) is the inspired F_{IO_2}:

$$\frac{220 \; (O_2)}{500 \; (V_T)} = F_{IO_2} \text{ of } 0.44. \tag{3}$$

e. *It must be kept in mind that the F_{IO_2} listed for each low flow system is purely speculative and that the F_{IO_2} is totally dependent on the patient's ventilatory pattern.*
7. Using similar calculations for other low flow systems, the following estimates of the delivered F_{IO_2} are calculated (RR = 20, I:E ratio = 1:2, V_T = 500 cc). It should be remembered that these are purely estimates and vary considerably from patient to patient.
   a. *O_2 cannula*
      (1) 1 L/min F_{IO_2}: 0.24
      (2) 2 L/min F_{IO_2}: 0.28
      (3) 3 L/min F_{IO_2}: 0.32

    (4) 4 L/min FI_{O_2}: 0.36

    (5) 5 L/min FI_{O_2}: 0.40

    (6) 6 L/min FI_{O_2}: 0.44

b. *Simple O₂ mask:* Should be run between 5 and 8 L/min to insure flushing and prevent CO_2 buildup in face mask. This flow will result in an FI_{O_2} between 0.40 and 0.60, *depending on patient's ventilatory pattern.*

c. *O₂ mask with bag* (partial rebreathing mask): Should be run between 7 and 10 L/min. Flow must be adequate to insure that bag deflates only about one-third during inspiration and to prevent CO_2 buildup in system. This flow will result in an FI_{O_2} between 0.70 and 0.95, *depending on patient's ventilatory pattern.*

d. *Non-rebreathing mask:* Must be run with sufficient flow to prevent bag from collapsing during inspiration. Non-rebreathing masks are difficult to use properly on patients with a high minute volume. A high flow cascade set-up is more practical for 1.0 FI_{O_2} administration. If a non-rebreathing mask is functioning properly, the FI_{O_2} is 0.90 to 1.0, *depending on patient's ventilatory pattern.*

BIBLIOGRAPHY

Bendixen, H. H., et al.: *Respiratory Care* (St. Louis: C. V. Mosby Co., 1965).

Burton, G. G., Gee, G. N., and Hodgkin, J. E.: *Respiratory Care: A Guide to Clinical Practice* (Philadelphia: J. B. Lippincott Co., 1977).

Egan, D. F.: *Fundamentals of Respiratory Therapy* (3d ed.; St. Louis: C. V. Mosby Co., 1977).

McPherson, S. P.: *Respiratory Care Equipment* (St. Louis: C. V. Mosby Co., 1977).

Safar, P. (ed.): *Respiratory Therapy* (Philadelphia: F. A. Davis Co., 1965).

Shapiro, B. A., Harrison, R. A., and Trout, C. A.: *Clinical Application of Respiratory Care* (Chicago: Year Book Medical Publishers, Inc., 1975).

Young, J. A., and Crocker, D.: *Principles and Practice of Respiratory Therapy* (2d ed.; Chicago: Year Book Medical Publishers, Inc., 1976).

19 / Intermittent Positive Pressure Breathing (IPPB)

I. Physiologic Effects on the Respiratory System
   A. Positive pressure breathing reverses the normal intrathoracic and intrapulmonary pressure relationship. With IPPB, the mean intrathoracic pressure is most positive during inspiration and least positive during expiration. Figures 6–1 and 6–2 depict normal intrathoracic and intrapulmonary pressure curves. These pressure curves are considerably altered during IPPB and may cause decreases in venous return and cardiac output (Fig 19–1).
   B. Mechanical bronchodilation is accomplished by increasing intraluminal to extraluminal pressure difference. The greater this difference the greater the degree of dilatation.
   C. Work of breathing with properly applied IPPB treatment may be significantly decreased. Since IPPB provides the ventilatory power, the work of the patient's ventilatory muscles is reduced.
      1. This allows the same degree of alveolar ventilation with far less expenditure of muscular energy.
      2. Decreased work of breathing occurs only during therapy, unless significant areas of atelectasis are reversed or a significant volume of secretions is mobilized.
   D. I:E ratios may be manipulated during properly applied IPPB treatment. This is accomplished by restoring a more efficient ventilatory pattern. Under most circumstances, this pattern is maintained only during therapy.
   E. The tidal volume (VT) may be increased by three to four times the patient's resting spontaneous tidal exchange during IPPB therapy.
   F. Secretions are more effectively mobilized during IPPB treatment. This is accomplished by improved distribution of inspired gas and mechanical dilatation of the airway.
   G. Pa_{O_2} normally is increased and P_{CO_2} normally is decreased *during* IPPB treatment. Improved alveolar ventilation during therapy may result in better gas exchange.

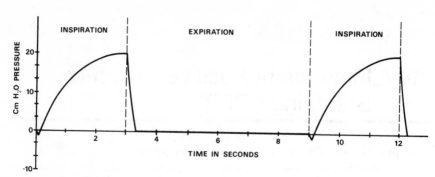

Fig 19–1.—Ideal intrapulmonary pressure curve associated with administration of intermittent positive pressure breathing (IPPB).

II. Indications for IPPB
   A. Primary indication: Inability to cough and/or deep breathe adequately.
      1. The efficiency of coughing and deep breathing is markedly decreased if patient is unable to perform a vital capacity (VC) maneuver of greater than three times his predicted VT.
      2. If patient's VC falls below the value in 1. and there is evidence of pulmonary congestion or poor distribution of ventilation IPPB therapy appears to be indicated.
III. Goals
   A. To provide a significantly deeper breath with more physiologic I:E ratios than patient can produce with spontaneous ventilation
   B. To improve and promote cough mechanism
      1. Optimal peripheral distribution of air through a slow, deep inspiration with an end inspiratory pause.
      2. Mechanical provision of necessary power.
   C. To improve distribution of ventilation
      1. In patients with ventilation/perfusion inequalities.
      2. Incidence of postoperative atelectasis and pneumonia is potentially decreased and already atelectatic alveoli may be re-expanded.
   D. To deliver medication
      1. Only if no means other than IPPB (hand-held nebulizer) can safely and conveniently deliver the medication. The mechanical advantages of IPPB have been overshadowed by its use to deliver medication.

IV. Administration
  A. Efficacy of IPPB treatment is greatly dependent on the therapist.
  B. Requirements for ideal administration of effective IPPB treatment
    1. Knowledgeable, well-trained therapist completely familiar with operation, maintenance and clinical application of equipment.
    2. Relaxed, informed, cooperative patient.
    3. Concise concept of therapeutic goals by physician, therapist and patient.
    4. Pressure-limited machine.
    5. Appropriate cough and breathing instruction.
    6. Honest appraisal by therapist of benefits from therapy for particular patient.
V. Hazards
  A. Hyperventilation
    1. Incorrect administration of IPPB often causes rapid, deep ventilation leading to acute alveolar hyperventilation.
      a. Possible results
        (1) Dizziness
        (2) Loss of consciousness
        (3) Tetany
    2. Decreased cerebrovascular PCO_2 during hyperventilation causes vasoconstriction and decreased cerebral blood flow.
  B. Excessive oxygenation
    1. When driven with oxygen, pneumatically powered, pressure-limited machines give excessively high oxygen concentrations. These high concentrations are potentially harmful to COPD patients who are breathing on a "hypoxic drive."
    2. The high oxygen concentration can be avoided by using machines powered by air compressors or by using a compressed air source.
  C. Increased air trapping
    1. Causes
      a. Excessive ventilation of partially obstructed areas in patients with severe COPD.
      b. Posttreatment an increase in difficulty of ventilation due to increased FRC

D. Decreased cardiac output
1. Spontaneous ventilation normally facilitates venous return. Increasingly negative intrathoracic pressure on inspiration widens the pressure gradient between abdominal viscera and thoracic cavity. This enhances venous return via inferior vena cava and is called the thoracoabdominal pump.
2. IPPB ablates the thoracoabdominal pump by causing a less negative or possible positive mean intrathoracic pressure during inspiration.
3. Proper I:E ratios in conjunction with minimal airway pressures help to minimize the above.
4. Clinical signs of decreased cardiac output
a. Tachycardia
b. Dyspnea
c. Distended neck veins
d. Anxiety
E. Increased intracranial pressure
1. Cranial venous drainage is potentially impeded by increased mean intrathoracic pressure.
2. This results in an increase in intracranial pressure, since more blood is contained in the cranium and the volume of the cranium is fixed.
F. Pneumothorax
1. IPPB mouth pressures of 20 cm H_2O seldom result in excessive alveolar pressures. These pressures by themselves normally are not high enough to cause a "bleb" to rupture.
2. IPPB may result in better distribution of ventilation and gas entering poorly ventilated lung area (e.g., a bleb), during IPPB treatment. With a good cough, increased intra-alveolar pressure could rupture a bleb, resulting in pneumothorax.
3. Possible complaints of chest pain with or after coughing should be anticipated.
4. If pneumothorax occurs, IPPB should be discontinued until chest decompression is accomplished.
G. Hemoptysis
1. May occur due to increase in cough effectiveness that follows IPPB.
2. Usually the result of bronchial venous bleeding; may be secondary to a tumor or to blood vessel rupture.

VI. Absolute Contraindication
   A. Untreated tension pneumothorax
      1. Tension is increased with positive pressure due to one-way check-valve mechanism.
      2. IPPB treatment should not be initiated until chest decompression is performed.

BIBLIOGRAPHY

Burton, G. G., Gee, G. N., and Hodgkin, J. E.: *Respiratory Care: A Guide to Clinical Practice* (Philadelphia: J. B. Lippincott Co., 1977).

Egan, D. F.: *Fundamentals of Respiratory Therapy* (3d ed.; St. Louis: C. V. Mosby Co., 1977).

Noehren, T. H.: Is positive pressure breathing overrated? Chest 57:507, 1970.

Noehren, T. H., et al.: Intermittent positive pressure breathing for the prevention and management of postoperative pulmonary complications, Surgery 43:658, 1958.

Safar, P. (ed.): *Respiratory Therapy* (Philadelphia: F. A. Davis Co., 1965).

Shapiro, B. A., Harrison, R. A., and Trout, C. A.: *Clinical Application of Respiratory Care* (Chicago: Year Book Medical Publishers, Inc., 1975).

Young, J. A., and Crocker, D.: *Principles and Practice of Respiratory Therapy* (2nd ed.; Chicago: Year Book Medical Publishers, Inc., 1976).

20 / Aerosol Therapy

An aerosol is a suspension of liquid or solid particles in a gas such as smoke or fog.

I. Stability: Tendency of particles to remain in suspension.
   A. Factors governing stability
      1. Size: The smaller the aerosol particle the greater the tendency toward stability. The larger the particle the greater the tendency to rain out of suspension.
      2. Concentration: The greater the concentration of particles the greater the tendency for individual particles to coalesce into larger particles and rain out of suspension.
      3. Humidity: The greater the relative humidity of the gas carrying the aerosol the greater the stability of the aerosol.

II. Penetration and Deposition
   A. Penetration refers to the depth within the respiratory tract that an aerosol reaches. Deposition is the rain-out of aerosol particles within the respiratory tract.
   B. Depth of penetration and volume of deposition depend on
      1. Gravity: Gravity decreases penetration and increases premature deposition but has minimal effect on particles in the therapeutic range of $1-5\,\mu$ (Table 20-1).
      2. Kinetic energy: The greater the kinetic energy of the gas carrying the particles the greater the tendency for premature deposition. This is because coalescence and impaction are increased.
      3. Inertial impaction: Deposition of particles is increased at any point of directional change or increased airway resistance. Thus the smaller the airway diameter the greater the tendency for deposition.

III. Ventilatory Pattern
   A. This is the most important variable that can be controlled to insure maximum penetration and deposition of aerosol particles.
      1. Patients should be instructed to breathe with a large, slowly inspired tidal volume.

TABLE 20–1.—PENETRATION AND DEPOSITION VS. PARTICLE SIZE

PARTICLE SIZE (μ)	DEPOSITION IN RESPIRATORY TRACT
> 100	Do not enter respiratory tract
100 – 10	Trapped in mouth
100 – 5	Trapped in nose
5 – 2	Deposited proximal to alveoli
2 – 1	Can enter alveoli, 95 – 100% of particles 1μ in size settling
1 – 0.25	Stable, with minimal settling

     2. Incorporating a momentary inspiratory hold and a slow respiratory rate will aid in penetration and deposition.

  B. This pattern cannot be assumed by all patients, but an attempt to achieve it should always be made.

IV. Clearance of Aerosols

  A. Inhaled particles are removed from the respiratory tract by three mechanisms.

     1. Primary mechanism: Mucociliary escalator, which moves about 100 ml of secretions to the oropharynx per day (see Chapter 3, Section I – C).

     2. Normal cough mechanism.

     3. Phagocytosis by type III alveolar cells.

V. Goals of Therapy

  A. Improve bronchial hygiene

     1. Hydrate dried retained secretions.

     2. Improve efficiency of cough mechanism.

     3. Restore and maintain normal function of mucociliary escalator.

  B. Humidify gases delivered to patients with artificial airways.

  C. Deliver medications.

VI. Hazards of Therapy

  A. Precipitation of bronchoconstriction

     1. Most common in asthmatic patients.

     2. May follow administration of certain drugs (i.e., acetylcysteine).

  B. Increased airway obstruction because of swelling of dried retained secretions

     1. Usually a problem with ultrasonic nebulizers more frequently than with mechanical aerosols.

     2. Seen primarily in debilitated patients with a poor cough mechanism.

C. Systemic fluid overload
  1. Primarily a problem with neonates and infants.
  2. Associated with use of ultrasonic nebulizers more frequently than of mechanical nebulizers.
D. Cross contamination
VII. Mechanical Aerosol Generators
  A. These generators use the Venturi effect to produce an aerosol and entrain a second gas.
  B. A system of baffles is utilized to impact out large particles.
  C. These generators are commonly used in delivery of medications and for humidification of inspired gases.
VIII. Ultrasonic Aerosol Generators
  A. The frequency range − 1 – 2 megacycles per second − for ultrasonic sound waves of ultrasonic nebulizers is governed by the Federal Commerce Commission. All ultrasonic nebulizers produced and sold in the United States have preset frequencies in this range.
  B. Ultrasonic nebulizers function by transforming standard household current into ultrasonic sound waves.
  C. The ultrasonic sound waves are applied to a quartz crystal or ceramic disc, causing it to vibrate at the same frequency as the ultrasonic waves. This is referred to as the piezoelectric quality of the disc.
  D. The crystal or disc transfers its vibratory energy to the fluid to be nebulized, creating an aerosol.
  E. These nebulizers incorporate an amplitude control that varies the intensity of ultrasonic waves, allowing varying aerosol (medication) outputs.
  F. Ultrasonic nebulizers are principally used in maintenance of bronchial hygiene.
IX. Comparison of Mechanical and Ultrasonic Nebulizers
  A. Total volume of aerosol output
    1. Mechanical nebulizers: Up to 1 – 1.5 cc/min.
    2. Ultrasonic nebulizers: Up to 6 cc/min.
  B. Particle size
    1. Mechanical nebulizers: 55% of particles produced fall in therapeutic range of $1-5\,\mu$
    2. Ultrasonic nebulizers: 97% of particles produced fall in therapeutic range of $1-5\,\mu$
X. Individual Model Specifications
  A. DeVilbiss

1. Model 900
   a. Frequency: 1.35 megacycles/sec
   b. Couplant: Distilled H_2O
   c. Output: Up to 3 cc/min
   d. Blower: 24 L/min
2. Model 800
   a. Frequency: 1.35 megacycles/sec
   b. Couplant: Distilled H_2O
   c. Output: Up to 6 cc/min
   d. Blower: 24 L/min
3. Models 35 and 35A
   a. Frequency: 1.35 megacycles/sec
   b. Couplant: Tap H_2O
   c. Output: Up to 3 cc/min
   d. Blower: 24 L/min

B. Monaghan
1. Model 670
   a. Frequency: 1.65 megacycles/sec
   b. Couplant: Same as medication
   c. Output: Up to 3 cc/min
   d. Blower: 21 L/min
2. Model 675
   a. Frequency: 1.65 megacycles/sec
   b. Couplant: Same as medication
   c. Output: Up to 6 cc/min
   d. Blower: 35 L/min

C. Mistogen
1. Models 140, 143 and 145
   a. Frequency: 1.40 megacycles/sec
   b. Couplant: Tap H_2O
   c. Output: Up to 6 cc/min
   d. Blower: 24 L/min

BIBLIOGRAPHY

Bendixen, H. H., et al.: *Respiratory Care* (St. Louis: C. V. Mosby Co., 1965).

Burton, G. G., Gee, G. N., and Hodgkin, J. E.: *Respiratory Care: A Guide to Clinical Practice* (Philadelphia: J. B. Lippincott Co., 1977).

Egan, D. F.: *Fundamentals of Respiratory Therapy* (3d ed.; St. Louis: C. V. Mosby Co., 1977).

McPherson, S. P.: *Respiratory Therapy Equipment* (St. Louis: C. V. Mosby Co., 1977).

Miller, W.: Fundamental principles of aerosol therapy, Respir. Care 17:295, 1972.

Safar, P. (ed.): *Respiratory Therapy* (Philadelphia: F. A. Davis Co., 1965).

Shapiro, B. A., Harrison, R. A., and Trout, C. A.: *Clinical Application of Respiratory Care* (Chicago: Year Book Medical Publishers, Inc., 1975).

Young, J. A., and Crocker, D.: *Principles and Practice of Respiratory Therapy* (2d ed.; Chicago: Year Book Medical Publishers, Inc., 1976).

21 / Chest Physiotherapy

I. Postural Drainage
   A. Postural drainage is a method of removing pooled secretions by positioning the patient so as to allow gravity to assist in movement of secretions. The patient is placed with the dependent lung segment as vertical as possible.
   B. Indications
      1. Excessive accumulation of secretions, as seen in many acute or chronic pulmonary diseases.
      2. Retained secretions caused by dehydration and pulmonary disease.
      3. Prophylactic care of preoperative patient with history of pulmonary problems or potential postoperative pulmonary problems.
   C. Standard postural drainage positions
      1. *Apical segments of right upper lobes:* Patient in semi-Fowler's position with head of the bed raised 45 degrees.
      2. *Anterior segments of both upper lobes:* Patient supine with the bed flat.
      3. *Posterior segments of right upper lobe:* Patient one-quarter turn from prone with the right side up, supported by pillows with head of the bed flat.
      4. *Apical-posterior segment of left upper lobe:* Patient one-quarter turn from prone with the left side up, supported by pillows with head of the bed elevated 30 degrees.
      5. *Medial and lateral segments of right middle lobe:* Patient one-quarter turn from supine with right side up and foot of the bed elevated 12–14 inches.
      6. *Superior and inferior segments of lingula:* Patient one-quarter turn from supine with left side up and foot of the bed elevated 12–14 inches.
      7. *Superior segments of both lower lobes:* Patient prone with head of the bed flat and pillow under abdominal area.
      8. *Anteromedial segment of left lower lobe and anterior segment of right lower lobe:* Patient supine, with foot of the bed elevated 18–20 inches.

      9. *Lateral segment of right lower lobe:* Patient directly on left side with right side up and foot of the bed elevated 18–20 inches.

    10. *Lateral segment of left lower lobe:* Patient directly on right side, with left side up and foot of the bed elevated 18–20 inches.

    11. *Posterior segment of both lower lobes:* Patient prone with foot of the bed elevated 18–20 inches.

  D. *The standard positions listed are not always feasible due to the patient's overall medical condition. If a position is medically unsafe or causes increased patient discomfort, the position must be modified to suit the clinical situation.*

  E. General precautions
1. Empyema
2. Pulmonary embolus
3. Open wounds, skin grafts, burns
4. Untreated tension pneumothorax
5. Flail chest
6. Frank hemoptysis
7. Orthopedic procedures
8. Acute spinal cord injuries

  F. Precautions and relative contraindications to head-down positioning
1. Unstable cardiac status
2. Hypertension
3. Head injuries
4. Thoracic surgery
5. Abdominal surgery
6. Diaphragmatic surgery
7. Tracheal-esophageal surgery
8. COPD
9. Obesity
10. Recent meals or tube feeding

II. Percussion

  A. Percussion is a technique of rhythmically tapping the chest wall with cupped hands. It is designed to loosen secretions in the area underlying the percussion by the air pressure that is generated by the cupped hand on the chest wall. Percussion is performed during inspiration and expiration.

  B. Indications (same as those for postural drainage, Section I, B)

  C. Precautions and relative contraindications
1. Cancer with known metastatic changes

2. Anticoagulant therapy
3. Tuberculosis
4. Petechiae
5. Osteoporotic changes
6. Empyema
7. Pulmonary embolus
8. Wounds, skin grafts, burns
9. Untreated tension pneumothorax
10. Flail chest
11. Frank hemoptysis
12. Acute spinal cord injuries
13. Limited patient tolerance
14. Chest tubes
15. Unstable cardiac status
16. Thoracic surgery

III. Vibrations
   A. Vibrations are performed by placing one hand on top of the other over the affected area and tensing the shoulders, keeping the arms straight and applying a vibrating action from shoulder to hand.
   B. Vibrations are intended to move secretions into larger airways.
   C. Vibrations are applied only during exhalation.
   D. Indications (same as those for postural drainage, Section I, B).
   E. Precautions and relative contraindications are similar to those for percussion.

IV. Breathing Retraining
   A. These techniques are designed to assist patients with muscular weakness, postoperative pain or chronic pulmonary disease to assume an efficient ventilatory pattern.
   B. Goals
      1. To increase and improve ventilation
      2. To strengthen respiratory musculature
      3. To prevent development of atelectasis
      4. To decrease work of breathing
   C. Specific techniques
      1. Diaphragmatic breathing exercises
         a. Therapist and patient locate the xiphoid process. Patient is instructed to "sniff" to determine location of diaphragm.
         b. Patient is relaxed, supported with a pillow and directed to inspire by contracting the abdomen slowly and

completely to allow a normal inspiratory pattern, i.e., diaphragm contracting, lateral chest expansion and then upper chest expansion.

    c. Patient is encouraged to exhale slowly and completely. Therapist may assist exhalation by a slight inward and upward pressure below xiphoid process.

  2. Lateral costal expansion exercises

    a. Therapist places his hands over patient's lower rib cage with the thumbs just above the xiphoid process.

    b. Patient is encouraged to relax and inspire against a slight pressure exerted by therapist's hands. Patient is instructed to try to expand area located under therapist's hands.

    c. Exhalation should be passive but complete. Therapist can assist exhalation by applying an inward and downward pressure during exhalation.

  3. Localized expansion exercises are designed to direct gas flow to specific area of lung.

    a. Therapist places his hands over problem area and instructs patient to inspire against a slight pressure exerted by therapist.

    b. Exhalation should be passive, complete and assisted by therapist. Therapist exerts an inward and downward force during exhalation following the natural contours of the rib cage.

V. Cough Instruction

  A. Normal cough

    1. A deep inspiration.

    2. Closure of glottis.

    3. Contraction of abdominal muscles, building up intrapulmonary pressure.

    4. Opening of glottis and a rapid forceful exhalation.

  B. Cough assistance indicated in the patient who cannot develop a forceful cough.

    1. Therapist places his hands on the sides of rib cage and pushes inward and downward during forced exhalation.

    2. Care should be taken to follow normal anatomical movement of chest.

  C. "Huffing" (in patients with ineffective cough)

    1. Patient is instructed to perform short, steplike coughs consisting of small volumes.

D. "Panting"
1. Patient is instructed to follow normal cough sequence but tongue is kept forward to prevent swallowing of secretions.

VI. Incentive Spirometry
A. Incentive spirometry: Use of a visual aid in coaching patients to take deep breaths.
B. Primary indication: Postoperative patient who is able to inspire deeply but requires visual encouragement and a regimented program.
C. Primary goal: Prophylactic prevention of alveolar collapse.
D. Requisites for success
1. Proper instruction in use of specific spirometer
2. Motivation
3. Follow-up procedure

BIBLIOGRAPHY

Bartlett, R. H., Gazzaniza, A. B., and Gerahty, T. R.: Respiratory maneuvers to prevent postoperative pulmonary complications, J.A.M.A. 22:1017, 1973.

Bendixen, H. H., et al.: *Respiratory Care* (St. Louis: C. V. Mosby Co., 1965).

Gaskell, D. V., and Webber, B. A.: *The Brompton Hospital Guide to Chest Physiotherapy* (Philadelphia: J. B. Lippincott Co., 1974).

Harris, J. A., and Jerry, B. A.: Indications and procedures for segmental bronchial drainage, Respir. Care 20:1164, 1975.

Ingwersen, U.: *Respiratory Physical Therapy and Pulmonary Care* (New York: John Wiley & Sons, Inc., 1976).

Safar, P. (ed.): *Respiratory Therapy* (Philadelphia: F. A. Davis Co., 1965).

Shapiro, B. A., Harrison, R. A., and Trout, C. A.: *Clinical Application of Respiratory Care* (Chicago: Year Book Medical Publishers, Inc., 1975).

Shearer, M., Joyce, M., and Banks, B. S.: Lung ventilation during diaphragmatic breathing, Am. Phys. Ther. Assoc. 52:139, 1972.

Thacker, E. W.: *Postural Drainage and Respiratory Control* (Chicago: Year Book Medical Publishers, Inc., 1973).

Wheeler, S. M. M., et al.: Respiratory Physical Therapy Manual (Chicago: Northwestern Memorial Hospital, 1978).

Young, J. A., and Crocker, D.: *Principles and Practices of Respiratory Therapy* (2d ed.; Chicago: Year Book Medical Publishers, Inc., 1976).

22 / Fluidics

I. Fluidic Gas Flow Systems
   A. These systems do not require moving parts for normal function.
   B. Fluidic systems incorporate "innate logic," which allows predictability of direction of gas flow.
   C. Innate logic is essentially determined by actual physical design of the system.
   D. Changes in direction of flow are accomplished by *amplification,* the control of direction of a large flow of gas by a small flow of gas.
      1. Normally, amplification flow enters the system perpendicular to the main gas flow.
      2. Upon entering the main gas flow, the amplification flow causes the main gas flow to alter its direction.
   E. The basic phenomenon responsible for the overall fluidic mechanism is the *Coanda effect.*
      1. The Coanda effect is based on the fact that a free-flowing gas system will create a subatmospheric pressure at its periphery.
      2. If a wall is placed near the source of gas, the stream of gas will adhere to the wall. Adherence is caused by subatmospheric pressure.
      3. When this phenomena is incorporated in a fluidic system, it is referred to as a wall attachment fluidic element and may be used to alter direction of gas flow.
II. Bistable Fluidic Element* (Fig 22–1)
   A. Gas entering the element at P_S is stable in either leg of the system O_1 or O_2. Both legs in the system are symmetric in design.
   B. Once gas enters a leg of the system, it will remain stable in that leg until acted upon by an external force.
   C. Amplification may occur from C_1 (or C_2), causing flow to move from O_1 to O_2 (or O_2 to O_1).

---

*Fluidic elements are used in many IPPB machines and are incorporated in the operation of the Monaghan 225 ventilator.

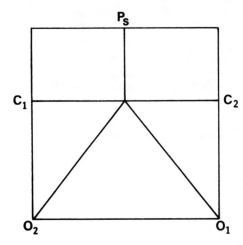

Fig 22–1. – Basic bistable fluidic element. Gas entering the element is stable in either leg of the system O_1 or O_2. Amplification from C_1 will force the main gas down leg O_1. Amplification from C_2 will force the main gas down leg O_2.

D. A negative pressure created at O_1 also will cause gas to move in a stable manner down its leg.

E. As pressure begins to increase at O_1 to a predetermined level, it will then move the flow to O_2 and remain stable there until it is acted upon by an external force.

F. This type of system allows a pressure limit and sensitivity control to be incorporated.†

G. This type of fluidic element is often referred to as a *flip-flop valve with a memory.*

III. Monostable Fluidic Element* (Fig 22 – 2)

A. This system is slightly asymmetric in design.

B. The asymmetric design is a result of positioning one of the systems legs off center. This is accomplished by the location of the *separator* (see Fig 22 – 2).

C. A *foil* may be incorporated into the system to assist in wall attachment down the monostable leg of the system.

1. A turbulent negative pressure area is developed just distal to the foil.

2. This negative pressure causes the gas to adhere to its wall.

D. In Figure 22 – 2 gas will normally proceed from P_S to O_1 as a result of the separator. Gas flow will be stable in O_1 until an external force causes movement to leg O_2.

---

†Seen in the Mine Safety Appliance Company fluidic IPPB machine.
*Fluidic elements are used in many IPPB machines and are incorporated in the operation of the Monaghan 225 ventilator.

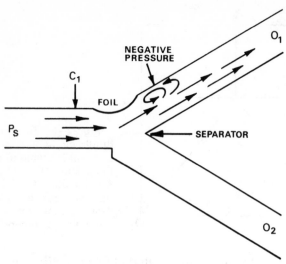

Fig 22–2. – Monostable fluidic element. Gas entering the system is stable only in leg O_1. Gas movement down O_2 will occur only during amplification from C_1 or as a result of back pressure at O_1.

    E. As gas moves to O_1, additional gas will be entrained from O_2, thus increasing the volume exiting at O_1.

    F. Gas flow will move to leg O_2 only under the following circumstances:

        1. If back pressure were generated at O_1 great enough to overcome the attachment at the foil.

        2. If amplification were to occur at point C_1, the main flow of gas would be directed down leg O_2.

           a. The flow from C_1 needs to be directed perpendicular to the main gas flow.

           b. The amplification flow must enter the system on a side opposite to that where it is directing the main gas flow.

    G. Once the back pressure is removed or the amplification flow is stopped, the main flow will return to its original path, O_1.

IV. AND/NAND Fluidic Element* (Fig 22–3)

    A. The flow is always stable from P_S to O_2 unless acted upon by an external force (monostable element).

    B. In order for flow to move from O_2 to O_1, amplification must occur from both C_1 and C_3.

---

*Fluidic elements are used in many IPPB machines and are incorporated in the operation of the Monaghan 225 ventilator.

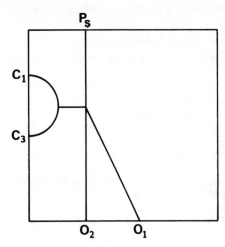

Fig 22–3. — AND/NAND fluidic element. Flow is normally stable from P_s to O_2. In order for flow to be diverted to O_1, amplification must originate from both C_1 and C_3.

C. If gas were to enter only from C_1, it would exit at C_3 without affecting the main gas flow. The same type of situation occurs if gas enters only from C_3.

D. Once amplification flow is stopped, flow will revert to O_2 and again remain stable.

V. OR/NOR Fluidic Element* (Fig 22–4)

A. The flow is always stable from Ps to O_2 unless acted upon by an external force.

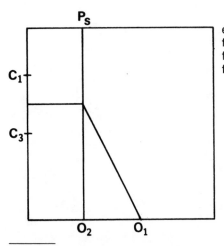

Fig 22–4. — OR/NOR fluidic element. Flow normally is stable from P_s to O_2. Flow may be diverted from O_2 to O_1 with amplification from either C_1 or C_3 or both.

---

*Fluidic elements are used in many IPPB machines and are incorporated in the operation of the Monaghan 225 ventilator.

B. In order for flow to move from O_2 to O_1, amplification must occur from C_1 or C_3 or both.

C. Amplification can result from three different effects.

D. Once amplification is stopped, flow will revert to O_2 and again remain stable.

BIBLIOGRAPHY

Angrist, S.: Fluid control devices, Sci. Am. 211:80, 1964.

Egan, D. F.: *Fundamentals of Respiratory Therapy* (3d ed.; St. Louis: C. V. Mosby Co., 1977).

McPherson, S. P.: *Respiratory Therapy Equipment* (St. Louis: C. V. Mosby Co., 1977).

Monaghan Product Information, Fluidics and Monaghan Volume Ventilators (Schaumburg, Ill.: Monaghan Co., A Division of Sandoz, Inc.).

Reba, I.: Application of the Coanda effect, Sci. Am. 214:84, 1966.

Respiratory Products Bulletin, Retec X70/IPPB (Portland, Ore., Retec Development Laboratory).

23 / Airway Care

I. General Indications for Use of Artificial Airways
   A. To prevent or relieve upper airway obstruction.
   B. To protect the airway from aspiration.
   C. To facilitate tracheal suction.
   D. To provide a sealed, closed system for mechanical ventilation.
II. General Classification of Artificial Airways
   A. Oral pharyngeal airway
      1. Used to relieve upper airway obstruction caused by the tongue.
      2. Used to prevent inadvertent laceration of tongue in the incoherent or seizuring patient.
      3. Used as a bite block with oral endotracheal tubes.
      4. Poorly tolerated in alert patient due to stimulation of gag reflex.
   B. Nasal pharyngeal airway
      1. Used to relieve upper airway obstruction caused by tongue and/or soft palate.
      2. Better tolerated than oral pharyngeal airway.
   C. Oral endotracheal airway
      1. Airway of choice in an emergency.
      2. Ideally used for short-term intubation of not more than 24 hours.
      3. Poorly tolerated in semiconscious or conscious patient.
      4. Difficult to stabilize in patient's mouth.
      5. Inadvertent extubation is common.
      6. Bite blocks usually are necessary.
      7. Vagal stimulation may result.
      8. Difficult to suction due to position and curvature of airway.
   D. Nasal endotracheal airway
      1. Advantages over oral endotracheal airway for long-term intubation
         a. Easier to stabilize.
         b. Easier to suction.
         c. Better tolerated.
         d. Safer for equipment attachment.

279

2. Problems associated with nasotracheal airway
   a. Movement of tip of tube when patient's head position changes.
   b. Possible pressure necrosis in area of the alae nasi.
   c. Possible obstruction of sinus drainage and acute sinusitis.
   d. Possible obstruction of eustachian tube drainage and otitis media.
   e. Significant increase in incidence of vocal cord damage after 72 hours (also seen with oral endotracheal airways).
   f. Possible vagal stimulation, but less frequently than with oral endotracheal tube.

E. Tracheostomy tube
   1. Advantages over endotracheal airway
      a. No complications with upper airway or glottis
      b. Easier to suction
      c. Easier to stabilize
      d. Best tolerated of all airways
   2. Problems associated with tracheostomy tube
      a. Immediate complications
         (1) Bleeding
         (2) Pneumothorax
         (3) Air embolism
         (4) Subcutaneous and mediastinal emphysema
      b. Late complications
         (1) Infection of surgical wound
         (2) Hemorrhage
         (3) Airway obstruction (secondary to complications such as cuff problems, mucous plugging)
         (4) Tracheoesophageal fistula
      c. Tracheostomy tubes need not be changed so long as they are functioning appropriately, the airway is being properly humidified and no infectious process is present in the airway or tracheostomy wound.

F. Esophageal obturator
   1. The obturator is used only as an emergency airway.
   2. The obturator is a mask attached to a blind endotracheal tube, which has perforations along its length and a cuff at tip of tube.
   3. The obturator is inserted into esophagus, and cuff is inflated.

4. The patient is ventilated by forcing gas into obturator. Gas will move out of perforations in tube and is forced into trachea.
5. Problems associated with esophageal obturator
    a. Intubation of trachea during insertion
    b. Regurgitation on removal of airway
G. Fenestrated tracheostomy tube
    1. Fenestration is located in outer cannula only.
    2. Inner cannula is similar in design to normal tracheostomy tube.
    3. Requisites for proper use
        a. Removal of inner cannula
        b. Deflation of cuff
        c. Corking of outer cannula
    4. Patient is forced to ventilate via upper airway through fenestration in outer cannula of tracheostomy tube and around tube.
    5. Problem associated with fenestrated tube
        a. Possible formation of granular tissue at site of fenestration
H. Tracheal buttons
    1. These are used to maintain patency of tracheal stoma.
    2. Inner lip of button lies on internal anterior tracheal wall, outer lip on tissue of the neck.
    3. Tracheal buttons allow patient to ventilate completely from upper airway without tracheal obstruction.
    4. In an emergency, patient may be suctioned and/or ventilated via the tracheal button.
III. Airway Cuffs
   A. Uses
      1. To mechanically ventilate patient
      2. To protect airway from aspiration
   B. If pressure in cuff is maintained above 20 mm Hg, capillary blood flow normally is stopped and may result in
      1. Ischemia
      2. Tracheal necrosis
      3. Tracheal malacia
      4. Tracheal stenosis
   C. Cuff inflation technique (minimal leak technique)
      Only minimum amount of air to allow optimum sealing of airway with minimum pressure on tracheal wall should be used.

  1. Technique
    a. Insertion of enough air into cuff to prevent any leaks.
    b. While positive pressure applied to airway, gas should be withdrawn from the cuff until a slight leak develops. Leak should not be so great as to overcome purpose of cuff. At this point pilot tube should be clamped.
 D. Cuff deflation technique
  1. Complete suctioning of lower airway.
  2. Complete suctioning above cuff.
  3. Deflation of cuff while positive pressure is applied in order to direct the pooled secretions above cuff up and out of airway.
 E. Special cuffs
  1. Kamen-Wilkinson cuff
    a. Made of polyurethane foam.
    b. Inflated by atmospheric pressure.
    c. No positive pressure added to cuff.
    d. Minimum pressures normally applied to tracheal wall.
    e. Deflation of cuff with syringe before insertion, allowing re-expansion by atmospheric pressure and vice versa.
  2. Lanz cuff
    a. Dynamic cuff theoretically will allow only 20 cm H_2O pressure to be developed in cuff.
    b. Valve assembly on pilot tube maintains constancy of intracuff pressure by allowing gas movement from pilot balloon to cuff.
IV. Suctioning of Airway
 A. Complications of airway suctioning
  1. Hypoxemia
  2. Arrhythmias
  3. Hypotension
  4. Lung collapse
 B. Requisites of suction catheters
  1. Constructed of a material that will cause minimal irritation and trauma to tracheal mucosa.
  2. Minimal frictional resistance when passing through artificial airway is essential.
  3. Sufficiently long to easily pass tip of artificial airway.
  4. Should have smooth, molded ends and side holes to prevent mucosal trauma.
  5. Catheter diameter should be only one-half that of artificial airway.

C. Suctioning technique
   1. Technique completely sterile.
   2. Preoxygenation of patient.
   3. Insertion of catheter without vacuum until an obstruction is met and then slight retraction.
   4. Application of suction while catheter is rotated between thumb and forefinger during removal.
   5. Duration of suction catheter in airway no longer than 10–15 seconds.
   6. Reoxygenation and/or ventilation.
   7. In event of catheter adherence to wall of airway, release of suction, withdrawal of catheter and reapplication of suction.
   8. To minimize airway trauma, use of suction pressure of −80 mm Hg to −120 mm Hg.

BIBLIOGRAPHY

Applebaum, E. L., and Bruce, D. L.: *Tracheal Intubation* (Philadelphia: W. B. Saunders Co., 1976).

Bendixen, H. H., et al.: *Respiratory Care* (St. Louis: C. V. Mosby Co., 1965).

Burton, G. G., Gee, G. N., and Hodgkin, J. E.: *Respiratory Care: A Guide to Clinical Practice* (Philadelphia: J. B. Lippincott Co., 1977).

Egan, D. F.: *Fundamentals of Respiratory Therapy* (3d ed.; St. Louis: C. V. Mosby Co., 1977).

Safar, P. (ed.): *Respiratory Therapy* (Philadelphia: F. A. Davis Co., 1965).

Shapiro, B. A., Harrison, R. A., and Trout, C. A.: *Clinical Application of Respiratory Care* (Chicago: Year Book Medical Publishers, Inc., 1975).

Young, J. A., and Crocker, D.: *Principles and Practice of Respiratory Therapy* (2d ed.; Chicago: Year Book Medical Publishers, Inc., 1976).

24 / Continuous Mechanical Ventilation

I. Physiologic Effects of Positive Pressure in Relation to Continuous Mechanical Ventilation
  A. Increased mean airway pressure and increased mean intrathoracic pressure (see Chap. 19).
  B. Decreased work of breathing (see Chap. 19)
  C. Mechanical bronchodilatation (see Chap. 19)
  D. Manipulation of the mechanical ventilatory pattern including I:E ratio, mechanical ventilatory rate, inspiratory time, inspiratory flow rate and application of airway maneuvers
  E. Manipulation of tidal volume and improved distribution of ventilation (see Chap. 19)
  F. Potential decrease in cardiac output (see Chap. 19)
  G. Potential increase in intracranial pressure (see Chap. 19)
  H. Potential decrease in urinary output may occur as a result of two mechanisms:
    1. Decreased cardiac output results in decreased renal blood flow, which alters renal filtration pressures and diminishes urine formation.
    2. The decreased right atrial pressure associated with positive pressure ventilation is interpreted by the body as a state of hypovolemia. As a result, the pituitary gland increases its production of Antidiuretic Hormone (ADH), causing retention of fluid.
  I. An altered emotional state may be associated with increased stress of continuous mechanical ventilation. This emotional state may be manifested as
    1. Apprehension
    2. Depression
    3. Frustration
    4. Fear
    5. Anxiety
    6. Insomnia
    7. Stress ulcers

II. Indications for Continuous Mechanical Ventilation
   A. Apnea
   B. Acute ventilatory failure
   C. Impending ventilatory failure
      1. Progressive deterioration of the arterial blood gas values that seems to be heading toward acute ventilatory failure.
      2. Increase in the work of breathing.
      3. Decrease in cardiopulmonary reserve.
      4. Clinical situations frequently leading to ventilatory failure
         a. Flail chest
         b. Drug overdose
         c. Neuromuscular or neurologic disease
         d. Status asthmaticus
   D. Poor oxygenation
      1. This is due to increased oxygen consumption and work of breathing. It is responsive neither to conventional oxygen therapy nor to PEEP therapy unless continuous mechanical ventilation also is initiated.
      2. Bases for clinical assessment
         a. Arterial blood gas picture
         b. Pathophysiology of the disease
         c. Cardiovascular status
         d. Pulmonary status
            (1) Ventilatory reserve
            (2) Work of breathing
      3. Specific examples of poor oxygenation
         a. Adult respiratory distress syndrome (ARDS): The work involved in attempting to maintain adequate oxygenation is excessive. With improved distribution of ventilation, mechanical bronchodilatation and decreased work of breathing accomplished by the ventilator, arterial oxygenation may improve.
         b. Massive pulmonary emboli: The ventilator can accomplish the excessively high minute volumes more efficiently and with much less cardiopulmonary stress than can spontaneous ventilation.
III. Guidelines for Ventilator Commitment
   A. Establish artificial airway.
   B. Manual support of ventilation until mechanical ventilator is prepared for attachment.

C. Correction of hypotension and cardiac arrhythmias to insure cardiovascular stability.

D. Record of baseline values
1. Arterial blood gases
2. Vital signs

E. Appropriate monitoring of cardiovascular system
1. ECG
2. Central venous pressure
3. Swan-Ganz catheter

F. Establishment of ideal ventilatory pattern
1. Tidal volumes of between 12 and 15 ml/kg of ideal body weight.
2. Respiratory rate limited to a minimum that will achieve adequate alveolar ventilation but will minimize mean intrathoracic pressures—about 8 to 12 for most adults.
3. Appropriate I:E pattern to insure cardiovascular stability
   a. I:E ratio of at least 1:2 in the control mode.
   b. Inspiratory time between 0.5 and 2 seconds in any mode.
4. Oxygen concentration dependent on arterial blood gas analysis
5. Adjustment of peak flow to insure proper I:E ratio
   a. Increasing flow rate will decrease inspiratory time.
   b. Decreasing flow rate will increase inspiratory time.
6. Sedation of patient as indicated by overall clinical condition.

IV. Guidelines for Monitoring the Ventilator Patient
A. Establishment of baseline readings
1. Effective dynamic compliance should be determined and monitored frequently to indicate changes in compliance of lung-thorax system (see Chapter 2, Section XII).
2. Shunt and deadspace studies
   a. These studies should be performed after the patient is stabilized on the ventilator.
   b. Results will indicate changes in actual functional lung parenchyma and pulmonary blood flow (see Chapter 10).
3. Arterial blood gas analysis
   a. Blood gases should be monitored closely until the

    patient is stabilized. After patient has stabilized, blood gases every 4–8 hours normally are adequate.

    b. After a change has been made in any of the ventilatory parameters, a blood gas analysis should be performed.

B. Recommended continuous monitors of ventilator system
1. Patient disconnect alarm (low inspiratory pressure alarm)
2. High inspiratory pressure alarm
3. Tidal volume monitor and alarm
4. Adverse I:E ratio alarm
5. Machine failure alarm (electric or mechanical)
6. Low oxygen and compressed air source pressure alarm

C. Monitoring of cardiovascular system (see Chapter 8, Section XI) and fluid and electrolyte balance

D. Clinical monitoring of patient's overall condition

E. Ventilator adjustments
1. Only one parameter should be changed at a time, followed by blood gas evaluation in 15–20 minutes.
2. After blood gas results are assessed, additional parameters may be individually altered.
3. If more than one variable is adjusted simultaneously and poor blood gas results are received, the cause of the poor results is difficult to determine.

F. Maintenance of appropriate bronchial hygiene
1. Aerosol therapy by inline ultrasonic nebulizer may be used.
2. Chest physiotherapy, as tolerated, may be used. For safety and maneuverability during chest physiotherapy, a manual ventilator should be employed.
3. The fiberoptic bronchoscope may be of therapeutic value in certain clinical situations.

G. Techniques for maintaining proper Pa_{CO_2} levels
1. In the control mode
    a. If Pa_{CO_2} is increased
      (1) Decrease mechanical deadspace or
      (2) Increase tidal volume or
      (3) Increase respiratory rate.
    b. If Pa_{CO_2} is decreased:
      (1) Increase mechanical deadspace or

      (2) Decrease respiratory rate or

      (3) Decrease tidal volume.

2. In the IMV (intermittent mandatory ventilation) or IDV (intermittent demand ventilation) mode: The patient's spontaneous parameters in conjunction with the ventilator's parameters will determine the effective alveolar ventilation. The following techniques will potentially manipulate Pa_{CO_2} levels:

   a. If Pa_{CO_2} is increased

      (1) Increase tidal volume or

      (2) Increase ventilator's respiratory rate.

   b. If Pa_{CO_2} is decreased

      (1) Decrease ventilator's respiratory rate or

      (2) Decrease tidal volume.

3. In the assist or assist/control mode: The patient's spontaneous parameters, in conjunction with the ventilator's parameters and the ventilator's cycling mechanism, will determine the effective alveolar ventilation. Particularly in these modes, the patient's spontaneous respiratory rate should be stable and regular and the patient should have an intact CNS. The following techniques will potentially manipulate Pa_{CO_2} levels:

   a. If Pa_{CO_2} is increased

      (1) When volume cycled, increase tidal volume or increase the ventilator's respiratory rate.

      (2) When time cycled, increase the inspiratory time.

      (3) When pressure or flow cycled, increase the inspiratory pressure.

   b. If Pa_{CO_2} is decreased

      (1) When volume cycled, decrease the ventilator's respiratory rate or tidal volume.

      (2) When time cycled, decrease the inspiratory time.

      (3) When pressure or flow cycled, decrease the inspiratory pressure ceiling.

H. Maintenance of adequate oxygenation

  1. Pa_{O_2} levels between 60 and 90 mm Hg.

  2. Adequate hemoglobin content.

  3. Normal acid–base balance.

  4. Adequate tissue perfusion.

  5. Prevent patient from fighting the ventilator.

      6. Use of positive end expiratory pressure when hypoxemia is refractory to oxygen therapy.

  I. Common clinical complications associated with continuous mechanical ventilation.

      1. Machine failure
      2. Airway obstruction
      3. Machine disconnection
      4. Atelectasis
      5. Hypotension
      6. Infection
      7. Pneumothorax
      8. Gastrointestinal malfunction
      9. Renal malfunction
    10. Emotional trauma

V. Guidelines for Ventilator Discontinuance

  A. Initiation of discontinuance

      1. Evidence of reversal or improvement of disease process that led to ventilator commitment is documented.

        a. Adequate ventilatory ability

          (1) Tidal volume

            (a) Normal V_T is 3–4 ml per pound of ideal body weight.

            (b) V_T on discontinuance should be about 50% of predicted

          (2) Vital capacity

            (a) VC of three times the patient's predicted V_T is considered adequate for effective coughing and deep breathing.

            (b) A VC of one and a half to two times patient's predicted V_T (minimally acceptable for discontinuance).

          (3) Respiratory rate: Between 12 and 35 spontaneous breaths per minute.

          (4) Negative inspiratory force (NIF)

            (a) NIF is a useful method of assessing ventilatory ability in the comatose or uncooperative patient (i.e., a substitute method for VC determination).

            (b) A negative 20 cm H_2O pressure generated in 20 seconds indicates that the patient *should have* a VC of about three times his predicted V_T.

        b. Adequate cardiopulmonary ability assessed during continuous ventilation.

           (1) Arterial blood gases that can be maintained within an acceptable range for the particular patient.

           (2) Shunt study of less than 20% (relatively normal).

           (3) Shunt study of between 20% and 30% (may be acceptable depending on overall clinical picture).

           (4) Deadspace to V_T ratio less than 60% (relatively normal).

           (5) Deadspace to V_T ratio of 60–80% (may be acceptable depending on overall clinical picture).

        c. Cardiovascular assessment should reveal a stable status.

        d. No active pulmonary infections should be present.

    B. Actual disconnection from ventilator

        1. The patient should be prepared psychologically.

        2. The same oxygen concentration and/or PEEP levels used on the ventilator should be maintained while the patient is ventilating spontaneously and until he is adequately stabilized.

        3. The patient should be manually ventilated to allow smooth transition from ventilator to spontaneous ventilation.

        4. The patient must be monitored extremely closely during the initial discontinuance phase, with frequent blood gas assessments.

  VI. Auxiliary Airway Maneuvers

    A. Hazards of airway maneuvers

        1. Increased mean intrathoracic pressure

        2. Potential decrease in venous return

        3. Potential barotrauma (lung rupture)

    B. Sigh

        1. This is the delivery of a periodic deep breath larger than that of the set normal V_T.

        2. It is incorporated to prevent patchy microatelectasis that may develop during constant volume ventilation.

    C. Inflation hold (Fig 24–1)

        1. The delivered volume is maintained in patient's airway for a determined period.

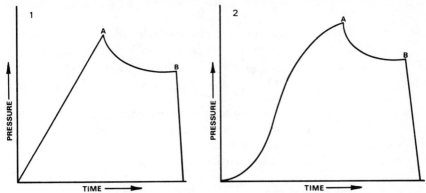

Fig 24–1. — Ideal pressure curves for **(1)** square wave flow pattern with inflation hold and **(2)** sine wave flow pattern with inflation hold. The pressure drop from *A* to *B* indicates equilibrium between mouth and alveolar pressures during inflation hold period.

    2. Effects
       a. Improves distribution of the inspired volume.
       b. Helps to eliminate microatelectasis.
    3. Continuous use of an inflation hold maneuver may cause increased mean intrathoracic pressure.
  D. Expiratory retard (Fig 24–2)
    1. This is an expiratory maneuver in which resistance is maintained in the airway during exhalation.
    2. Airway pressure takes an extended period of time to return to atmospheric (baseline).

Fig 24–2. — Ideal pressure curves for **(1)** square wave flow pattern with expiratory retard and **(2)** sine wave flow pattern with expiratory retard. *Dotted line* illustrates "normal" return of pressure to baseline.

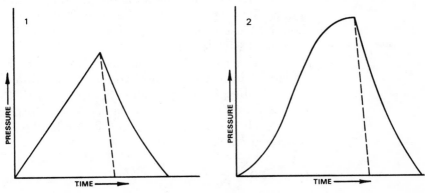

   3. This maneuver is used to minimize air trapping and to
      insure complete exhalation.
 E. Positive end expiratory pressure (PEEP)
   1. This is an expiratory maneuver in which airway pres-
      sure is not allowed to return to atmospheric at end
      exhalation.
   2. Physiologic effects
      a. Increased mean intrapulmonary pressure
      b. Increased mean intrathoracic pressure
      c. Increased FRC
      d. Decreased work of breathing
      e. Improved oxygenation
   3. Indications
      a. Refractory hypoxemia that results from collapsing
         of alveoli during exhalation (i.e., respiratory dis-
         tress syndrome [RDS]) is the primary indication
         for use of PEEP.
      b. Acute diffuse lung parenchymal restrictive diseases
         (1) Pulmonary edema
         (2) IRDS
         (3) ARDS
         (4) Chest trauma
   4. Goals of PEEP
      a. Restoring FRC to normal level.
      b. Improving oxygenation to an acceptable level by
         (1) Maintaining Pa_{O_2} greater than 50 mm Hg
         (2) Maintaining FI_{O_2} less than 0.50
      c. Accomplishing the above with minimal cardiovas-
         cular embarrassment.
   5. Evaluation of PEEP levels
      a. Various methods provide an approximation of the
         optimal level of PEEP; none is definitive and
         should be used purely as a clinical guideline for
         assessing PEEP levels.
         (1) Effective dynamic compliance (CED) is deter-
             mined by dividing the expired tidal volume
             (ETV) by plateau pressure (Pei) minus PEEP
             pressure. The plateau is obtained at end inspi-
             ration by incorporation of an inflation hold (see
             Chapter 2, Section XII):

$$C_{ED} = \frac{ETV}{Pei - PEEP}. \tag{1}$$

(a) As PEEP is applied, pulmonary compliance progressively improves until a point of hyperinflation is reached. At this point of hyperinflation, total compliance begins to decrease. The optimal PEEP level correlates well with the point of greatest compliance.

(b) PEEP is subtracted from plateau pressure in the calculation because this resultant *change* in pressure from the PEEP baseline is the amount of pressure necessary to create lung tissue expansion for the specified volume change.

(2) Mixed venous partial pressure levels ($P\bar{v}_{O_2}$) are directly related to optimal PEEP. With application of PEEP, the $P\bar{v}_{O_2}$ will begin to increase up to the optimal. If PEEP levels increase excessively, the $P\bar{v}_{O_2}$ will begin to decrease as a result of cardiovascular embarrassment. Thus optimal PEEP levels correlate well with maximum $P\bar{v}_{O_2}$.

(3) Total physiologic shunt levels correlate well with optimal PEEP. When there is a stable cardiac output and consistent rate of oxygen consumption, as the PEEP is increased, the percent measured shunt normally will decrease. This will occur up to optimal PEEP. Once optimal PEEP levels are exceeded, there will be an increase in percent measured shunt. Thus optimal PEEP levels are associated with the lowest percent measured shunt.

(4) Arterial partial pressure (Pa_{O_2}) and alveolar–arterial partial pressure differences ($A - aDO_2$) correlate well with optimal PEEP levels. This correlation occurs if the FI_{O_2}, oxygen consumption rate, cardiac output and mechanical minute ventilation are stable. Under these conditions, as PEEP is increased, the Pa_{O_2} will increase and $A - aDO_2$ will decrease. Once optimal PEEP levels are exceeded, the Pa_{O_2} will begin to decrease and the $A - aDO_2$ will increase. Thus optimal PEEP correlates with maximum Pa_{O_2} and minimum $A - aDO_2$.

6. Methods of applying PEEP to patient's airway
  a. Continuous positive airway pressure (CPAP) (Fig 24–3)
    (1) CPAP is a method of applying PEEP to the spontaneously ventilating patient.
    (2) Indications for the use of CPAP: Same as those for PEEP, with the additional criterion that the patient can ventilate spontaneously.
    (3) The primary factor in maintaining a nonfluctuating PEEP during spontaneous inspiration is flow. As with all high flow systems, the flow is maintained at least three times the patient's spontaneous minute volume and is measured distal to the PEEP device.
    (4) PEEP may be maintained by
      (a) Water columns
      (b) Spring-loaded valves
      (c) Magnetic valves
      (d) Balloon diaphragms
      (e) Adjustable diaphragms
      (f) Varying orifices
  b. Expiratory Positive Airway Pressure (EPAP) (Fig 24–4)
    (1) As with CPAP, EPAP is a method of applying PEEP to the spontaneous ventilating patient.

Fig 24–3. — Intrapulmonary pressure curve with application of 10 cm H_2O PEEP via a CPAP system. This curve is theoretically identical to the normal intrapulmonary pressure curve except that the baseline is shifted from 0 to 10 cm H_2O (see Fig 6–2).

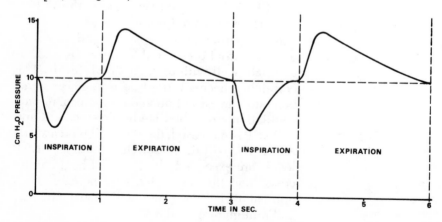

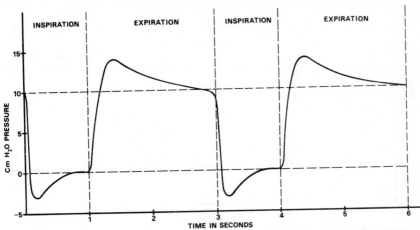

Fig 24–4. —Intrapulmonary pressure curve with application of 10 cm H$_2$O PEEP via an EPAP system. During expiration, the pressure is maintained above 10 cm H$_2$O but, during inspiration, the pressure reverts to subatmospheric, as seen with normal spontaneous ventilation.

(2) The primary difference between CPAP and EPAP is that with CPAP the above-atmospheric pressure is applied throughout the entire respiratory cycle; with EPAP the above-atmospheric pressure is applied only during exhalation.

(3) Technical operation of EPAP

(a) One method of accomplishing an EPAP system is to incorporate a low resistance one-way valve between a nonpressurized inspiratory circuit and a pressurized expiratory circuit.

(b) During inspiration the patient opens the one-way valve, which allows him to inhale gas from the inspiratory circuit. The inspiratory circuit is an open high flow system, which runs parallel to the expiratory circuit. Airway pressure must return to a subatmospheric level before opening the one-way valve. A deadspace volume of gas between the airway and the one-way valve must be decompressed. This deadspace volume depends on the construction of the circuit. The

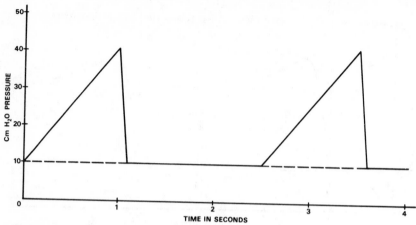

Fig 24–5. — Ideal intrapulmonary pressure curve seen with a square wave flow pattern and application of 10 cm H_2O PEEP on a CPPV system.

amount of work necessary to accomplish this decompression is minimal but is greater than that of a closed CPAP system. Thus the work of breathing may be manipulated by changing the amount of deadspace tubing.

    (c) At expiration the one-way valve closes and the patient passively exhales against the PEEP. PEEP is maintained by one of the PEEP devices previously described.

  c. Continuous Positive Pressure Ventilation (CPPV) (Fig 24–5)

    (1) This system is the application of PEEP to a patient during continuous mechanical ventilation.

    (2) PEEP may be placed on most positive pressure ventilators in *any* mode of ventilation.

    (3) PEEP is applied by mechanisms available on the machine or via those devices used to create PEEP with CPAP set-ups.

VII. Twelve-Point Classification System for all Mechanical Ventilators

  A. Positive or negative pressure

    1. Positive pressure ventilators use an above-atmospheric pressure to cause delivery of the patient's VT.

    2. Negative pressure ventilators use a subatmospheric pressure applied to the thorax to cause delivery of the patient's VT.

B. Powering mechanism
   1. Source of the physical energy that provides the power to the driving mechanism of the ventilator.
   2. Three powering mechanisms for all ventilators
      a. Electric: Normally uses household current.
      b. Pneumatic: Normally uses a 40–60 psi gas source.
      c. Combined electric/pneumatic: Both mechanisms must be activated for proper machine function.
C. Driving mechanism
   1. Provides the mechanical force that produces the flow of gas necessary for delivery of the VT.
   2. Basic characteristic types of driving systems
      a. Pneumatic systems: Driven by a compressed gas source (either internal or external to ventilator) regulated by electronic or mechanical devices inside the ventilator.
         (1) Pneumatic clutches and valves
         (2) Electronic Servo mechanisms
         (3) Electronic and mechanical solenoids
         (4) Preset and adjustable regulators
         (5) Fluidic regulation
      b. Piston systems: Driven by devices exhibiting
         (1) Linear motion
         (2) Rotary motion (i.e., exponential or logarithmic acceleration)
      c. Bellows systems: Driven by a compressed gas source (either internal or external to ventilator) generated from
         (1) Compressor (i.e., turbine)
         (2) Fluidic system
         (3) Pneumatic system
D. Number of circuits
   1. A circuit is the path that the gas flow follows inside the ventilator.
   2. A single circuit means that only one pressurized gas volume is produced (or maintained) within the ventilator. This pressurized gas volume is the same as that delivered to the patient (i.e., the same gas that is produced by the ventilator's driving mechanism is delivered to the patient).
   3. A double circuit means that two separate pressurized gas volumes are produced (or maintained) within the ventilator. One gas source is used to compress the sec-

ond gas. This latter compressed gas is the volume delivered to the patient (i.e., one gas powers the driving mechanism and another gas is delivered to the patient). So, two distinct gas flow systems are involved in the delivery of gas to the patient.

E. Modes of ventilation

1. A mode of ventilation is the manner in which inspiration is initiated. Traditionally, modes are divided into three categories

    a. Control mode: The machine is totally responsible for initiation of the inspiratory phase.

    b. Assist mode: The patient is totally responsible for initiation of the inspiratory phase.

    c. Assist/control mode: The patient normally initiates the inspiratory phase but, if this spontaneous rate falls below predetermined levels, the machine will take over the initiation of inspiration.

2. Intermittent mandatory ventilation (IMV)

    a. System by which the patient breathes spontaneously from a high flow system or from the ventilator via a nonpressurized flow of gas. At intermittent predetermined intervals, the ventilator delivers a control positive pressure inspiration.

    b. Clinical indications

        (1) Weaning of a patient from a controlled ventilatory state to a spontaneous ventilatory state

            (a) The transition from mechanical to spontaneous ventilation may be facilitated by use of IMV.

            (b) IMV allows the patient's ventilatory muscles to accommodate slowly to spontaneous breathing.

            (c) IMV allows the patient the psychologic support necessary to overcome ventilator dependence.

        (2) Maintenance of a patient who is spontaneously ventilating but is in need of sustained ventilatory support

            (a) IMV minimizes the use of some pharmacologic agents (diazepam [Valium], morphine, pancuronium [Pavulon], curare).

            (b) IMV minimizes the psychologic trauma

involved in ventilator maintenance (e.g., improves morale, minimizes emotional dependence).

(c) IMV allows the patient to progressively assume more of the work of breathing.

c. Problems associated with IMV

(1) Fighting or bucking uncoordinated positive pressure breaths.

(2) All other hazards involved in mechanical positive pressure ventilation.

d. The main technical advantage of IMV is its adaptability to any ventilator capable of giving low control respiratory rates.

3. Intermittent demand ventilation (IDV)

a. System by which the patient breathes spontaneously from a high flow or nonpressurized system. At intermittent predetermined intervals or after a specific number of spontaneous breaths, the ventilator delivers an assisted positive pressure breath. Therefore, these positive pressure breaths will be synchronized with the patient's inspiratory efforts.

b. IDV is also described as

(1) Intermittent augmented ventilation (IAV)

(2) Synchronized intermittent mandatory ventilation (SIMV)

c. Clinical indications: The same as for IMV.

d. Advantages of IDV over IMV

(1) The assisted breath normally is coordinated with the patient's inspiratory efforts.

(2) Patients normally do not fight the assisted breath.

(3) The coordinated pattern theoretically minimizes changes in mean intrathoracic pressures.

F. Cycling parameter

1. The physical parameter that, when reached, will result in termination of inspiration.

2. Four basic parameters are involved in the delivery of gas to any patient. One or more of these will always be the cycling parameter.

a. Volume

b. Pressure

c. Time

d. Flow

3. A cycling parameter that has been reached normally does *not* activate an audiovisual or audio alarm.
   a. An alarm being activated with each inspiration indicates an inappropriate condition for continuous mechanical ventilation.
   b. Some alarms that signal the end of inspiration for a particular parameter have been designed to allow deliberate deactivation. Such alarms allow this physical parameter to become a cycling parameter, if so desired (e.g., high airway pressure limit and alarm on the Bennett MA – 1).

G. Limit
   1. A limit is one of the four physical parameters of the ventilator (flow, time, pressure, volume) that cannot be exceeded and that is not the cycling mechanism. These limiting parameters may be divided into three categories.
      a. Limits that are preset with adjustable controls on the ventilator.

         Examples:

         (1) Peak flow control on the MA – 1
         (2) Normal pressure limit control on the Bourns Bear I
         (3) Pressure relief on the Emerson Post-Op
      b. Limits that are the result of two preset adjustable controls.

         Examples:

         (1) Inspiratory time on the MA – 1 $\left(\dfrac{V_T}{\text{flow}}\right)$

         (2) Volume on the Veriflo CV 2000 $\left(\dfrac{\text{flow}}{\text{inspiratory time}}\right)$
      c. Some limits also may serve as a secondary means of ending inspiration.
         (1) All limiting factors that end inspiration should have simultaneous audio or audiovisual alarms.

            Examples:
            (a) Normal pressure limit on the MA – 1
            (b) I : E ratio limit on the Bourns Bear I

H. Flow pattern
   1. Square wave flow pattern (Fig 24–6): The flow is non-varying during the entire inspiratory phase. This flow pattern normally will result in a rectilinear pressure curve. Most ventilators do not consistently maintain a square flow in the face of back pressure. This results in a decreasing (decelerating) flow toward the end of inspiration, depicted by the dotted line in Figure 24–6.
   2. Sine wave flow pattern (see Fig 24–6): The flow varies throughout the entire inspiratory phase. The greatest volume delivery occurs at the point of peak flow.

      Examples:
      a. Emerson Post-Op: A ventilator that has a sine wave flow pattern created by a rotary driven piston. This flow pattern creates a sigmoidal pressure curve.
      b. Engström 300: A ventilator that has a modified sine wave flow pattern (Fig 24–7). This creates a sigmoidal pressure curve with a plateau effect.
   3. Accelerating flow pattern (see Fig 24–7): Flow progressively increases during inspiration until a preset limit is reached, at which time the flow plateaus to a square wave.
   4. Decelerating flow patterns: The flow begins at a maximum and, at some point during the inspiratory phase, the flow decreases to the completion of inspiration.
      a. Square wave with flow taper pattern (Fig 24–8): Peak flow is maintained at a maximum during the beginning of inspiration but decreases as a result of the flow taper as the inspiratory phase ends.

Fig 24–6.—Graph **1** depicts ideal square wave flow pattern. *Dotted line* indicates actual flow pattern seen with most square wave ventilators as a result of back pressure. Graph **2** depicts a normal sine wave flow pattern.

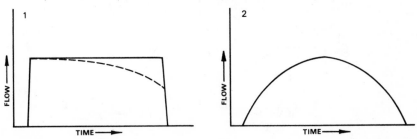

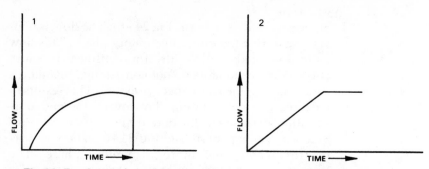

Fig 24–7.—Graph **1** depicts a modified sine wave flow pattern, as seen with the Engström ventilator. Graph **2** depicts an ideal accelerating flow pattern where flow increases initially, then converts to a square wave pattern.

b. Decaying flow pattern (see Fig 24–8): Flow begins at its peak level but rapidly and progressively decreases to a terminal level during the final portion of the inspiratory phase.

I. Pressure pattern

1. *The pressure patterns generated during inspiration are the result of the type of flow pattern delivered to the patient.*

a. Rectilinear pressure pattern (Fig 24–9) seen with square wave flows.

b. Sigmoidal pressure pattern (see Fig 24–9) seen with sine wave flow.

c. Modified sigmoidal pressure pattern (Fig 24–10) seen with modified sine wave flows.

d. Initially linear and terminally decelerating pres-

Fig 24–8.—Graph **1** depicts an ideal square wave flow pattern with a flow taper. Graph **2** depicts a decaying flow pattern, as seen with the Bennett PR series.

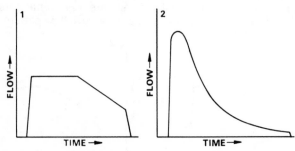

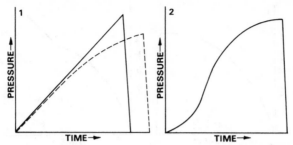

Fig 24–9. – Graph **1** depicts a rectilinear pressure curve associated with a square wave flow pattern. *Dotted line* indicates actual curve seen with most square wave flow patterns. Graph **2** depicts sigmoidal pressure curve associated with a sine wave flow pattern.

        sure pattern (see Fig 24–10) seen with a square wave with flow taper flow.

    e. Parabolic pressure pattern (Fig 24–11) seen with decaying flow.

    f. Nonlinear (exponential) increasing pressure pattern (see Fig 24–11) seen with an accelerating flow.

  J. Internal resistance

    1. The ability of a machine's driving mechanism to maintain its programmed flow pattern in the face of increasing back pressure

    2. Internal resistance ratings

      a. High: Increasing back pressure has no effect on the programmed flow pattern (e.g., Emerson and Engstrom).

Fig 24–10. – Graph **1** depicts a modified sigmoidal pressure pattern associated with a modified sine wave flow pattern. Note built-in inflation hold. Graph **2** depicts an initially linear and terminally decelerating pressure pattern seen with a square wave flow with flow taper.

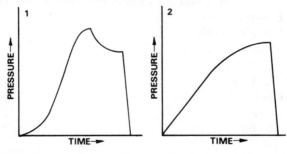

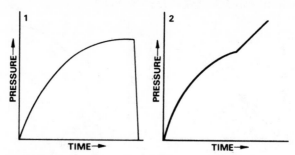

Fig 24–11.—Graph **1** depicts a parabolic pressure pattern associated with a decaying flow pattern. Graph **2** depicts a nonlinear (exponential) increasing pressure pattern associated with an accelerating flow pattern.

b. Medium: Increasing back pressure will cause a moderate decrease in the preset flow rate and so alter the programmed flow pattern (e.g., Bennett MA – 1 and Ohio 560).

c. Low: Increasing back pressure will cause a pronounced alteration in flow pattern and significantly decrease flow rate (e.g., Bennett PR – 2 and Bird Mark 7).

K. Auxiliary airway maneuvers (those that come standard with the ventilator)
   1. Sigh
   2. Inflation hold
   3. Expiratory retard
   4. PEEP
L. Alarm system: A listing of the various alarm mechanisms that are standard with the machine.

VIII. Ventilator: Bennett PR Series
   A. Pressure: Positive
   B. Powering mechanism: Pneumatic
   C. Driving mechanism: Pneumatic system regulated by the Bennett valve
   D. Circuit: Single
   E. Modes
      1. Assist
      2. Assist/control
   F. Cycling parameters
      1. Flow
      2. Time

    G. Limit (preset): Pressure

    H. Flow pattern: Decaying

    I. Pressure pattern: Parabolic

    J. Internal resistance: Low

    K. Airway maneuvers

       1. CPPV

    L. Alarm: None

       1. Optional Bennett spirometer

IX. Ventilator: Bird Mark 7 and 8

    A. Pressure: Positive

    B. Powering mechanism: Pneumatic

    C. Driving mechanism: Pneumatic system regulated by pneumatic clutch and peak flow needle valve

    D. Circuit: Single

    E. Modes

       1. Assist

       2. Assist/control

       3. Control

    F. Cycling parameter: Pressure

    G. Limit (preset): Flow

    H. Flow patterns

       1. Decaying in airmix

       2. Square in 100% source delivery

    I. Pressure patterns

       1. Parabolic with airmix

       2. Rectilinear with 100% source delivery

    J. Internal resistance: Low

    K. Airway maneuvers

       1. CPPV

    L. Alarm: None

X. Ventilator: Bennett MA – 1

    A. Pressure: Positive

    B. Powering mechanism: Electric

    C. Driving mechanism: Bellows system driven by compressed gas from electric compressor

    D. Circuit: Double

    E. Modes

       1. Control

       2. Assist/control

       3. Assist

    F. Cycling parameters

       1. Volume

       2. Pressure

G. Limits (preset)
   1. Flow
   2. Pressure
   3. Volume
H. Flow pattern: Square
I. Pressure pattern: Rectilinear
J. Internal resistance: Medium
K. Airway maneuvers
   1. CPPV
   2. Expiratory retard
L. Alarms
   1. High airway pressure
      a. For normal tidal volume
      b. For sigh volume
   2. Low oxygen source pressure
   3. Power failure
   4. I : E ratio
   5. Bennett spirometer (optional)
      a. Patient disconnect (low ETV) alarm
      b. Expired tidal volume monitor

XI. Ventilator: Emerson Post-Operative
A. Pressure: Positive
B. Powering mechanism: Electric
C. Driving mechanism: Piston system driven via rotary motion by electric motor
D. Circuit: Single
E. Mode: Control
F. Cycling parameter: Combined volume/time
G. Limit (preset): Pressure (relief/pop-off)
H. Flow pattern: Sine wave
I. Pressure pattern: Sigmoidal
J. Internal resistance: High
K. Airway maneuvers
   1. CPPV
   2. Sigh
L. Alarms
   1. None standard
   2. Optional devices from Emerson
      a. Emerson spirometer for ETV
      b. Low airway pressure

XII. Ventilator: Engström 300
A. Pressure: Positive

B. Powering mechanism: Electric
C. Driving mechanism: Piston system driven via rotary motion by electric motor
D. Circuit: Double
E. Mode: Control
F. Cycling parameter: Time (Fixed I : E at 1 : 2)
G. Limits (preset)
    1. Volume
    2. Pressure (relief/pop-off)
H. Flow pattern: Modified sine wave
I. Pressure pattern: Modified sigmoidal
J. Internal resistance: High
K. Airway maneuvers
    1. CPPV
    2. Expiratory retard
    3. Inflation hold (mandatory)
L. Alarms:
    1. Low airway pressure
    2. Power failure

XIII. Ventilator: Ohio 550
A. Pressure: Positive
B. Powering mechanism: Pneumatic
C. Driving mechanism: Bellows system driven by compressed gas regulated by fluidic mechanism
D. Circuit: Double
E. Mode: Assist/control
F. Cycling parameter: Volume
G. Limits (preset)
    1. Flow
    2. Pressure (relief/pop-off) optional
H. Flow pattern: Square
I. Pressure pattern: Rectilinear
J. Internal resistance: Medium
K. Airway maneuver: CPPV
L. Alarms
    1. Low airway pressure
    2. Failure to cycle

XIV. Ventilator: Ohio 560
A. Pressure: Positive
B. Powering mechanism: Electric
C. Driving mechanism: Bellows system driven by compressed gas from an electric compressor (turbine)

    D. Circuit: Double
    E. Modes
        1. Control
        2. Assist/control
    F. Cycling parameter: Volume
    G. Limits (preset)
        1. Flow
        2. Pressure (relief/pop-off)
    H. Flow pattern: Square
    I. Pressure pattern: Rectilinear
    J. Internal resistance: Medium
    K. Airway maneuvers
        1. CPPV
        2. Inflation hold
        3. Sigh
    L. Alarms
        1. Low airway pressure
        2. High airway pressure
        3. Low oxygen source pressure
        4. Failure to cycle
        5. Power failure
XV. Ventilator: Ohio 570 CCV (Critical Care Ventilator)
    A. Pressure: Positive
    B. Powering mechanism: Electric
    C. Driving mechanism: Bellows system driven by compressed gas from an electric compressor
    D. Circuit: Double
    E. Modes
        1. Control
        2. IMV
        3. Assist/control
    F. Cycling parameter: Volume
    G. Limits (preset)
        1. Flow
        2. Pressure (relief/pop-off)
    H. Flow pattern: Square
    I. Pressure pattern: Rectilinear
    J. Internal resistance: Medium
    K. Airway maneuvers
        1. CPPV
        2. Inflation hold
        3. Sigh

L. Alarms
   1. Low airway pressure
   2. High airway pressure
   3. Low oxygen source pressure
   4. Power failure
   5. Failure to cycle

XVI. Ventilator: Searle VVA
  A. Pressure: Positive
  B. Powering mechanism: Electric
  C. Driving mechanism: Piston system driven by a spring-loaded mechanism
  D. Circuit: Single
  E. Modes
    1. Control
    2. IDV (optional)
    3. Assist/control
  F. Cycling parameter
    1. Volume
    2. Pressure
  G. Limits (preset)
    1. Pressure (ends inspiration)
    2. Flow
    3. Time
  H. Flow patterns (adjustable)
    1. Square
    2. Square with flow taper
  I. Pressure patterns (variable)
    1. Rectilinear
    2. Initially linear, terminally decelerating
  J. Internal resistance: High
  K. Airway maneuvers
    1. CPPV
    2. Inflation hold
    3. Sigh
    4. CPAP (optional)
  L. Alarms
    1. Low airway pressure
    2. High airway pressure
    3. Low oxygen source pressure
    4. Short exhalation (inspiration greater than exhalation)
    5. Failure to cycle
    6. Power failure

       7. High end expiratory pressure
       8. Apnea (adjustable)
       9. Fan

XVII. Ventilator: Servo 900 B
    A. Pressure: Positive
    B. Powering mechanism: Combined electric/pneumatic
    C. Driving mechanism: Pneumatic system regulated by servo mechanisms
    D. Circuit: Single
    E. Modes
       1. Assist/control
       2. IDV
       3. Control
    F. Cycling parameters
       1. Combined volume/time
       2. Pressure
       3. Time
    G. Limits (preset)
       1. Pressure (ends inspiration or will plateau)
       2. Inspiratory time
       3. Volume
    H. Flow patterns
       1. Square
       2. Accelerating
    I. Pressure patterns
       1. Rectilinear
       2. Nonlinear exponentially increasing
    J. Internal resistance: High
    K. Airway maneuvers
       1. CPPV
       2. Inflation hold (pause time %)
       3. Sigh
       4. Expiratory retard (maximum expiratory flow)
       5. CPAP
    L. Alarms
       1. Low expired minute volume
       2. High expired minute volume
       3. High airway pressure
       4. Power failure

XVIII. Ventilator: Gill I
    A. Pressure: Positive
    B. Powering mechanism: Electric

    C. Driving mechanism: Piston system driven by force (weight) of gravity

    D. Circuit: Single

    E. Modes
   1. Control
   2. Assist/control
   3. Assist

    F. Cycling parameter: Volume

    G. Limits (preset)
   1. Flow
   2. Pressure (ends inspiration)
      a. Normal tidal volume
      b. Sigh volume

    H. Flow pattern: Square wave with flow taper

    I. Pressure pattern: Initially linear, terminally decelerating

    J. Internal resistance: Medium

    K. Airway maneuvers
   1. CPPV
   2. Inflation hold
   3. Sigh

    L. Alarms
   1. Low airway pressure
   2. High airway pressure
   3. Low oxygen percent
   4. Power failure
   5. Failure to cycle (improper cycle)
   6. Fill humidifier

XIX. Ventilator: Veriflo CV 2000

    A. Pressure: Positive

    B. Powering mechanism: Pneumatic

    C. Driving mechanism: Pneumatic system regulated by pneumatic relays and balanced diaphragm mechanism

    D. Circuit: Single

    E. Modes
   1. Control
   2. IDV
   3. Assist/control

    F. Cycling parameter: Time

    G. Limits (preset)
   1. Flow
   2. Pressure (relief/pop-off)

    H. Flow pattern: Square

      I.   Pressure pattern: Rectilinear
      J.   Internal resistance: High
     K. Airway maneuvers
         1. CPPV
         2. Sigh
      L. Alarms
         1. Low airway pressure
         2. High airway pressure
         3. Low oxygen/air source pressure

XX. Ventilator: Bourns Bear I
     A. Pressure: Positive
     B. Powering mechanisms: Electric
     C. Driving mechanism: Pneumatic system regulated by solenoids and regulators
     D. Circuit: Single
     E. Modes
         1. Control
         2. IDV
         3. Assist/control
     F. Cycling parameter
         1. Volume
         2. Pressure
         3. Time
     G. Limits (preset)
         1. Pressure (ends inspiration)
         2. Inspiratory time (ends inspiration when inspiration greater than exhalation)
         3. Flow
     H. Flow patterns
         1. Square
         2. Square with flow taper
      I. Pressure patterns
         1. Rectilinear
         2. Initially linear, terminally decelerating
      J. Internal resistance: Medium
     K. Airway maneuvers
         1. CPPV
         2. Inflation hold
         3. Sigh
         4. CPAP
     L. Alarms
         1. Low airway pressure

2. High airway pressure
3. Low oxygen source pressure
4. Low air source pressure
5. Low exhaled tidal volume
6. Apnea
7. I : E ratio
8. Power failure
9. Failure to cycle (ventilator inoperative)
10. Low PEEP/CPAP

XXI. Ventilator: Monaghan 225
   A. Pressure: Positive
   B. Powering mechanism: Pneumatic
   C. Driving mechanism: Bellows system driven by compressed gas from fluidic mechanism
   D. Circuit: Double
   E. Modes
      1. Control
      2. IDV
      3. Assist/control
      4. Assist
   F. Cycling parameters
      1. Volume
      2. Pressure
      3. Time
   G. Limits (preset)
      1. Pressure
      2. Flow
      3. Volume
      4. Time (ends inspiration)
   H. Flow pattern: Square
   I. Pressure pattern: Rectilinear
   J. Internal resistance: High
   K. Airway maneuver: CPPV
   L. Alarms
      1. High airway pressure (visual only)
      2. Time cycle/inverse I : E ratio (visual only)
      3. Optional Monaghan monitor
         a. High exhaled tidal volume
         b. Low exhaled tidal volume
         c. High respiratory rate
         d. Low respiratory rate
         e. High minute volume
         f. Low minute volume

XXII. Ventilator: Foregger 210
   A. Pressure: Positive
   B. Powering mechanism: Pneumatic
   C. Driving mechanism: Pneumatic system regulated by sole-
      noids, flow control valve and regulators
   D. Circuit: Single
   E. Modes
      1. IMV
      2. Assist/control
      3. Control
   F. Cycling parameter: Time
   G. Limits (preset)
      1. Flow
      2. Pressure
   H. Flow pattern: Square
   I. Pressure pattern: Rectilinear
   J. Internal resistance: High
   K. Airway maneuvers
      1. CPPV
      2. Inflation hold
      3. Sigh
   L. Alarms
      1. High airway pressure (normal and sigh tidal volume)
      2. Low air/oxygen source pressure
      3. High minute volume
      4. Low minute volume
      5. Apnea
      6. Failure to cycle
XXIII. Ventilator: Baby Bird
   A. Pressure: Positive
   B. Powering mechanism: Pneumatic
   C. Driving mechanism: Pneumatic system regulated by a
      servo mechanism
   D. Circuit: Single
   E. Mode: IMV
   F. Cycling parameter: Time
   G. Limits (preset)
      1. Flow
      2. Pressure (relief/pop-off or plateaus)
   H. Flow pattern: Square
   I. Pressure pattern: Rectilinear
   J. Internal resistance: High

        K. Airway maneuvers
             1. CPPV
        L. Alarms
             1. Long inspiratory time
             2. Low oxygen source pressure (in blender)
             3. Low air source pressure (in blender)

XXIV. Ventilator: Bourns LS 104–150
        A. Pressure: Positive
        B. Powering mechanism: Electric
        C. Driving mechanism: Piston system driven via linear motion by electric motor
        D. Circuit: Single
        E. Modes
             1. Control
             2. IMV
             3. Assist/control
             4. Assist
        F. Cycling parameters
             1. Volume
             2. Pressure
        G. Limits (preset)
             1. Flow
             2. Pressure (relief/pop-off or ends inspiration)
        H. Flow pattern: Square
        I.   Pressure pattern: Rectilinear
        J.   Internal resistance: High
        K. Airway maneuvers
             1. CPPV
             2. Inflation hold
             3. Sigh
        L. Alarms
             1. Low airway pressure
             2. High airway pressure
             3. Apnea (forces assist mode to change into assist/control mode also)

XXV. Ventilator: Bourns BP 200
        A. Pressure: Positive
        B. Powering mechanism: Combined electric/pneumatic
        C. Driving mechanism: Pneumatic system regulated by solenoids and regulators
        D. Circuit: Single
        E. Modes: IMV

    F. Cycling parameter: Time
    G. Limits (preset)
        1. Flow
        2. Inspiratory time
        3. Pressure (relief/pop-off)
    H. Flow pattern: Square
    I. Pressure pattern: Rectilinear
    J. Internal resistance: High
    K. Airway maneuver: CPPV
    L. Alarms
        1. Low oxygen/air source pressure
        2. Excessive inspiratory time (visual)
        3. Insufficient expiratory time (visual)
        4. Power failure

BIBLIOGRAPHY

ACCP-ATS Joint Committee on Pulmonary Nomenclature: Pulmonary terms and symbols, Chest 67:583, 1975.

Ashbough, D. G., et al.: Continuous positive pressure breathing (CPPB) in adult respiratory distress syndrome, J. Thorac. Cardiovasc. Surg. 57:31, 1969.

Ayers, S. M.: Assisted PEEP: Helpful or disastrous? Respir. Care 19:410, 1974.

Barach, A. L., Bickerman, H. A., and Petty, T. L.: Perspectives in pressure breathing, Respir. Care 20:627, 1975.

Baratz, R., et al.: Urinary output and plasma levels of antidiuretic hormone during intermittent positive pressure breathing in the dog, Anesthesiology 32:17, 1970.

Berman, L. S., et al.: Optimum levels of CPAP for tracheal extubation, J. Pediatr. 89:109, 1976.

Bowser, M. A., et al.: A systematic approach to ventilator weaning, Respir. Care 20:959, 1975.

Breivik, H., et al.: Normalizing low arterial CO_2 tension during mechanical ventilation, Chest 63:525, 1973.

Civetta, J. M., Barnes, T. A., and Smith, L. O.: "Optimal PEEP" and intermittent mandatory ventilation in the treatment of acute respiratory failure, Respir. Care 20:551, 1975.

Crossman, P. F., Bushnell, L. S., and Hedley-Whyte, J.: Deadspace during artificial ventilation: Gas compression and mechanical deadspace, J. Appl. Physiol. 28:94, 1970.

Demers, R. R., Irwin, R. S., and Braman, S. S.: Criteria for optimum PEEP, Respir. Care 22:596, 1977.

Desautels, D. A.: Answering service, Respir. Care 22:1230, 1977.

Desautels, D. A., Sanderson, R. R., and Klein, E. F., Jr.: A unified approach to pulmonary ventilation terminology, Respir. Care 23:42, 1978.

Downs, J. B., et al.: Intermittent mandatory ventilation: A new approach to weaning patients from mechanical ventilators, Chest 64:331, 1973.

Editorial: The difference between PEEP, CPPB, and CPAP, Respir. Care 19: 14, 1974.

Egan, D. F.: *Fundamentals of Respiratory Therapy* (3d ed.; St. Louis: C. V. Mosby Co., 1977).

Feeley, T. W., and Hedley-Whyte, J.: Weaning from controlled ventilation and supplemental oxygen, N. Engl. J. Med. 292:903, 1975.

Fratto, C.: Positive end expiratory pressure (PEEP): An overview, Md. State Med. J. 22: (11):78, 1973.

Gjerde, G. E.: A method for spontaneous breathing with expiratory positive pressure, Respir. Care 20:839, 1975.

Greenbaum, D. M., et al.: Use of continuous positive airway pressure (CPAP) without tracheal intubation in spontaneously breathing patients, Chest 69: 685, 1976.

Gregory, G. A., et al.: Continuous positive airway pressure with spontaneous respiration: A new method of increasing arterial oxygenation in the respiratory distress syndrome, Pediatr. Res. 4:469, 1970 (abstract).

Gregory, G. A., et al.: Treatment of the idiopathic respiratory distress syndrome with continuous positive airway pressure, N. Engl. J. Med. 284:1333, 1971.

Hodgkin, J., et al.: Respirator weaning, Crit. Care Med. 2:96, 1974.

Kumar, A., et al.: Continuous positive-pressure breathing ventilation in acute respiratory failure, N. Engl. J. Med. 283:1430, 1970.

Leftwich, E. I., Witorsch, R. J., and Witorsch, P.: Positive end expiratory pressure in refractory hypoxemia, Ann. Intern. Med. 89:187, 1973.

McPherson, S. P.: *Respiratory Therapy Equipment* (St. Louis: C. V. Mosby, Co., 1977).

Modell, J. H.: Weaning patients from mechanical ventilation, Respir. Care 20: 373, 1975.

Mushin, W. W., et al.: *Automatic Ventilation of the Lungs* (2d ed.: Philadelphia: F. A. Davis Co., 1969).

Nicotra, M. B., et al.: Physiologic evaluation of positive end expiratory pressure ventilation, Chest 64:10, 1973.

Operating Instructions, Bennett PR–2 Respiration Unit, Form 2131 H (Santa Monica, Calif.: Bennett Respiration Products, Inc., 1975).

Operating Instructions, Bennett PR–I Respiration Unit, Form 1693 G (Santa Monica, Calif.: Bennett Respiration Products, Inc., 1975).

Operating Manual, Bourns Adult Volume Ventilator BEAR I, Form P/N 50000–10500, Bourns Inc. (Riverside, Calif.: Life System Division).

Operating Instructions, IPPB Therapy Unit Models TV–2P, PV–3P, and T V–4, Form 1008-B (Santa Monica, Calif.: Bennett Respiration Products, Inc., 1969).

Operating Manual, Model CV–2000, Veriflo Adult Ventilator (Irvine, Calif: McGaw Respiratory Therapy Products).

Operating Manual, Model 210, Foregger Adult Ventilator (Irvine, Calif.: McGaw Respiratory Therapy Products).

Operating Manual, Monaghan 225 Volume Ventilator, Form 13929–01 5m (Littleton, Colo.).

Operating Manual, Emerson Post-op Ventilator, Form 3–PV–1 (Cambridge, Mass.: J. H. Emerson Co., 1969).

Operating Manual, Siemens-Elema Servo Ventilator 900, ME 461/5098.101,

1974 and Servo Ventilator 900B, Preliminary supplement to operating manual (Solna, Sweden: Siemens-Elema, AB, 1975).

Operating Manual, VVA Volume Ventilator Adult, OMI–4, Form 12125–B (Haywood, Calif.: Searle Cardio-Pulmonary Systems, Inc., 1976).

Operating and Repair Manual, Model 560 Respirator, Form 1887 (Madison, Ohio: Ohio Medical Products, 1970).

Petty, T. L., Bigelow, D. B., and Broughton, J. O.: A new volume cycled ventilator, Respir. Ther. 2:33, 1972.

Radford, E. P., Jr.: Ventilation standards for use in artificial respiration, J. Appl. Physiol. 7:451, 1955.

Service Manuals, Engström Respirator Systems, ER–300 (Rockville, Md.: LKB Medical, Inc.).

Shapiro, B. A., Harrison, R. A., and Trout, C. A.: *Clinical Application of Respiratory Care* (Chicago: Year Book Medical Publishers, Inc., 1975).

Shapiro, B. A., et al.: Intermittent mandatory ventilation (IDV): A new technique for supporting ventilation in critically ill patients, Respir. Care 21: 521, 1976.

Sladen, A., et al.: Pulmonary complications and water retention in prolonged mechanical ventilation, N. Engl. J. Med. 279:448, 1968.

Stevens, P. M.: Positive end-expiratory pressure breathing, (Basics of RD) Am. Thorac. Soc. News, vol. 5, no. 3, 1977.

Suter, P. M., Fairley, H. B., and Isenberg, M. D.: Optimum end expiratory airway pressure in patients with acute pulmonary failure, N. Engl. J. Med. 292:284, 1975.

Suwa, K., and Bendixen, H. H.: Change in Pa_{CO_2} with mechanical deadspace during artificial ventilation, J. Appl. Physiol. 24:556, 1968.

Whittenberger, J. L. (ed.): *Artificial Respiration: Theory and Applications* (New York: Paul B. Hoeber Co., 1962).

25 / Microbiology

I. Classification of Microorganisms by Cell Type
   A. Eukaryotic cell type higher Protista
      1. Algae (except blue-green)
      2. Protozoa
      3. Fungi
      4. Slime molds
   B. Prokaryotic cell type lower Protista
      1. Blue-green algae
      2. Bacteria
      3. Rickettsiae
      4. Mycoplasmas
II. Eukaryotic Cell Structure
   A. Well-defined nucleus
      1. Well-defined control center of cell for growth and development.
      2. Chromosomes maintained within nucleus.
      3. Nuclear membrane continuous with endoplasmic reticulum.
   B. Numerous free-floating cytoplasmic structures
      1. Endoplasmic reticulum: Responsible for manufacture and secretion of cellular protein.
      2. Mitochondria: Contain enzymes for Krebs' cycle and electron transport chain (seen in animal cells).
      3. Chloroplasts: Contain enzymes for photosynthesis.
      4. Ribosomes: Distinct structures that may be attached to the endoplasmic reticulum; involved with synthesis and secretion of proteins.
      5. Lysosomes: Contain proteolytic enzymes for metabolism of ingested organic material.
   C. Surface layers
      1. Cell membrane: Lipoprotein
      2. Cell wall: Polysaccharide
   D. Motility organelles
      1. Cilia or flagella
      2. Structurally similar but flagella longer

III. Prokaryotic Cell Structure
  A. Poorly defined nucleus
    1. No nuclear membrane.
    2. No mitotic apparatus.
    3. Free existence of chromosomes in protoplasm with attachment to cell membrane.
  B. Absence of cytoplasmic structures
    1. Enzymes for Krebs' cycle and electron transport chain located on inside of cell membrane.
    2. Various cell nutrients stored by the many cytoplasmic granules.
    3. Ribosomes: Exist freely in the protoplasm.
  C. Surface layers
    1. Cell membrane: Lipoprotein
    2. Cell wall: Very rigid
      a. Gram-positive bacteria
        (1) Major component: Mucopeptide
        (2) Secondary components: Teichoic acids or mucopolysaccharides
      b. Gram-negative bacteria: Three distinct layers
        (1) Inner layer: Mucopeptide
        (2) Middle layer: Lipopolysaccharides
        (3) Outer layer: Lipoprotein
  D. Motility organelles: Primarily flagella
IV. Necessary Growth Conditions
  A. Internal environment is equivalent to a 10–20% sucrose solution.
  B. Water is essential for survival of vegetative cells.
  C. Some microorganisms require oxygen (aerobic) while others cannot survive with oxygen (anaerobic).
  D. Light: Ultraviolet and blue light are destructive to bacteria.
  E. Essential nutrients: Water, carbon, hydrogen, nitrogen, sulfur, phosphorus and amino acids.
  F. pH: Optimal pH for most bacteria is between 6.0 and 8.0.
  G. Temperature: Optimal temperature for most bacteria is between 30 C and 40 C.
  H. Microorganisms are obligate (survive only in very specific environment) or facultative (easily adapt to new environmental conditions).
V. Microbial Reproduction (Binary Fission)
  A. Division process in which two daughter cells result from single parent cell division (asexual reproductive process).

    B. Chromosome: Normally only one present, which is about 1 mm long.

    C. Normal chromosome replication.

VI. Growth Pattern

    A new culture of bacteria will develop similar to growth curve seen in Figure 25–1.

    A. Lag phase: Adaptation to new environment; little reproduction.

    B. Exponential phase: Stage of rapid cell growth.

    C. Stationary phase: Coincidence of death and growth rate.

    D. Death phase: Depletion of culture nutrients and build-up of toxic waste. Death rate exceeds growth rate.

VII. Measurement of Growth

    A. Cell concentration: Expressed as number of viable cells.

    B. Cell density: Expressed as dry weights.

VIII. Microbial Relationships

    A. Autotroph: Organism capable of using simple inorganic matter as nutrients (nonpathogenic).

    B. Heterotroph: Organism capable of using organic matter to survive (pathogenic).

        1. Saprophyte: Organism that lives on dead organic matter.

        2. Parasite: Organism that lives on or in another organism and that benefits from but does not benefit the host organism.

        3. Symbiosis: Two dissimilar organisms existing together.

            a. Commensalism: Two species existing together—one benefiting, the other not affected.

            b. Antibiosis: Association between two dissimilar organisms that is harmful to one or both.

Fig 25–1.–Growth pattern of a new, closed culture. *A* is the lag phase, *B* the exponential phase, *C* the stationary phase, *D* the death phase.

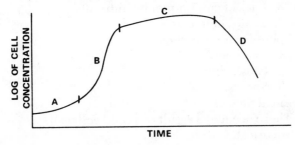

      c. Ammensalism: Two dissimilar organisms existing with no effect on each other.

      d. Synnecrosis: Two dissimilar organisms existing together to the detriment of both.

      e. Mutualism: Two dissimilar organisms existing together, each benefiting from the association and unable to survive without it.

IX. Capsule
  A. This is a structure secreted by the cell, which surrounds and encloses the vegetative cell.
  B. Many pathogenic organisms are capable of producing capsules.
  C. Functions
    1. To prevent phagocytosis
    2. To prevent virus attachment
  D. Causative factors
    1. Presence of high sugar concentration
    2. Presence of blood serum in culture
    3. Microorganism living in host organism
  E. Composition: Secreted slime
    1. Polypeptides
    2. Dextran
    3. Polysaccharides
    4. Cellulose

X. Spore
  A. This structure develops inside a bacterial cell in response to adverse environmental conditions.
  B. Will regenerate to an active vegetative cell when environmental conditions improve.
  C. Metabolically active; contains enzymes necessary for the Krebs cycle.
  D. Extremely resistant to
    1. Heat
    2. Drying
    3. Lack of environmental nutrients
    4. Toxic chemicals
  E. Spore-forming genera
    1. Bacillus
    2. Clostridium
    3. Sporosarcina

XI. Microbial Shapes
  A. These occur as a result of a rigid cell wall.
  B. Spherical: Coccus

    C. Rod-shaped: Bacillus
    D. Spiral: Spirillum
XII. Gram Staining
    A. All bacteria can be separated into two general categories
       (gram-positive or gram-negative) by virtue of their stain-
       ing properties. Variation in staining is determined by cell
       wall construction.
    B. Staining sequence
       1. Basic dye: Crystal violet
       2. Grams iodine
       3. Alcohol wash
       4. Counterstain: Red dye safranin
    C. Gram-positive bacteria: Stain blue or violet
    D. Gram-negative bacteria: Stain red or pink
       1. More virulent
       2. Necrotic infections
       3. Difficult to treat with antibiotics
XIII. Acid-Fast (Ziehl-Neelsen's) Stain
    A. Identifies bacteria of genus Mycobacterium
    B. Acid-fast bacteria: stain red
    C. Staining sequence
       1. Carbol-fuchsin (red)
       2. Hydrochloric acid in alcohol wash
       3. Water wash
       4. Counterstain: Methyl blue
XIV. Definitions
    A. Inflammation: Specific tissue response to stress by living
       agents or to electric, chemical or mechanical trauma,
       evidenced by vascular dilatation, fluid exudation, accumu-
       lation of leukocytes or any combination of the three.
    B. Contamination: Presence of a microorganism in otherwise
       sterile environment.
    C. Infection: Inflammation caused by multiplication of patho-
       genic microorganisms.
    D. Pathogen: Any disease-producing microorganism.
    E. Virulence: Heightened ability of an organism to produce
       infection in its host.
    F. Immunity: Level of resistance of a body to effects of a del-
       eterious agent (e.g., pathogenic microorganism).
    G. Superinfection: Infection developed primarily in the de-
       bilitated or immunosuppressed patient previously treated
       with antibiotics.
    H. Pyrogenic: Fever-inducing inflammatory process.

I. Nosocomial infection: Hospital-acquired infection.
J. Aerobic: Growing only in presence of oxygen.
K. Anaerobic: Growing only in absence of oxygen.
L. Toxins: Poisonous substances produced by bacteria
    1. Exotoxin
       a. Primarily produced by gram-positive bacteria.
       b. Is protein and normally is diffused by bacteria into surrounding media.
       c. Some are extremely lethal.
    2. Endotoxin
       a. Primarily produced by gram-negative bacteria.
       b. Is a lipopolysaccharide and normally is released when the bacterial cell is destroyed.
M. Vegetative cell: Metabolically active form of a bacterium in which reproduction can occur.
XV. Frequently Encountered Gram-Positive Pathogenic Genera
  A. Bacillus
    1. Large gram-positive aerobic rods arranged in chains.
    2. All species spore forming.
    3. Usually saprophytic.
    4. *Bacillus anthracis*
       a. Enters via injured skin or by inhalation.
       b. May cause
          (1) Skin infections
          (2) Septicemia
          (3) Pneumonia (Woolsorters' disease)
          (4) Enteritis
          (5) Meningitis
       c. Secretes potent exotoxin.
    5. Antibiotic susceptibility: Penicillin.
  B. Clostridium
    1. Large gram-positive anaerobic rod
    2. Spore forming
    3. Secretes potent exotoxins
    4. Generally a localized infection
    5. *Clostridium botulinum* (botulism)
       a. Produces highly toxic exotoxins.
       b. Disease produced by ingesting infected food.
       c. Treatment: Antitoxins.
    6. *Clostridium perfringens*
       a. Produces gas gangrene
       b. Secretes potent exotoxins

    c. Treatment
      (1) Surgical debridement
      (2) Hyperbaric oxygen
      (3) Penicillin
      (4) Antitoxins
  7. *Clostridium tetani* (tetanus)
    a. Produces potent exotoxin that acts on nerve tissue of spinal cord and peripheral nerves.
    b. Treatment
      (1) Surgical debridement
      (2) Antitoxins
      (3) Penicillin
C. Corynebacterium
  1. Gram-positive aerobic rod with club-shaped appearance.
  2. Often arranged in a palisade pattern.
  3. Some species are normal flora of upper respiratory tract.
  4. *Corynebacterium diphtheriae* (Klebs-Loeffler bacillus)
    a. Causes diphtheria.
    b. Produces a potent exotoxin.
    c. Produces a pseudomembrane covering pharynx and larynx.
    d. Treatment
      (1) Antitoxin
      (2) Penicillin
      (3) Erythromycin
D. Diplococcus (also called pneumococcus)
  1. Gram-positive aerobic coccus existing as encapsulated diplococcus.
  2. Normal flora of upper respiratory tract in 30–70% of population.
  3. *Diplococcus pneumoniae*
    a. Most common pathogen causing bacterial pneumonia.
  4. May also cause
    a. Sinusitis
    b. Meningitis
    c. Endocarditis
    d. Bacteremia
    e. Septic arthritis
    f. Osteomyelitis

     5. Factors predisposing to infection
       a. Respiratory tract abnormalities
       b. Alcohol or drug intoxication
       c. Abnormal circulatory dynamics
       d. Malnutrition
     6. Antibiotic susceptibility: Penicillin

E. Staphylococcus
     1. Gram-positive aerobic coccus.
     2. Arranged in irregular clusters.
     3. Pigment: White to yellow in culture.
     4. Part of normal flora of skin and respiratory and gastrointestinal tracts.
     5. Many resistant strains.
     6. *Staphylococcus aureus*
       a. Normally produces pimples, abscesses or boils.
       b. May produce pneumonia, wound infection, empyema or septicemia.
       c. Infections: Suppurative.
     7. Antibiotic susceptibility: Penicillin, tetracycline.

F. Streptococcus
     1. Gram-positive aerobic coccus.
     2. Arranged in chains.
     3. Widely distributed in nature.
     4. Can cause disease in almost every organ.
     5. Classification of species and infections
       a. Group A, β-hemolytic streptococci: Septicemia, tonsillitis, scarlet fever, pneumonia, nasopharyngitis, middle ear infections, rheumatic fever, endocarditis, glomerulonephritis.
       b. Group B, β-hemolytic streptococci: Female genital tract infections; may cause endocarditis, meningitis, neonatal sepsis.
       c. Group C, β-hemolytic streptococci erysipelas: Throat infections and opportunistic infections.
       d. Group D, β-hemolytic streptococci: Urinary tract infections and endocarditis.
     6. Antibiotic susceptibility: Penicillin.

G. Mycobacterium
     1. Gram-positive aerobic rod.
     2. Acid-fast positive.
     3. Saprophytes.
     4. Pathogenic species

a. *Mycobacterium tuberculosis*
b. *Mycobacterium leprae* (Hansen's bacillus)
5. May cause pulmonary tuberculosis, spinal tuberculosis, urinary tract tuberculosis and leprosy.
6. Antibiotic susceptibility: Isoniazid (INH), ethambutol, rifampin and streptomycin.
XVI. Frequently Encountered Gram-Negative Pathogenic Genera
A. Proteus
1. Gram-negative aerobic rod.
2. Part of normal fecal flora.
3. May cause chronic urinary tract infections, pneumonia, gastroenteritis and bacteremia.
4. Pathogenic species
a. *Proteus mirabilis*
b. *Proteus vulgaris*
5. Opportunistic pathogen.
6. Antibiotic susceptibility: Gentamicin, penicillin, ampicillin.
B. Pseudomonas
1. Gram-negative aerobic rod.
2. Widely distributed in nature.
3. Frequent infection
a. Debilitated individuals
b. Patients on prolonged antimicrobial therapy
4. *Pseudomonas aeruginosa*
a. Pigmentation usually green to brown
b. Opportunistic pathogen
c. Frequently cultured from nebulizers
d. Predominantly causes
(1) Pneumonia
(2) Wound infection
(3) Urinary tract infection
(4) Empyema
(5) Meningitis
(6) Septicemia
5. Antibiotic susceptibility: Carbenicillin, gentamicin, polymyxins, chloramphenicol.
C. Serratia
1. Gram-negative aerobic rod.
2. *Serratia marcescens*
a. Widely distributed in nature.
b. Pigmentation red.

    c. May cause serious pneumonia.

    d. May cause

       (1) Empyema

       (2) Septicemia

       (3) Wound infections

    e. May cause hospital epidemics.

  3. Antibiotic susceptibility: Gentamicin.

D. Escherichia

  1. Gram-negative aerobic rod.

  2. Normal flora of gastrointestinal tract.

  3. Pathogenic species: *Escherichia coli*

    a. Cause of urinary tract infections.

    b. Can cause septicemia, endocarditis, meningitis, wound infections, diarrhea and pneumonia.

       (1) Pneumonias: Very necrotic

  4. Antibiotic susceptibility: Primarily gentamicin.

E. Klebsiella

  1. Short gram-negative aerobic rod

  2. *Klebsiella pneumoniae* (Friedlander's bacillus)

    a. Normal flora of nose, mouth and intestines.

    b. May cause pneumonia, lung abscess, upper respiratory tract infections, endocarditis and septicemia.

       (1) Pneumonias: Very necrotic.

    c. Produces characteristic "red currant jelly" sputum.

    d. Infection often hemolytic.

  3. Antibiotic susceptibility: Primarily gentamicin

F. Haemophilus

  1. Minute gram-negative aerobic rod.

  2. Normal flora of upper respiratory tract.

  3. Commonly produces infections in children, rarely in adults.

  4. Pathogenic species

    a. *Haemophilus influenzae* (Pfeiffer's bacillus)

       (1) Normal flora of respiratory tract.

       (2) *Most common cause of epiglottitis in children.*

       (3) Can cause meningitis, laryngitis, sinusitis, croup and subacute bacterial endocarditis.

    b. *Haemophilus haemolyticus*

       (1) Normal flora of respiratory tract.

       (2) Can cause pharyngitis.

    c. *Haemophilus parainfluenzae*

       (1) Normal flora of respiratory tract.

       (2) May cause bacterial endocarditis.

5. Antibiotic susceptibility: Chloramphenicol and ampicillin.
G. Salmonella
   1. Gram-negative aerobic rod.
   2. Resistant to freezing and releases potent endotoxins.
   3. May produce mild enteritis, gastroenteritis and septicemia.
   4. Transmitted orally from contaminated milk; turtles; eggs; shell fish; and undercooked chicken, fish and pork.
   5. Pathogenic species
      a. *Salmonella typhi* (typhoid fever)
      b. *Salmonella enteritidis*
   6. Antibiotic susceptibility: Chloramphenicol, ampicillin.
XVII. Mycoplasma
   A. Gram-negative aerobic highly pleomorphic organism.
   B. *Does not* contain a rigid cell wall.
   C. Similar to bacteria in all other aspects.
   D. May be isolated from saliva, sputum, blood, pleural fluid and genitourinary tract.
   E. Pathogenic species
      1. *Mycoplasma hominis*
         a. May cause pharyngitis, tonsillitis or pelvic inflammatory disease.
         b. Specific antibodies against this organism produced by many adults.
      2. *Mycoplasma pneumoniae* (also called Eaton agent, primary atypical pneumonia or pleuropneumonia-like organism [PPLO])
         a. Normally causes a self-limiting respiratory syndrome characterized by
            (1) Malaise
            (2) Cough
            (3) Fever
            (4) Pulmonary infiltrate
         b. May be asymptomatic.
   F. Antibiotic susceptibility: Inhibited by tetracycline or erythromycin.
XVIII. Rickettsiae
   A. Very small obligate intracellular parasite
   B. Considered true bacterium.
   C. Normally inhabits arthropods.

    D. Pleomorphic short rod or coccus.
    E. Occurs singly, paired, chained or in filaments.
    F. Special staining techniques needed for identification.
    G. Typical diseases
       1. Typhoid fever
       2. Rocky Mountain spotted fever
       3. Q fever
       4. Trench fever
    H. Clinical findings
       1. Fever
       2. Headache
       3. Malaise
       4. Prostration
       5. Skin rash
       6. Enlargement of liver and spleen
    I. Antibiotic susceptibility
       1. Para-aminobenzoic acid
       2. Chloramphenicol
       3. Tetracycline
XIX. Viruses
    A. Obligate intracellular parasites.
    B. Do not possess metabolic enzymes.
    C. Contain either a single DNA or RNA molecule.
    D. Do not contain a cell wall.
    E. Reproduction by intracellular replication, relying on protein systems of host.
    F. No antibiotic susceptibility.
    G. Pathogenic species
       1. Respiratory syncytial virus (RSV)
          a. Single most important agent causing infantile bronchiolitis and pneumonia.
       2. Influenza virus
          a. Causes an acute respiratory tract infection characterized by chills, malaise, fever, muscular aches, prostration, cough and sputum production.
       3. Parainfluenza virus
          a. *Primary cause of croup in children and also may cause other upper respiratory problems.*
       4. Adenovirus
          a. Commonly causes both upper and lower respiratory infections, pharyngitis, rhinitis, otitis and laryngitis.

5. Rhinovirus
   a. Primary agent causing the common cold.
XX. Fungi
   A. Structurally a complex formation of hyphae, a series of branching filaments developing into mycelium.
   B. Reproduce by asexual budding.
   C. Disease: Hypersensitive reaction induced by chemical constituents of the fungus.
   D. Infection: Systemic, superficial or subcutaneous.
      1. Systemic infection
         a. Chronic granuloma with varying degrees of necrosis and abscess.
      2. Superficial infection
         a. Tinea pedis (athlete's foot)
         b. Tinea corporis (ringworm)
         c. Tinea capitis (ringworm of scalp)
   E. *Candida albicans*
      1. Normal flora of respiratory, gastrointestinal and female genital tracts.
      2. In the debilitated patient, immunosuppressed patient or an individual receiving excessive antibiotic therapy, this fungus may cause septicemia, thrombophlebitis, endocarditis or infection in other organs.
   F. *Histoplasma capsulatum* (histoplasmosis)
      1. Causes infection via respiratory tract.
      2. Found in bird feces transmitted via dust from housing pigeons or chickens or from silos.
         a. Pulmonary disease results in small inflammatory or granulomatous foci, which heal or calcify.
         b. Systemic disease may cause high fever, anemia and high mortality.
   G. *Coccidioides immitis* (coccidioidomycosis)
      1. Causes infection through inhalation of airborne spores.
         a. Initially, symptoms are similar to influenza and may be self-limiting.
         b. Of infected individuals, 1% may develop highly fatal granulomas.
         c. Endemic to the southwest.
   H. *Aspergillus fumigatus* (aspergillosis)
      1. Immunosuppressed patients or individuals with leukemia or those receiving intensive corticosteroid

therapy are particularly susceptible to this organism.
2. The organism normally enters via the respiratory tract, producing pneumonia, hemorrhagic pulmonary infarction or granulomas.
    a. Infection may disseminate to other organs, with granuloma formation.

XXI. Normal Flora
  A. Skin
    1. Staphylococci
    2. Streptococci
    3. Coliform bacteria
    4. Enterococci
    5. Diphtheroids (aerobic and anaerobic)
    6. Proteus species
    7. Pseudomonas species
    8. Bacillus species
    9. Fungi (lipophilic)
  B. Respiratory tract
    1. Staphylococci
    2. Streptococci
    3. Diphtheroids
    4. Neisseria species
    5. Haemophilus species
    6. Pneumococci
    7. Spirochetes
    8. Actinomycetes
    9. *Candida albicans* and other fungi
  C. Gastrointestinal tract
    1. Coliform bacteria
    2. Enterococci
    3. Clostridium species
    4. Proteus species
    5. Yeasts
    6. Penicillium species
    7. Enteroviruses
    8. *Pseudomonas aeruginosa*
    9. Streptococci
   10. Staphylococci
   11. *Alcaligenes faecalis*
   12. Bacteroides species
   13. Lactobacillus species

BIBLIOGRAPHY

Brock, T. D.: *Biology of Microorganisms* (Englewood Cliffs, N. J.: Prentice-Hall, Inc., 1970).

Griggs, B. M., and Reinhardt, D. T.: *Fundamentals of Nosocomial Infections Associated with Respiratory Therapy* (New York: Projects in Health, Inc., 1975).

Jawetz, E., Melinick, J. L., and Adelberg, E. A.: *Review of Medical Microbiology* (12th ed.; Los Altos, Calif.: Lange Medical Publications, 1976).

Mikat, D. M., and Mikat, K. W.: *A Clinician's Guide to Bacteria* (2d ed.; Indianapolis: Eli Lilly and Co., 1975).

Shapiro, B. A., Harrison, R. A., and Trout, C. A.: *Clinical Application of Respiratory Care* (Chicago: Year Book Medical Publishers, Inc., 1975).

Smith, L. A.: *Principles of Microbiology* (7th ed.; St. Louis: C. V. Mosby Co., 1973).

Walton, J. R., et al.: Serratia bacteremia from mean arterial pressure monitors, Anesthesiology 43:113, 1975.

26 / Sterilization

I. Definitions
   A. *Sterilization:* Complete destruction of all types of microorganisms.
   B. *Germicide:* Chemical or physical agent used to destroy all types of microorganisms.
   C. *Disinfectant:* Germicidal agent used on inanimate objects.
   D. *Bactericide:* Chemical or physical agent used to destroy bacteria in nonspore-forming states.
   E. *Sporicide:* Chemical or physical agent used to destroy spores.
   F. *Bacteriostatic:* Chemical or physical agent used to inhibit bacterial growth.
   G. *Antiseptic:* Chemical agent used to destroy or inhibit the growth of microorganisms on living tissue.
   H. *Asepsis:* Removal and/or prevention of recontamination with microorganisms.
   I. *Decontamination:* Process of removing a contaminant by chemical or physical means.
   J. *Sanitization:* Any process that reduces total bacterial contamination to a level consistent with safety.
II. Preparation for Sterilization
   A. Equipment must be washed clean of all organic matter.
      1. Use an alkaline soap to prevent formation of curds on the equipment.
      2. Hand wash small items with a brush.
      3. Ultrasonic washers may be used for large items.
   B. Rinsing should be complete.
   C. Air-dry
   D. Package appropriately for the sterilization process to be used.
III. Mechanisms of Action of Various Agents
   A. Denaturation and coagulation of protein
      1. Denaturation: Chemical alteration of a protein's structure, causing it to lose some or all of its unique or specific characteristics.
      2. Coagulation: Solidification of protoplasmal protein into a gelatinous mass.

B. Surface tension alteration
   1. Lowering aqueous plasma surface tension increases plasma membrane permeability, allowing an influx of fluid.
   2. The increased permeability causes cellular lysis.
C. Interference with intracellular metabolic pathways
   1. Normally either the cell is destroyed or multiplication is inhibited.

IV. Sterilization by Heat
  A. The mechanism of action is by denaturation and coagulation.
  B. Efficiency of heat sterilization is determined by the heat capacity of the gas involved in the sterilization process.
  C. Heat capacity of water at any temperature significantly exceeds the heat capacity of air.
  D. Steam has a heat capacity seven times that of water at the same temperature due to the latent heat of vaporization of water molecules.
  E. Heat capacity of steam increases logarithmically with increasing pressure.
  F. Order of efficiency of sterilization by heat
   1. Steam under pressure (autoclave)
   2. Steam at atmospheric pressure
   3. Boiling water
   4. Dry heat under pressure
   5. Dry heat at atmospheric pressure
   6. Water below its boiling point (pasteurization)
  G. Autoclaving
   1. Uses steam and pressure to produce the most efficient method of sterilization.
   2. Sterilization occurs as a result of heat transfer from the condensation and evaporation of steam on the surface of the substance being sterilized.
   3. Equipment is packaged in material that allows steam to enter but prevents microorganisms from entering.
     a. Muslin
     b. Linen cloth
     c. Kraft paper
     d. Nylon
     e. Brown paper
     f. Crepe paper
     g. Vegetable parchment
   4. Variables involved in proper autoclaving
     a. Temperature

    b. Pressure

    c. Concentration of steam

  5. The holding time is the minimum amount of time necessary to kill spores at a specific pressure.

  6. The actual sterilization time is one and a half times the holding time.

  7. Examples of autoclaving cycles:

    a. 121 C at 15 psi for 15 minutes

    b. 126 C at 20 psi for 10 minutes

    c. 134 C at 29.4 psi for 3 minutes

  8. Heat-sensitive indicators are applied to all equipment to be autoclaved.

    a. These indicate that the equipment has been exposed to conditions necessary for sterilization.

    b. *They do not indicate sterilization.*

  9. Biologic indicators are used to insure that actual sterilization has been accomplished.

    a. *Bacillus stearothermophilus* spores are specifically used because of their high heat resistance.

    b. Capsules containing 10^6 spores should be placed in at least one load per day and inspected for viable cells.

H. Dry heat

  1. Efficiency is considerably lower than steam heat.

  2. In general, dry heat should be used only on materials in which moist heat would be deleterious to or unable to permeate the product being sterilized.

  3. Temperature-time relationships

    a. 170 C:　60 minutes

    b. 160 C: 120 minutes

    c. 150 C: 150 minutes

    d. 140 C: 180 minutes

    e. 121C: Overnight

I. Pasteurization

  1. Equipment is submerged in medium hot water for certain periods of time.

  2. Pasteurization is effective only in the destruction of vegetative cells.

  3. Equipment is immersed in water at a temperature of 75 C for 10 minutes.

  4. When the equipment is removed from the pasteurization unit, it must be dried and packaged.

V. Ethylene Oxide Sterilization (ETO; $[CH_2]_2O$)
  A. Characteristics of ETO
    1. A gas at room temperature but liquefies readily under moderate pressure.
    2. Has a pleasant ethereal odor.
    3. Causes irritation of tissues, especially the mucous membranes.
    4. ETO is flammable and explosive in all concentrations in air.
    5. Normally is used in 10–12% mixtures with carbon dioxide or halogenated hydrocarbons (e.g., dichlorodifluoromethane [Freon 12], which act as a damping agent).
       a. These mixtures are nonflammable at temperatures up to 55 C.
  B. Mechanism of action
    1. Alkylation occurs at specific enzyme sites, which interrupts normal metabolism and reproduction.
    2. The moisture increases sensitivity of both vegetative cells and spores to ETO.
    3. Coordination of the following factors is necessary for proper sterilization:
       a. Gas concentration
       b. Humidity
       c. Temperature
       d. Time
    4. Sterilization proceeds most rapidly at relative humidities of 30% and slows progressively below or above that level.
    5. Other factors being equal, the effectiveness of the gas doubles for each 10 C rise in temperature up to 60 C.
    6. Pressure for carbon dioxide mixtures is between 20 and 30 psi and for hydrocarbon mixtures between 5 and 7 psi.
    7. Typical systems
       a. Temperature of 54.4 C, relative humidity of 30–60% and 5–7 psi with 450 mg of $(CH_2)_2O$ per liter of air will sterilize in 6 hours.
       b. If the concentration of $(CH_2)_2O$ is raised to 850 mg per liter, a 3-hour exposure will suffice.
    8. The packaging material should be permeable to humidity and $(CH_2)_2O$, but not to microorganisms.
       a. Wrapping paper

b. Cloth
c. Muslin
d. Polyethylene
e. Nylon film

9. The use of indicator tape will identify exposure to gas but not sterility of equipment.

10. A biologic indicator is used to insure that conditions necessary for sterility have been achieved. Cultures of *Bacillus subtilis* var. globigii should be used daily.

11. Aeration time
    a. Most materials require at least a 24-hour aeration time in a well-ventilated area (aeration chambers can significantly decrease this time).
    b. Substances made of neoprene rubber or polyvinyl chloride require extended aeration times — up to 7 days depending on thickness — as a result of their tendency to absorb $(CH_2)_2O$ efficiently.

12. ETO residues
    a. Substances that have been previously gamma irradiated, especially polyvinyl chloride, react with $(CH_2)_2O$ to form ethylene chlorhydrin, which is very irritating to tissue.
    b. If the material to be sterilized is not dry, the water on it reacts with $(CH_2)_2O$ to form ethylene glycol (this usually results in a very sticky residue on the material).

VI. Gamma Irradiation
   A. Gamma waves are very short wavelength light waves possessing extremely high energy and having the ability to ionize a substance.
   B. Ionization of water molecules will inactivate DNA molecules by increasing the rate of reaction of DNA with hydrogen and hydroxyl ions.
   C. Advantages
      1. High efficiency
      2. Negligible temperature change
      3. Equipment may be prepackaged and sealed.
   D. Disadvantages
      1. Sterilization time prolonged 48 to 72 hours.
      2. Polyvinyl chloride may release chlorine gas.
      3. Feasible only on a large scale industrial level.

VII. Liquid Disinfectants
  A. Alcohol
    1. Ethyl alcohol: 50–70% most efficient.
    2. Isopropyl alcohol: 75–100% most efficient.
    3. Effective against vegetative cells.
    4. Ineffective against viruses and spores.
  B. Formaldehyde
    1. Formaldehyde: Formalin in a 37% solution.
    2. It is used in disinfectant solutions.
    3. Formalin is very effective when used in combination with isopropyl alcohol or hexachlorophene.
    4. It is sporicidal with prolonged exposures of 6–12 hours.
    5. It is toxic to tissues and has a pungent, penetrating, irritating odor.
  C. Phenol and related compounds
    1. Considerable variation in concentration
    2. Some preparations virucidal
    3. No sporicidal properties
    4. Irritating to tissue
  D. Iodine and related compounds
    1. Concentrations variable
    2. Efficient bactericidal activity
    3. No sporicidal activity
  E. Mercurial compounds
    1. Concentrations variable
    2. Poor germicides
    3. Normally considered bacteriostatic only
    4. Rapidly inactivated by organic substances
  F. Quaternary ammonium compounds
    1. Selective bactericidal activity.
    2. Not destructive to tuberculosis bacillus spores or enteroviruses.
    3. Rapid loss of potency, especially in the presence of protein.
  G. Glutaraldehyde
    1. Cidex (activated alkaline glutaraldehyde, pH 7.5–8.5)
      a. The equipment should be completely washed and partially dried.
      b. Cidex is effective in the presence of protein material if immersion is complete.
      c. A 10-minute exposure is germicidal.

      d. A 10-hour exposure is sporicidal.

      e. Cidex is toxic to tissue.

      f. The product must be rinsed completely after exposure, left to air dry and packaged in a sterile manner.

      g. Maximum solution life is 14 days.

  2. Sonacide (acid glutaraldehyde, pH 2.7 – 3.7)

      a. The equipment should be completely washed and partially dried.

      b. A 10-minute exposure is germicidal except for Mycobacterium.

      c. A 20-minute exposure is completely germicidal.

      d. Heated sonacide (60 C) is sporicidal after 1 hour.

      e. It is extremely toxic to tissue.

      f. The product must be rinsed completely after exposure, left to air dry and packaged in a sterile manner.

      g. Maximum solution life is 28 days.

BIBLIOGRAPHY

AMA Z – 79, Subcommittee on Ethylene Oxide Sterilization: Ethylene oxide sterilization: A guide for hospital personnel. Respir. Care 22:12, 1977.

Becker, K. O.: Decontamination area for inhalation therapy, J. Am. Hosp. Assoc. 45:68, 1971.

Becker, K. O.: Inhalation therapy department chooses ETO, J. Am. Hosp. Assoc. 45:681, 1971.

Block, S. S.: *Disinfection, Sterilization and Preservation* (2d ed.; Philadelphia: Lea & Febiger, 1977).

Haselhuhn, D. H., Brason, F. W., and Borick, P. M.: In-use study of buffered glutaraldehyde for cold sterilization of anesthesia equipment, Anesth. Analg. (Cleve) 46:468, 1967.

Masferrer, R., and Marguez, R.: Comparison of two activated glutaraldehyde solutions: Cidex solution and Sonacide, Respir. Care 22:257, 1977.

Nelson, E. J.: Respiratory therapy equipment contamination surveillance program – Part I. Techniques of Infection Control in Respiratory Therapy and Anesthesia, Series 5 1977 (Seattle: Olympic Medical Corp.).

Perkins, J. J.: *Principles and Methods of Sterilization in Health Sciences* (2d ed.; Springfield: Charles C Thomas, Publisher, 1969).

Rendell-Baker, L., and Roberts, R. B.: Safe use of ethylene oxide sterilization in hospitals, Anesth. Analg. (Cleve) 51:658, 1972.

Rubbo, S. D., and Gardner, J. F.: *A Review of Sterilization and Disinfection* (Chicago: Year Book Medical Publishers, Inc., 1965).

Starkey, D. H., and Himmelsbach, C. K.: On the avoidance of failures in sterilization, Hospitals 48:143, 1974.

Sykes, G.: *Disinfection and Sterilization* (London: E. and E. N. Spon. Ltd., 1958).

Sykes, M. K.: Sterilization of ventilators, Int. Anesthesiol. Clin. 10:131, 1972.

Synder, J. E.: Infection control, Hospitals 44:80, 1970.

Synder, R. W., and Cheatle, E. L.: Alkaline glutaraldehyde, an effective disinfectant, Am. J. Hosp. Pharm. 22:321, 1965.

Technical Standards and Safety Committee, AART: Recommendations for respiratory therapy equipment – Processing, handling and surveillance, Respir. Care 22:928, 1977.

Wilson, R. D., et al.: An evaluation of the acidemic decontamination system for anesthesia equipment, Anesth. Analg. (Cleve) 51:658, 1972.

Index